CRITICAL CARE NURSING OF CHILDREN AND ADOLESCENTS

by
The American Association of Critical-Care Nurses

Editor

ANNALEE R. OAKES, R.N., M.A., CCRN

Associate Professor and Instructor
Emergency/Critical Care Nursing
Seattle Pacific University
Seattle, Washington

W. B. SAUNDERS COMPANY   Philadelphia   London   Toronto   1981

W. B. Saunders Company: West Washington Square
Philadelphia, PA 19105

1 St. Anne's Road
Eastbourne, East Sussex BN21, 3UN, England

1 Goldthorne Avenue
Toronto, Ontario M8Z 5T9, Canada

Library of Congress Cataloging in Publication Data

American Association of Critical–Care Nurses.

Critical care nursing of children and adolescents.

1. Pediatric intensive care.   2. Pediatric nursing.   3. Intensive care
nursing.   I. Oakes, Annalee R.   II. Title. [DNLM: 1. Critical care–
In infancy and childhood–Nursing texts.   2. Critical care – In
adolescence–Nursing texts.   3. Pediatric nursing.   WY159 A512c]

RJ370.A47 1980   610.73'61   80–50296

ISBN 0-7216-1003-X

Front and back cover illustrations are modified from illustrations appearing in
Victorian Stained Glass Pattern Book, by Ed Sibbett, Jr.,
published by Dover Publications, Inc., New York, 1979.

Critical Care Nursing of Children and Adolescents   ISBN 0-7216-1003-X

Last digit is the print number: 9   8   7   6   5   4   3   2   1

CONTRIBUTORS

CARA QUIGLEY BROWN, R.N., M.S.

Formerly Instructor, School of Nursing, University of Washington, Seattle, Washington

ANGELA DELVECCHIO, R.N.

Formerly with the Burn Unit, Boston Shriners' Hospital, Boston, Massachusetts

KAY EIDAL, R.N., M.N.

Formerly with the Pediatric Intensive Care Unit, University of Oregon Health Center, Portland, Oregon

MARSHA ELIXSON, R.N.

Senior Staff Nurse, Cardiac/Surgical Intensive Care Unit, Children's Hospital Medical Center, Boston, Massachusetts

JUDY HUNTINGTON, R.N., B.S.

Head Nurse, Pediatric Intensive Care Unit, Children's Orthopedic Hospital and Medical Center, Seattle, Washington

ANNALEE R. OAKES, R.N., M.A., CCRN

Associate Professor and Instructor, Emergency/Critical Care Nursing, Seattle Pacific University, Seattle, Washington

PATRICIA PALKO, R.N.

Formerly Inservice Director, Outpatient Department, Children's Orthopedic Hospital and Medical Center, Seattle, Washington

DONALDA PARKES, R.N., B.Sc.N.

Staff Instructor, Intensive Care Unit, The Hospital for Sick Children, Toronto, Ontario, Canada

CAROLE SALAMAHA, R.N., M.S.N.

Clinical Specialist, Pediatric Intensive Care Unit, Denver General Hospital, Denver, Colorado

ANITA STOEPPEL, R.N., B.S.N., M.S.N.

Clinical Instructor, Nursing Education, Children's Hospital Medical Center, Cincinnati, Ohio

CARMELLE SYLVESTRE-SIMON, R.N., B.Sc.N.

Staff Instructor, Intensive Care Unit, The Hospital for Sick Children, Toronto, Ontario, Canada

JOAN ALESSIO VERNOSE, R.N., B.S.N.

Formerly with the Children's Hospital of Philadelphia, Philadelphia, Pennsylvania

JEANNE YOCKE, R.N., M.S.N.

Clinical Specialist, Pediatric Intensive Care, Denver General Hospital, Denver, Colorado

PREFACE

During the late 1950's, a new plan for giving intensive care to adults with the cardiac insults of myocardial infarction and arrhythmias became popular. Success in reducing mortality and morbidity spawned enthusiasm among other subspecialty groups for developing similar concentrated critical care delivery, and soon many adult units were functioning for these purposes. Little thought was given to a large segment in our society, children, and to creating separate critical care areas for them outside of general pediatric units.

Someone once said that a pediatric practice is simply caring for "little adults," and that is primarily how children were interspersed through adult intensive care units. Very soon, fortunately, a few medical and nursing personnel began to recognize the definite and unique nature of treating critically ill and injured children. But separate units, complete with staff who held degrees of advanced education in pediatric critical care, were extremely slow to form.

Twenty-five years of specialty care came and went, with a continued scarcity of written guidelines or educational programs to support pediatric critical care nurses. A small group of far-sighted critical care nurses, holding national board positions with the AACN, agreed to sponsor a text about pediatric and adolescent critical care nursing. An urgency was voiced by the AACN contingency to design a book that would provide a ready reference for nurses interested in providing the highest quality of critical care nursing to any pediatric patient regardless of geographic position in the hospital.

Since most nurses will not immediately recall every aspect of a child's normal growth and development, much less how critical illness or injury may disrupt these phenomena, the first section of *Critical Care Nursing of Children and Adolescents* offers a detailed description of this material, so that the reader may chronologically identify physiologic parameters as well as categorically recognize a wide range of conceptual data. Appropriate nursing interventions are provided that are commensurate with the child's physical and mental age.

The foundational section is followed by several chapters focusing on individual organ systems disruptions, including pathophysiology, diagnostic and assessment procedures and results, goals of care, medical/surgical/nursing interventions, complications, and special nursing needs. Several chapters include detailed information about supportive concepts within the general system presented, such as oxygen therapy and acid-base imbalances peculiar to children of various ages. The third section incorporates special disorders and problems that are prevalent among or unique to children; child abuse and craniofacial abnormalities, among others.

No text of this nature would be considered complete without some clinical integration, and this is provided by two case studies outlining separate stages and pathophysiologic states. Each one presents a sequential, day-by-day advance of problems and interventions.

The AACN Board of Directors, who originally conceived the idea of providing a clinical reference text about pediatric and adolescent critical care nursing, will not receive the final honors. Those joys belong to the many nurses who have committed themselves to putting into practice the content of this book. To them go the blessing and good wishes of the editor and contributors.

Special thanks must be extended to the many nurses, physicians, paramedical personnel, and personal colleagues who helped keep this text going even when it seemed destined to lag. It would never have reached your hands without Kathy Pitcoff, Nursing Editor at W.B. Saunders, and her outstanding crew, who are some of the most talented people with whom I have worked. Finally, I thank those who always stood by to encourage me in the hardest moments: my husband and three daughters, Alice, Joyce, and Anne. To them I dedicate this book.

A.R.O.

CONTENTS

CHAPTER 1
GROWTH AND DEVELOPMENT

Carole Salamaha, R.N., M.S.,
Jeanne Yocke, R.N., M.S.N.,
Kay Eidal, R.N., M.N., and
Annalee Oakes, R.N., M.A., CCRN

OBJECTIVES

1. Describe normal growth and development (physical and psychological). Name at least three physical characteristics for each of the various age groups listed.

2. Recognize deviations from normal growth and development by describing common abnormalities for each phase. Indicate how illness may alter the physical or behavioral growth.

3. Delineate appropriate coping mechanisms available to the child at various ages.

4. Describe the major components of a healthy parent-child interaction.

5. Recognize the abnormal parent-child interaction by providing examples from literature, experience, or both.

6. Outline the normal responses of a child at various ages to separation from the parent(s).

7. Identify individualized nursing interventions that can help the child and family cope with illness in the intensive care setting. Apply knowledge of developmental behavior to the nurse's expectations of the ill child.

8. Outline a plan to instruct parents regarding the possible effects of hospitalization on normal growth and development after discharge.

INTRODUCTION

In a critical care unit, the child's physical well-being is understood to be of primary importance. For example, a patent airway must not be sacrificed in order to prevent the trauma of being physically restrained for suctioning. However, it is hoped that the information contained in this chapter (Growth and Development) will help the nurse understand that the child has limited coping mechanisms and fewer resources than the adult.

Because of the large quantity of basic material available on growth and development, this section will be limited primarily to discussion of those aspects that pertain directly to the care of children in the critical care unit. Generally accepted facts and protocols are included, with the expectation that nurses practicing pediatric critical care will be alert to new and creative ways to implement these data. Some specific information is pertinent for parent teaching and for helping the nurse to choose appropriate toys and activities to occupy a child's time while confined to bed or hospital. "Play permits the child to respond to challenge, to influence his environment, to initiate action, and to observe the results. . . he acquires. . . confidence in his own powers. . . and a positive self image."[1]

NORMAL PHYSICAL AND PHYSIOLOGIC DEVELOPMENT

1 to 3 Months

1. Height
   a. Girls: 57 to 62 cm by 3 months
   b. Boys: 58 to 63 cm by 3 months
2. Weight
   a. Girls: 4.8 to 6.3 kg
   b. Boys: 5 to 6.5 kg
3. Fontanels
   a. Anterior: may be closed by 3 months; average age of closure is 18 months
   b. Posterior: usually closes by 2 months
4. Head circumference at 3 months
   a. Girls: 37 to 43 cm
   b. Boys: 38 to 44 cm (3rd to 97th percentile)
5. Reflexes disappear (stepping, rooting)
6. Pulse: 100 to 140/min; average 110/min
7. Respirations: 30/min
8. Blood pressure
   a. Systolic: 80±16 mm Hg
   b. Diastolic: 46±16 mm Hg
9. Stomach capacity: 90 to 150 ml at 1 month
10. Caloric requirements: 117 Cal/kg/day or 51 Cal/lb/day (0 to 5 months)*

---

*Recommended daily allowances established by Food and Nutrition Board, National Academy of Sciences, and The National Research Council, 1975.

     a. Fluid requirements: approximately 600 ml (20 oz) per day after 8 days of age; up to 1000 ml (1 qt) per day

     b. Plan 20 Cal per 30 ml (1 oz) of volume

11. Number of stools

     a. Bottle fed: 1 stool per day

     b. Breast fed: up to 3 per day

12. Urine output: 250 to 400 ml /day

13. Sleep patterns: may have a preference for sleeping position by 2 months of age

14. Blood

     a. Volume: 75 to 100 ml/kg

     b. Hematocrit: 35 to 49%

     c. Hemoglobin

        1) 1 month: 11 to 17 gm/dl

        2) 2 months: 11 to 14 gm/dl

        3) 3 months: 10 to 13 gm/dl

3 to 6 Months

1. Height

     a. Girls: 62.5 to 67.8 cm by 6 months

     b. Boys: 63.9 to 69.3 cm by 6 months

2. Weight: birth weight has doubled by 4 to 5 months

     a. Girls: 6.4 to 8.4 kg by 6 months

     b. Boys: 6.7 to 8.7 kg by 6 months

3. Head circumference

     a. Girls: 41 to 46 cm at 6 months (3rd to 97th percentile)

     b. Boys: 42 to 47 cm at 6 months (3rd to 97th percentile)

4. Reflexes

     a. All superficial reflexes should be present by 6 months

     b. Infant reflexes should disappear

5. Pulse: 100 to 140/min; average 110/min

6. Respirations: 30/min

7. Blood pressure: see 1 to 3 months and 6 to 12 months

8. Stomach capacity: average 200 ml

9. Caloric requirements: 110 Cal/kg/day

     a. Fluid requirements: 150 ml/kg/day, up to 1000 ml (1 qt) per day

10. Urine output: 250 to 400 ml/day (1–3 cc/kg/hr)

11. Sleep patterns

     a. Has a preferred sleeping position

     b. Has an established routine before sleeping, i.e., sucking fingers or toy, listening to music, crying

     c. At about 4 months, sleep habits include definite nap times during day

     d. At 4 to 5 months, sleeps through night

12. Blood

     a. Volume: 75 to 100 ml/kg

     b. Hematocrit: 35 to 50%

     c. Hemoglobin: 10.5 to 14.5 gm/dl at 6 months[13]

6 to 9 Months
1. Height by 9 months
    a. Girls: 67 to 73 cm
    b. Boys: 68.6 to 74 cm
2. Weight by 9 months
    a. Girls: 7.5 to 10.1 kg
    b. Boys: 8.0 to 10.3 kg
3. Head circumference at 9 months
    a. Girls: 43 to 49 cm
    b. Boys: 45 to 49 cm
4. Pulse: 90 to 140/min; average 110/min
5. Respirations: 30/min
6. Blood pressure
    a. Systolic: 89±29 mm Hg (6 to 12 months)
    b. Diastolic: 60±10 mm Hg (6 to 12 months)
7. Stomach capacity: average 200 ml
8. Caloric requirement: 108 Cal/kg/day or 47 Cal/lb/day
    a. Fluid requirement: 150 ml/kg/day
9. Urine output: 400 to 500 ml/day (1–3 cc/kg/hr)
10. Sleep patterns
    a. Usually sleeps through night, awakening later
    b. Usually continues to have two naps per day
11. Blood
    a. Volume: 75 to 100 ml/kg
    b. Hematocrit: 30 to 40%
    c. Hemoglobin: 10.5 to 14.5 gm/dl[13]

9 to 12 Months
1. Height: child grows 25 cm in first year of life
    a. Girls: 70.6 to 71 cm by 12 months
    b. Boys: 72.4 to 78 cm by 12 months
2. Weight: birth weight tripled by 1 year
    a. Girls: 8.3 to 11.25 kg by 12 months
    b. Boys: 8.8 to 11.5 kg by 12 months
3. Fontanels
    a. Anterior: usually closes between 10 and 14 months; average age is 18 months
4. Head circumference at 12 months
    a. Girls: 44 to 50 cm
    b. Boys: 46 to 51 cm
5. Pulse: 90 to 140/min; average 110/min
6. Respirations: 30/min
7. Blood pressure
    a. Systolic: 89±29 mm Hg
    b. Diastolic: 60±10 mm Hg
8. Stomach capacity: 210 to 360 ml at one year
9. Caloric requirements: 108 Cal/kg/day or 47 Cal/lb/day
    a. Fluid requirements: 150 ml/kg/day
10. Urine output: 400 to 500 ml/day

11. Sleep patterns
   a. Sleeps through night
   b. May continue with 2 naps per day but probably naps only in afternoon
12. Blood
   a. Volume: 75 to 100 ml/kg
   b. Hematocrit: 30 to 40%
   c. Hemoglobin: 11 to 15 gm/dl at 1 year[13]

12 to 18 Months

1. Height
   a. Girls: 76.8 to 84.5 cm
   b. Boys: 78.8 to 85 cm
2. Weight
   a. Girls: 9.6 to 12.8 kg
   b. Boys: 10 to 13 kg
3. Fontanels
   a. Anterior may remain open until 18 months
4. Head circumference at 18 months
   a. Girls: 46 to 51 cm
   b. Boys: 47 to 53 cm
5. Pulse: 90 to 110/min; average 95
6. Respirations: 25/min
7. Blood pressure
   a. Systolic: 96±30 mm Hg
   b. Diastolic: 66±25 mm Hg
8. Stomach capacity: 210–360 ml
9. Caloric requirements: 100 Cal/kg/day
   a. Fluid requirements: 125 ml/kg/day
10. Urine output: 500 ml/day
11. Sleep patterns
   a. Sleep requirements diminish to 10 to 14 hr/day
   b. Continues with afternoon nap
   c. May require additional "quieting down" at bedtime owing to increasing autonomy and "fighting sleep" behavior
12. Blood
   a. Volume: 75 to 100 ml/kg
   b. Hematocrit: 30 to 40%
   c. Hemoglobin: 11 to 15 gm/dl

1½ to 2 Years

1. Height: child grows 12.5 cm in second year of life
   a. Girls: 82 to 91 cm
   b. Boys: 84 to 91 cm
2. Weight: birth weight is quadrupled by end of second year
   a. Girls: 10.6 to 14.3 kg
   b. Boys: 11.2 to 14.4 kg
3. Head circumference at 2 years
   a. Girls: 46 to 52 cm
   b. Boys: 48 to 53 cm

4. Pulse: 80 to 110/min; average 95/min
5. Respirations: 25/min
6. Blood pressure
   a. Systolic: 99±25 mm Hg
   b. Diastolic: 64±25 mm Hg
7. Stomach capacity: approximately 500 ml at 2 years
8. Caloric requirements: 100 Cal/kg/day
   a. Fluid requirements: 125 ml/kg/day
9. Urine output: 500 to 600 ml/day
10. Sleep patterns
    a. Has set pattern for sleep, i.e., ritual of after-dinner bathing, bedtime stories, night light, and quiet play
    b. May physically object to sleep, climb out of bed with frequent falls, get out of bed and into dangerous activities
11. Blood
    a. Volume: 75 to 100 ml/kg
    b. Hematocrit: 30 to 40%
    c. Hemoglobin: 12 to 15 gm/dl
    d. BUN: 5 to 15 mg/dl[13]

2 to 3 Years

1. Height: child grows 7.5 to 10 cm in third year of life
   a. Girls: 90 to 101 cm
   b. Boys: 92 to 100 cm
2. Weight
   a. Girls: 12.5 to 16.9 kg
   b. Boys: 13 to 16.6 kg
3. Head circumference at 3 years
   a. Girls: 47 to 52 cm
   b. Boys: 49 to 54 cm
4. Pulse: 80 to 110 min; average 95/min
5. Respirations: 25/min
6. Blood pressure
   a. Systolic: 100±25 mm Hg
   b. Diastolic: 67±23 mm Hg
7. Stomach capacity: 750 to 900 ml
8. Caloric requirements: 100 Cal/kg/day
   a. Fluid requirements: 125/ml/kg/day
9. Urine output: 500 to 600 ml/day
10. Sleep patterns
    a. Continues bedtime ritual, with increasing self-control over preparatory activities
    b. May awaken crying and show "nightmare" fears
11. Blood
    a. Volume: 75 to 100 ml/kg
    b. Hematocrit: 30 to 40%
    c. Hemoglobin: 12 to 15 gm/dl[13]

4 to 6 Years

1. Height: child grows 6 to 8 cm (2.5 to 3.5 in) per year

      a.   Boys: 105 to 117 cm (41.5 to 46 in)
      b.   Girls: 105 to 115 cm (41.5 to 45 in)
2. Weight: child gains 2.0 kg (4.5 lb) per year
      a.   Boys: 16.23 kg (36 to 50 lb)
      b.   Girls: 16.22 kg (36 to 48 lb)
3. Head circumference
      a.   Boys: 51 to 56 cm
      b.   Girls: 49 to 54 cm
      c.   By 6 years, head is 90% of final adult size
4. Pulse: 80 to 90/min
5. Respirations: 24 to 25/min
6. Blood pressure
      a.   Systolic: 80 to 110 mm Hg
      b.   Diastolic: 50 to 60 mm Hg
7. Stomach capacity: 750 to 900 ml
      a.   Protuberant abdomen disappears
8. Caloric requirements: 1400 to 1800 Cal/day (or 90 Cal/kg)
      a.   Fluid requirements: 100 to 125 ml/kg/day
9. Urine output: 700 to 1000 ml/day
10. Sleep patterns
      a.   Sound sleeper, continues to sleep 10 to 12 hours at night
      b.   Relinquishes daytime naps
      c.   May begin reporting and describing nightmares
11. Blood
      a.   Volume: 75 to 100 ml/kg
      b.   Hematocrit: 31 to 43%
      c.   Hemoglobin (5 yr): 12 to 13 gm/dl
12. Body temperature: 37±0.2° C

6 to 12 Years

1. Height: child grows 6 to 8 cm (92 to 3 in) per year
      a.   At 7 years: boys   117 to 131 cm (46 to 51 in)
                      girls   117 to 129 cm (46 to 50 in)
      b.   At 11 years: boys   137 to 152 cm (54 to 60 in)
                      girls   137 to 153 cm (54 to 60.5 in)
      c.   Growth of bones is faster than increase in muscle and ligament strength[1]
2. Weight: child gains 3 to 3.5 kg (7 lb) per year
      a.   At 7 years: boys   20.7 to 29.2 kg (46 to 64 lb)
                      girls   20.2 to 27.8 kg (45 to 61 lb)
      b.   At 11 years: boys   30 to 45 kg (66 to 99 lb)
                      girls   28 to 45.5 kg (62 to 100 lb)
3. Head circumference
      a.   Average 51 to 54 cm (20 to 21 in)
      b.   Brain reaches adult size by 10 to 12 years
4. Pulse: 70 to 100/min; average 70 to 80/min
5. Respirations: 18 to 20/min

6. Blood pressure
   a. Systolic: 95 to 108 mm Hg
   b. Diastolic: 60 to 67 mm Hg
7. Stomach capacity: 750 to 900 ml
8. Caloric requirements
   a. At 7 years: 80 Cal/kg/day
   b. At 12 years: 70 Cal/kg/day
      1) Range: 1600 to 2800 Cal/day
   c. Fluid requirements: 75 ml/kg/day
      1) Range: 1500 to 3000 ml/day
9. Urine output: 700 to 1500 ml/day
10. Sleep patterns
    a. Continues to sleep 8 to 10 hours at night
    b. Describes dreams frequently and nightmares in detail
11. Blood
    a. Volume: 75 to 100 ml/kg
    b. Hematocrit 34 to 40%
    c. Hemoglobin: 13 to 14 gm/dl
12. Cardiac
    a. Murmurs: peak incidence of innocent ("functional")
       murmurs is 6 to 9 years of age
13. Body temperature: 36.8±0.2°C

12 to 18 Years (Puberty and Adolescence)

1. Height
   a. At 15 years: boys   158 to 177 cm (62 to 70 in)
                      girls   155 to 168 cm (61 to 66 in)
   b. By 17 years, average girl and boy both achieve 100% of mature
      height.
   c. Boys show rapid growth in muscular strength and coordination
2. Weight
   a. At 15 years: boys   45 to 67 kg (99 to 148 lb)
                      girls   44 to 63 kg (97 to 138 lb)
   b. In girls, most rapid weight gain occurs during the year prior
      to menarche
3. Pulse: 60 to 80/min
4. Respirations: 18 to 20/min
5. Blood pressure
   a. Systolic: 100 to 120 mm Hg
   b. Diastolic: 50 to 70 mm Hg
6. Caloric requirements
   a. Pubertal girls, moderately active: 2200 to 2800 Cal/day
   b. Pubertal boys, active: 3000 Cal/day
   c. 15% of calories should come from protein[13]
   d. Fluid requirements: 50 to 65 ml/kg/day[13]
7. Urine output: 700 to 1500 ml/day
8. Sleep patterns: resemble adult patterns

9. Blood
   a. Volume: 70 to 85 ml/kg
   b. Hematocrit: male   42 to 52%
                     female   37 to 47%
   c. Hemoglobin: male   14 to 18 gm/dl
                     female   12 to 16 gm/dl
10. Body temperature: 36.8±0.2°C
11. Sexual characteristics
    a. Definitions
       1) Pubescence: time span during which secondary sexual changes occur and reproductive functions begin to mature. [28,33]
       2) Puberty: period during which person reaches reproductive maturity; occurs approximately 2 to 3 years after pubescence. [33]
       3) Adolescence: period beginning with pubescence and ending when somatic growth and reproductive maturity are complete [25,33]
    b. Sequence of sexual maturation [5,16]
       1) Female: Pelvis contours; fat deposition
                     Breast enlargement; pigmentation of nipples
                     Initial appearance of straight pubic hair
                     Beginning of vaginal secretions
                     Kinky pubic hair, abundant
                     First menses
                     Growth of axillary hair
       2) Male: Growth of penis and testes
                     Hypertrophy, nodularity of breasts
                     Initial appearance of straight pubic hair
                     Voice changes
                     Continued rapid growth of penis and testes
                     Ejaculation
                     Kinky pubic hair, abundant
                     Disappearance of breast hypertrophy
                     Axillary hair
                     Facial hair
    c. Appearance of acne varies considerably in both male and female

NORMAL SOCIAL AND EMOTIONAL DEVELOPMENT

1 to 3 Months

1. Erikson's stage, "basic trust versus basic mistrust," predominates. Child develops sense of trust if close relationship is established with primary caregiver and if needs for food, warmth, love, and comfort are met. Mistrust develops if close relationship is absent or

sporadic.[9,15] Some infants at this state are happy only when being carried or in constant motion.[5]

a. *Critical care problems*
Infant is distressed because of unmet physical needs.

b. *Nursing interventions and coping skills*
Patient enjoys cuddling, rocking, fondling, and hearing voice of caretaker. Parent should be with the child at feeding times if possible.

2. Child is developing first emotionally related "attachment."[16,21] A variety of attachment behaviors (crying, fussing, smiling) may be manifested.

a. *Critical care problems*
Absent mother figure, multiple caregivers.

b. *Nursing interventions and coping skills*
Encourage liberal parental visiting.

3. Child will respond to a variety of people and objects (indiscriminate "attachment").[3]

a. *Critical care problems*
Multiple caregivers.

b. *Nursing interventions and coping skills*
Consistent mother image is not critical as long as needs are met.

4. Child awakens slowly.

a. *Nursing interventions and coping skills*
Approach sleeping child gently.

3 to 6 Months

1. "Basic trust versus mistrust" stage continues.[15]
2. "Attachment" begins to narrow. A one-to-one relationship with the mother is well established.[3]

a. *Critical care problems*
Multiple caregivers.

b. *Nursing interventions and coping skills*
Consistent mother image important

3. Smiles spontaneously.

a. *Nursing interventions and coping skills*
Play peek-a-boo. Repetition.

4. Mimics facial expressions.

a. *Nursing interventions and coping skills*
Smile, use facial expressions of happiness when talking with child.

5. Recognizes mother but enjoys other people.
6. Wakes up fast, gets going immediately.

   a. *Critical care problems*
   Numerous and frightening sounds.

   b. *Nursing interventions and coping skills*
   If rousing child for treatment, vital signs, or feeding, have everything ready first. Have play activity ready when treatments are completed.

6 to 9 Months

1. "Basic trust versus mistrust" stage continues.[15]
2. Child exhibits behaviors denoting separation anxiety. Cries when mother leaves. Substitute care-givers are less acceptable than mother.

   a. *Critical care problems*
   Short visitation periods bring about frequent episodes of separation.

   b. *Nursing interventions and coping skills*
   Unlimited visiting privileges for parents and/or significant others.

   No concept of parents' existence when out of sight. Dislikes bedtime, naptime, and inevitable separation. Attachment to parents is stronger than previously.[5]

   a. *Critical care problems*
   Child is mostly confined to bed or small space.

   b. *Nursing interventions and coping skills*
   Sit, snuggle in nurse's or parent's lap to give comfort and build trust.

3. Specific "attachment" begins and may be directed to inanimate objects (blanket, toys).[3]

   a. *Critical care problems*
   Absence of stable mother figure or parent.

   b. *Nursing interventions and coping skills*
   Encourage parent visitation. Provide inanimate objects for child's comfort. Allow child to keep his own blanket and to take it anywhere he must go; alert staff to its importance.

4. Stranger anxiety reflects ability to differentiate between familiar and unfamiliar people.[35]

   a. *Critical care problems*
   Multiple caregivers of varying appearances, i.e., different clothing or colors.

5. Stretches arms to loved adults.

    a. ***Critical care problems***
        Restraints.

6. Rudimentary independent behaviors (holding own bottle, turning over independently).

    a. ***Critical care problems***
        Intravenous lines, nasogastric feedings.

    b. ***Nursing interventions and coping skills***
        If possible, allow as much repositioning and self-movement as environment permits.

9 to 12 Months

1. "Basic trust versus mistrust" stage continues.[15]

    a. ***Critical care problems***
        Painful procedures.

    b. ***Nursing interventions and coping skills***
        Always follow treatments with much tender, loving care.

2. Father equals mother in importance.[21]

    a. ***Critical care problems***
        Working fathers unable to visit often.

    b. ***Nursing interventions and coping skills***
        Unlimited visiting for parents. Encourage mother and father to take turns visiting.

3. Child has beginning concept of social give and take (love pats, hugs, kisses).

    a. ***Critical care problems***
        Limited opportunity for touching, hugging, kissing.

    b. ***Nursing interventions and coping skills***
        Stroke and caress as much as condition permits.

4. Child responds positively to friends and strangers.

    a. ***Nursing interventions and coping skills***
        Allow other family and friends to visit as much as possible.

5. Child is increasingly aware of social world. Responds to facial expressions and sounds.

    a. ***Critical care problems***
        Possible isolation room. Limited visual contact if head is restrained.

    b. ***Nursing interventions and coping skills***
        Allow mother to be with child as much as possible, especially at feedings. Let patient see and hear you before touching him gently.

6. Child understands "no-no." Cries when scolded.

   a. Nursing interventions and coping skills
   Use soft voice when setting limits.

7. Child becomes egocentric, shows jealousy, anger, and fear.

   a. Critical care problems
   Invasive procedures, pain.

8. Child is upset by changes in household.

   a. Critical care problems
   Strange environment.

   b. Nursing interventions and coping skills
   Try to provide familiar objects from home, such as special
   or personal toys.

12 to 18 Months

1. "Attachment" again becomes more diffuse; may extend to include other family members (father, siblings, grandparents).[3]

   a. Critical care problems
   Changing staff and length of contact time.

   b. Nursing interventions and coping skills
   Allow siblings, grandparents to visit. Maintain same staff with
   patient.

2. Needs to explore but must return to mother periodically.

   a. Critical care problem
   Confined to bed or room.

3. "Basic trust versus mistrust" stage continues, but assertion and independence may begin.

   a. Critical care problems
   Illness and injury frequently do not allow independence even on same matters consistently.

   b. Nursing interventions and coping skills
   Try to maintain same staff with child so that one person on
   each shift can be relied upon.

18 to 24 Months

1. Beginning of Erikson's stage, "autonomy versus shame and doubt." Muscular maturation sets the stage for exploration and experimentation, which foster the child's independence and self-control. Suppression of these behaviors or lack of "basic trust" results in clinging dependence, self-consciousness (shame), and paranoic fear (doubt).

   a. Critical care problems
   Prolonged or catastrophic limitations such as traction, full body casts, massive or restrictive dressings.

    b. Nursing interventions and coping skills
    Let child explore through such material as books, building toys, "see-through" pictures, magic slates. Nurse may need to read or hold object as child identifies or mimics nurse's description or words.

2. Independence alternates with sudden dependence and the need for periodic cuddling and reassurance.
3. Negativism may be child's primary means of exhibiting control. "No" can sometimes mean "yes."

    a. Critical care problems
    Procedures are often directed "for" and "at" patient.

    b. Nursing interventions and coping skills
    Play games using "yes" and "no" in correct sequence, e.g., "Can John play in this corner?" "Yes." "Can John go night-night (or similar term) on the floor?" "No."

4. Temper tantrums, ritualistic behaviors, and breath-holding "spells" are common.[5]

    a. Critical care problems
    Frustration and anger because of painful procedures, physical restraint, confinements.

    b. Nursing interventions and coping skills
    Give kisses at bedtime; allow child to hug and caress nurse. If parent or loved one available, encourage touch interaction. Careful observation is important to differentiate apnea from breath-holding spells.

5. Obeys simple commands.
6. Imitates adult activities seen in the home.

2 to 3 Years

1. "Autonomy versus shame and doubt" stage continues.
2. Need to please may often conflict with wants. Child may threaten to alienate person on whom he is most dependent.

    a. Critical care problems
    Great dependency for comfort needs.

    b. Nursing interventions and coping skills
    Provide comfort and meet as many needs of this age as possible to decrease conflicts.

3. Negativism, ritualism (necessary for security), and dawdling increase. Thumb-sucking and temper tantrums decrease. Temper tantrums may occur with frustration, however.

    a. Critical care problems
    Different caregivers interrupt rituals.

    b. Nursing interventions and coping skills
    Anticipatory play may help. Bed-time rituals are most common.

4. Child is impatient; has strong desires and urgent demands but is willing to accept substitutes.[16]

   a. *Critical care problems*
   Delays and waiting intervals are common.

   b. *Nursing interventions and coping skills*
   Avoid criticism; provide acceptable alternatives.

5. Child is indecisive, unable to make choices. May have imaginary friends (good or bad).

   a. *Nursing interventions and coping skills*
   Do not expect decision-making except of obvious likes and dislikes. Do not frustrate by forcing decisions.

6. Child is unable to share possessions.

   a. *Critical care problem*
   Little opportunity for shared play because of confinement.

7. Child lives in the present, e.g., when mother leaves she no longer exists.

8. May seem to understand parent is going to leave, but is overwhelmed by first separation experience.[31]

   a. *Nursing interventions and coping skills*
   Play "going and coming."

9. This is a most endangered age. Child is no longer totally supported by parent, but is too young to use own reason or to accept verbal explanation. Needs mother to make hospitalization bearable.

   a. *Critical care problems*
   Restricted visiting.

   b. *Nursing interventions and coping skills*
   Encourage visiting, especially by mother or surrogate mother figure.

3 to 6 Years

1. Erikson's stage, "initiative versus shame and doubt" begins at about 4 years. Undertaking, planning, and attacking are added to autonomy already formulated. Guilt occurs when the child desires to remain dependent.[9,15]

   a. *Critical care problems*
   Dependency is necessary because of pain, course of disease, immobilization.

   b. *Nursing interventions and coping skills*
   Encourage independence whenever possible. Allow child to select time for bathing, snack, kind of juice, etc. Point to autonomous actions; as independency increases, identify new self-initiated controls.

2. Basic family remains significant; primary security is within family.

   a. *Critical care problems*
      Removal from family. Prolonged hospitalization.

   b. *Nursing interventions and coping skills*
      Invite siblings to accompany parents on special visits.

3. Interaction with others increases.

   a. *Critical care problem*
      Isolation.

4. Sharing capacity begins, as does sense of property rights.

   a. *Critical care problems*
      Limited contact with other children due to risk of infection, severity of illness or injuries.

   b. *Nursing interventions and coping skills*
      Use tape recorders to make and play "messages" of familiar voices.

5. Egocentricity continues along with a growing desire to make own decisions. May need to return to mother periodically, but less frequently as age 6 approaches.

6. Ritualism may continue, but child becomes increasingly flexible in routine.

   a. *Nursing interventions and coping skills*
      Introduce changes in the familiar pattern, keeping the same components. If a new function is introduced, try to surround it with familiar activities.

7. Oedipal conflict. Child begins identification with parent of the opposite sex and is in conflict with parent of the same sex.

   a. *Critical care problems*
      Female nurses outnumber male nurses.

   b. *Nursing interventions and coping skills*
      Have the more "acceptable" parent assist with care. Teach parents about phase child is going through.

8. Role playing and imitation of adult behavior.

6 to 12 Years

1. Erikson's stage, "industry versus inferiority" coincides with school entrance. The child attempts to bring a protective situation to completion and subsequently to win approval for his successes. Repeated failure promotes the child's sense of inferiority and inadequacy.[9,15]

   a. *Critical care problems*
      Child misses long intervals of education; may be set back by illness and complications.

b. *Nursing interventions and coping skills*
Incorporate word and math games for positive results. Be sure patient experiences success in answering.

2. Shows greater mastery of self and environment.

a. *Critical care problems*
Loss of control because of injury or illness.

3. Enormous curiosity, especially concerning adult activities.
4. Peer relationships and conformity are foremost; family ties are no longer paramount. Need for assured position in social group, e.g., gangs or secret clubs. Friendships usually confined to members of the same sex and similar age; sex antagonism may be acute.

a. *Critical care problems*
Is confined with children of several ages and varying kinds of severe injuries and illnesses.

b. *Nursing interventions and coping skills*
Try to consider personalities, age range, and degree of illness when making bed assignments.

5. Child meets dependency needs through relationships with significant adults other than parents. However, participation in family affairs remains important.

a. *Critical care problems*
Child's participation in decision making and therapeutic regime is frequently not possible.

b. *Nursing interventions and coping skills*
In addition to visits from parents, include messages from teachers and other significant adults.

6. Child is critical of adults; rebels at routines. Has opinions about everything, wants to be considered important.

a. *Critical care problems*
Procedures are routine. Child is not knowledgeable about severity of illness or injuries.

b. *Nursing interventions and coping skills*
Allow as much individualization and self-care as possible.

7. Behavior may be erratic or extreme; courtesy, congeniality, and affection may alternate with anti-social behavior to attract attention.[16, 24]

a. *Critical care problems*
Limited social contact; child immobilized by physical problems.

b. *Nursing interventions and coping skills*
Let child express thoughts about environment, procedures, and illness.

8. Teasing not well tolerated.
9. Desires group's attention; likes to take turns; abides by group decisions.

   a. *Nursing interventions and coping skills*
   Provide as much visual and verbal contact with other patients as possible.

10. Boasting and rivalry evidenced as child seeks prestige.

    a. *Critical care problems*
    Child is frequently stripped of personal belongings, peer recognition, and status of school achievements.

    b. *Nursing interventions and coping skills*
    Compliment child and show genuine interest in the small accomplishments of getting well. Focus on child, not body parts or things.

11. Defense mechanisms, such as repression, reaction-formation, sublimation, used in coping behavior.[21]
12. Responds to anxiety by inappropriate laughter, excessive talking, psychosomatic illness.

    a. *Critical care problems*
    Intubation inhibits ability to express anxiety.

    b. *Nursing interventions and coping skills*
    Encourage self-expression via handgrips, blinking eyes, tapping on bed rails.

12 to 18 Years

1. Erikson's stage, "identity versus role confusion," predominates during adolescence, a transitory time characterized by vacillations between dependence and independence, idealism and realism, confidence and uncertainty. Failure of the adolescent to integrate inner feelings with universal realities results in role confusion and vagueness regarding identity.

   a. *Critical care problems*
   Sensory stimulation and overload. Sleep deprivation, pain, and unfamiliar terminology and roles of personnel.

   b. *Nursing interventions and coping skills*
   Plan appropriate sleep intervals. Protect privacy of young males by staffing male nurses to provide care of genitalia. Drape and keep chest and genitalia covered as much as possible for females. Recognize and describe all elimination and excretion needs with familiar terms.

2. Desires to be useful to society; begins to prepare for vocation or career.
3. Conformity to peer standards and acquisition of group prestige is stronger than response to adult guidance.

    a.　*Critical care problems*
       Rigid rules for procedures and emergency care.

    b.　*Nursing interventions and coping skills*
       Assign young staff members for easier relationship. Identify expectations of patient in patient's own vocabulary. Set realistic standards of patient involvement in care plan.

4.　Acquisition of skills is required for successful group participation; adolescent is willing to practice in order to gain proficiency.
5.　Capable of making a commitment to concrete relationships and partnerships.
6.　Has one or two best friends.

    a.　*Critical care problems*
       Friend may have sustained injuries in same car with patient.

    b.　*Nursing interventions and coping skills*
       Be honest about involvement of others.

7.　Relationships initially confined to same sex, with energies devoted to attracting opposite sex (e.g., teasing).

    a.　*Nursing interventions and coping skills*
       Respect feelings of love and emotion for girlfriend or boyfriend.

8.　Identification continues with significant adult other than parent; teachers may be influential.

    a.　*Nursing interventions and coping skills*
       Encourage significant adult to visit and interact with patient; praise all attempts to cooperate in care.

9.　Cliques, fads, and unconventional attire predominate.

    a.　*Critical care problems*
       Unattractive hospital attire, sterile environment, need for frequent assessment of vital signs.

    b.　*Nursing interventions and coping skills*
       For girls, use becoming hair style to keep hair from face and away from secretions or wastes. Use deodorant or frequent cleansing to decrease offensive body odors.

10.　Has idealistic attitudes; demonstrates rebellion against established social and adult authority.
11.　Intensely emotional, especially while striving to understand social relationships.

    a.　*Nursing interventions and coping skills*
       Talk about friends. Encourage notes and cards. Respect feelings and emotions.

12.　Frequent "know-it-all" attitude.

SELF-CONCEPT FORMATION AND
SEX-ROLE IDENTIFICATION

1 to 3 Months
1. Unable to differentiate between self and rest of world.

    a. *Nursing interventions and coping skills*
    Snuggle and wrap closely to imitate security of womb.

3 to 6 months
1. Incorporative approach; puts everything into mouth to make it a part of self.

    a. *Critical care problems*
    Intravenous therapy, restraints.

    b. *Nursing interventions and coping skills*
    Allow hands, fingers, feet to be free as much as possible. Do not discourage fingers in mouth.

2. Inspection of upper parts of body and trunk indicates beginning of body awareness.

    a. *Critical care problems*
    Bandages, dressings.

    b. *Nursing interventions and coping skills*
    If possible, place intravenous lines in foot so baby will move, suck, and see hands.

6 to 9 Months
1. Acquires ability to separate self from other individuals and objects in the environment (self-awareness).
2. Differentiate mother's face from others, e.g., during feedings.

    a. *Critical care problems*
    Limited contact with mother.

    b. *Nursing interventions and coping skills*
    Have mother available for at least one feeding each day, preferably at same time.

3. Plays with feet and puts them in mouth.

    a. *Critical care problems*
    Restraints, casts.

4. Recognizes self in mirror.

    a. *Nursing interventions and coping skills*
    Use mobile, mirror at bed side, toys with mirror reflectors.

9 to 12 Months
1. Realizes the body is a continuous part of self (beginnings of body image concept).

   a. *Critical care problems*
       Pain, analgesics, nerve involvement in severe injuries.

   b. *Nursing interventions and coping skills*
       Play game of pointing to nose, eyes, mouth.

2. Listens to and recognizes own name.

   a. *Nursing interventions and coping skills*
       Use first name or nickname as appropriate.

12 to 18 Months
1. Body image formation continues.

18 to 24 Months
1. Child perceives self as good or bad depending upon how others respond to him.

   a. *Nursing interventions and coping skills*
       Assure child he is good as often as appropriate; avoid labeling him as bad.

2. Handles genitals (continued development of body awareness).

   a. *Critical care problems*
       Urinary catheters, bed pans, and urinals may be difficult to use.

   b. *Nursing interventions and coping skills*
       Place potty chair in bed if possible, or carry child to bathroom.

3. Kisses at bedtime.

   a. *Nursing interventions and coping skills*
       Have mother or loved one available as much as possible.

2 to 3 Years
1. Little awareness that he has weight or can be an obstacle.

   a. *Critical care problems*
       Complicated environment and many pieces of equipment.

2. Fascinated with own name; refers to self by name rather than by using pronouns.

   a. *Nursing interventions and coping skills*
       Refer to child by name, not by "honey" or "dear." Use own name (simple) and point to self.

3. Views his body as a hollow organ encased in skin, a reservoir for blood, food, wastes, and stomach.[16]

   a. *Critical care problems*
       Interruption of feeding and toileting procedures.

   b. *Nursing interventions and coping skills*
       Assimilate home functions as much as possible. Adhesive bandages important, may even be needed on imaginary scratches or hurts to help maintain body integrity.

4. Can name some external body parts, e.g., eye, nose, ear. Concerned with wholeness of body.

   a. *Critical care problems*
   Incisions, encasing of part in cast.

   b. *Nursing interventions and coping skills*
   Show body parts in mirror; touch and point to them.

5. Is aware of pain, but cannot point to it.
6. Is able to label himself or herself as "boy" or "girl" by about 3 years but is basically unaware of sex differences.
7. May begin to be curious about physical differences between sexes; exhibits desire to look at or touch parts of adults' body, especially female breasts.

   a. *Critical care problems*
   Co-ed rooms with other children.

   b. *Nursing interventions and coping skills*
   Answer questioning glances and pointing. Describe room partners with, "This is Jane, a little girl." "This is John, a little boy."

8. Expresses interest in different postures for urinating.[32]

3 to 6 Years
1. Increasingly accurate picture (body image) of physical self. Awareness of body functions extends to internal processes (heart, bowel movements, procreation).

   a. *Nursing interventions and coping skills*
   Use proper terminology for body functions, relate terms to familiar ones as noted on care plan or history.

2. Concern over body intactness; awareness of exterior body boundary.
3. Extends concept of self to include things that belong to him. Uses pronouns (I, my, mine) to demonstrate possessiveness.

   a. *Critical care problems*
   Restraints. Objects frequently removed from reach or awareness.

4. Is able to verbalize feelings about himself.

   a. *Critical care problems*
   Intubation restricts expression. Unfamiliar with objects and equipment invading body.

   b. *Nursing interventions and coping skills.*
   Ask questions about pain, repositioning, staying with him, playing with certain toy(s), and so on, so that yes or no answers will suffice. Use simple words to describe a limited number of materials to be used in care.

5. Is more aware of others' bodies and how they are different from his.
6. Preferences for sex-related toys and activities are evident.
7. Differences between sexes not associated with genital differences until about 5 to 6 years. Consistency of gender is conceptualized by child.

   a. *Critical care problems*
      Child may be naked with only a sheet covering.

8. Early in this period the Oedipal conflict is evident; the child identifies with the parent of the opposite sex and turns away from the parent of the same sex.

   a. *Nursing interventions and coping skills*
      Utilize parent of choice as much as possible. Interact with other parent to support understanding of patient's attitude.

9. Begins to wonder where he came from.

6 to 12 Years

1. Self-concept is stable if developmental progression unhindered.

   a. *Critical care problems*
      Education is interrupted.

2. Clear notion of own sex and of male and female roles. Uses labels to describe himself, i.e., boy, girl, cute.

   a. *Critical care problems*
      Caregivers are frequently female.

   b. *Nursing interventions and coping skills*
      If male child is embarrassed by female caregiver, try to respect feelings by having orderly or male nurse assist.

12 to 18 Years

1. Rapid physical maturation disrupts self-concept established in earlier years.
2. Heightened body awareness evident in attempt to promote acceptance of major physical changes.

   a. *Critical care problems*
      Invasive procedures: bladder catheter, rectal tubes. Frequent involuntary erections in males.

   b. *Nursing interventions and coping skills*
      Treat as adult if indicated. Do not talk or treat down. Involve parent of same sex if possible.

3. Meticulous concern over personal appearance; girls concerned about attractiveness (attire, hairstyles); boys concerned about physical appearance and strength.

   a. *Critical care problems*
      Clothing removed to expose entire body for assessment.

    b. *Nursing interventions and coping skills*
    Careful hair and face care for both sexes. Protect from undue
    exposure, drape, respect modesty.

4. Support and acceptance by peer group fosters security and a
strong self-concept; wants to be like peers but better.

    a. *Nursing interventions and coping skills*
    Allow as much self-help as feasible, given injuries or illness.

5. Sex roles solidifying; satisfactory heterosexual relationships are
important.

    a. *Critical care problems*
    Analgesia, sedation. Loss of body control. Care givers are
    frequently female.

    b. *Nursing interventions and coping skills*
    If patient indicates desire for significant friend to visit, allow
    short intervals of visitation. Prepare both patient and friend
    for unfamiliar sights or reactions.

_____ SENSORY AND PERCEPTIVE DEVELOPMENT _____

1 to 3 Months
1. Visual: responsive to complex, bright, mobile, or contrasting
visual objects; follows large, moving objects with both eyes and
head; eyes begin to converge; focuses best from approximately
8 inches away; ability to accommodate is limited; responds to
various features of an individual's face.[3,11]

    a. *Critical care problems*
    Sterile hospital environment, equipment, white walls and
    ceilings.

    b. *Nursing interventions and coping skills*
    Choose appropriate mobiles, toys, pictures in and around bed
    where they can be seen even if not touched.

2. Auditory: initial hearing response is at subcortical level; responds
to low-pitched sounds with decrease in motor activity and to
high-pitched sounds with alerting reactions; muscles particularly
respond to sound at about 2 months.

    a. *Critical care problems*
    Habituation due to excessive noise.

    b. *Nursing interventions and coping skills*
    Alternate periods of quiet rest with periods of meaningful
    auditory stimulation (music boxes, soothing voices, singing).
    Inform parents about possibility of decreased response to
    stimuli at home after discharge.

3. Olfactory: will turn away from unpleasant odors.
4. Taste: taste buds located primarily on tip of tongue in early childhood; infant has different responses to sweet and bitter tastes.

    a. **Critical care problems**
    Unpleasant-tasting medications.

    b. **Nursing interventions and coping skills**
    Insert oral medications inside cheek area to avoid tip of tongue.

5. Tactile: infant senses pressure, pain, and temperature; sensation is heightened in face (especially mouth), hands, and soles of feet. Touch and oral modes of stimulation are sources of gratification.

    a. **Critical care problems**
    Child may have nothing orally, or feedings may be limited.

    b. **Nursing interventions and coping skills**
    Caressing important; hold, touch, pat. Use pacifier. Don't try to prevent thumbsucking. If feeding is taken quickly, allow infant to dawdle with nipple or suck fingers or pacifier. May need up to 4 hours a day of extra sucking.[20]

6. Mature pain receptors in viscera; proprioceptive receptors in muscles, joints, and tendons.

    a. **Critical care problems**
    Child unable to verbalize pain sensation. Caregivers unfamiliar with child's usual responses.

    b. **Nursing interventions and coping skills**
    Nurse must be aware of pain and give sedation or analgesics appropriately.

3 to 6 Months

1. Visual: visual acuity 20/300 to 20/200; binocular vision improving; hand-eye coordination appears. Child fixates immediately on small objects less than 1 to 2 feet away; shows interest in stimulus greater than 3 feet away; inspects own hand; shows greater interest in complex objects with sharp contours.

    a. **Critical care problems**
    Sterile appearance of hospital environment. White or dull colors on walls and ceiling.

    b. **Nursing interventions and coping skills**
    Put mobiles and other toys within reach.

2. Tactile: touch and oral stimulation are gratifying.[21]

    a. **Critical care problems**
    Nothing by mouth.

>   b. *Nursing interventions and coping skills*
>   *Use pacifier; don't try to prevent thumbsucking. If feeding is taken quickly, allow to dawdle with nipple or suck fingers or pacifier.*

6 to 9 Months

1. Visual: binocular fixation; beginning depth perception. Attracted to two and three dimensional objects; responds more readily to familiar than unfamiliar faces.

>   a. **Critical care problems**
>   Limited visual field, may be able to see only the ceiling.

2. Tactile: need for sucking begins to decrease although touch and oral stimulation continue to be gratifying.[32] Bites and mouths objects[5]; rubs gums to decrease pain of teething.

>   a. **Critical care problems**
>   Hospital regimen may prolong the need to continue sucking.

>   b. *Nursing interventions and coping skills*
>   *Avoid hand restraints if possible. Provide objects that child may suck or bite.*

9 to 12 Months

1. Visual: vision 20/200. Interested in tiny objects; prefers three-dimensional objects to two-dimensional ones.

>   a. **Critical care problems**
>   Small, possibly sharp objects used at bedside.

>   b. *Nursing interventions and coping skills*
>   *Remove needles and syringes from visual field immediately.*

2. Auditory: music boxes have great appeal.

>   a. **Critical care problems**
>   General noises from large ward units; other extraneous noises.

>   b. *Nursing interventions and coping skills*
>   *Use music and music boxes; talk to baby.*

3. Tactile: touch and oral stimulation remain sources of gratification.

>   a. **Critical care problems**
>   Limited amount of time for procedures and care.

>   b. *Nursing interventions and coping skills*
>   *Pat and caress lovingly. Use soft voice and patience.*

4. Often has trouble unwinding;[16] will practice during sleep.

>   a. *Nursing interventions and coping skills*
>   *Parent education regarding dreams.*

12 to 18 Months
1. Visual: vision 20/180; discriminates between simple geometric forms; likes pictures.

   a. ***Critical care problems***
   Visual field limited to ceiling and upper walls.

18 to 24 Months
1. Visual: vision 20/40; accommodation well-developed.

   a. ***Nursing interventions and coping skills***
   Have large books that nurse can hold; show pictures; have musical and detailed mobiles available.

2 to 3 Years
1. Visual: vision 20/30.
2. Tactile: if blindfolded, no systematic way of exploring unidentified objects.[11]

   a. ***Critical care problems***
   Eyes patched.

   b. ***Nursing interventions and coping skills***
   Must have familiar or personal toy or object (e.g., blanket) to feel.

3 to 6 Years
1. Vision: 4- to 5-year old can distinguish open from closed letters (e.g., O from C); 5-year-old can distinguish straight from curved lines (e.g., U from V), upright from inverted letters (e.g., M from W), and directionality (e.g., b from d). By 6 years vision is 20/20. Critical period for development of three-dimensional perception.[11]

   a. ***Critical care problems***
   Visual fields limited if child is restrained or immobilized.

   b. ***Nursing interventions and coping skills***
   Hang large pictures and familiar objects on overhead frame. Provide ceiling movies, flash pictures and stories, or television if possible.

2. Auditory: complete maturation of auditory function (i.e., at cortical level).

   a. ***Critical care problems***
   Noises from hardware such as monitors and respirators.

   b. ***Nursing interventions and coping skills***
   Provide radio with music or familiar programs.

3. Taste and smell: has voluntary control; reacts accurately.

   a. ***Critical care problems***
   Intravenous and nasogastric feedings. Hospital food.

4. Tactile: blindfolded child is able to identify unknown objects by systematic exploration of contours.[11]

   a. *Nursing interventions and coping skills*
   Place necessary personal objects within reach. Allow patient to feel where they all are.

6 to 12 Years
1. Visual: eyeball reaches adult size; hyperopia may occur.

   a. *Critical care problems*
   Diplopia occurs in some head injuries or with certain medications.

   b. *Nursing interventions and coping skills*
   Place familiar personal objects within reach. Identify their placement. Remind patient that you know he sees two of everything; assure him that this will pass.

12 to 18 Years
1. Individual differences in style of perceptual exploration, dependent upon previous experiences, are evident.[3]

   a. *Critical care problems*
   Head restraints cause one-sided visual field. Head tongs, cervical collars.

   b. *Nursing interventions and coping skills*
   Use of beds or frames that allow for turning and expanded visual fields.

MOTOR DEVELOPMENT

1 to 3 Months
1. Gross motor: when prone, raises head and chest with fairly good head control;[4, 20] midline arm coordination developing; almost continuous arm and leg movement when awake; bats at objects with hands; makes reaching movements while lying on back.

   a. *Critical care problems*
   Child restrained on back; extremity restrained.

   b. *Nursing interventions and coping skills*
   Allow as much movement and turning as possible.

2. Fine motor: holds objects for brief inspection; hand-to-mouth organization of movement; hand grasp now deliberate (initially reflexive).

   a. *Critical care problems*
   Intravenous lines.

   b. *Nursing interventions and coping skills*
   If possible, put IV in foot so baby will be free to move, suck, and see hands. Provide appropriate toys within reach.

3 to 6 Months

1. Gross motor: enjoys sitting up when propped; back is becoming straight; holds head erect when supported in sitting position; controls head when leaning forward; may be too active for infant chair; may only be happy when in motion (e.g., carried); reaches for objects out of reach; may roll from supine to prone position.

    a. *Critical care problems*
        Casts, splints, bandages, restraints.

    b. *Nursing interventions and coping skills*
        Use infant seat as much as possible; weight bottom so it won't topple. Keep toys within reach. Keep side rails up.

2. Fine motor: shakes and bangs rattles; opposes thumb when grasping; manipulates and chews small objects.

    a. *Critical care problems*
        Mitten restraints.

    b. *Nursing interventions and coping skills*
        Provide appropriate toys. Allow child to "gum" toys. Use arm restraints if absolutely imperative to immobilize child. Keep fingers free.

6 to 9 Months

1. Gross motor: sits without support; rolls over easily; can support weight for short periods; may crawl; may pull self to sitting or standing position.

    a. *Critical care problems*
        Bed restraints. Supine position. Infant chair inadequate.

    b. *Nursing interventions and coping skills*
        Allow supervised crawling on floor mat. Allow to pull self up on nurse's finger.

2. Fine motor: holds object in one hand while other is active, holds own bottle; feeds self with fingers, both hands have equal importance (no dominance shown);[6] thumb-finger grasp present. May refuse feeding by others.[4,5]

    a. *Nursing interventions and coping skills*
        Provide appropriate toys. Provide finger foods.

9 to 12 Months

1. Gross motor: establishes upright posture; crawls by about 9 months; stands alone at about 11 months; walks holding onto furniture or hand and alone by about 12 months; sits from standing position without assistance; strong urge to become upright and mobile, making even naps intolerable; maintains balance while turning from side to side.

    a. **Critical care problems**
    Bed restraint. Supine position. Confinement to bed or very small area.

    b. **Nursing interventions and coping skills**
    High side rails. Allow parent to "walk" child around crib or preferably by bed. Nurse should allow ambulation, even with IV therapy, under supervision.

2. Fine motor: hand dominance may appear; more proficient at self-feeding with fingers; uses cup well; picks up small objects with fingers; can bend, grasp, and manipulate objects; holds crayon but pounds with it instead of drawing; in periods immediately before and after walking, likes to have object in one or both hands for sense of support.[16]

    a. **Critical care problems**
    Intravenous lines, nasogastric feedings.

    b. **Nursing interventions and coping skills**
    Provide easy-to-grasp toys and objects with handles. Provide finger foods if possible, or small, flexible objects such as straws or rubber tubes.

12 to 18 Months

1. Gross motor: walking characterized by wide stance and short steps; pushes and pulls toys while walking; climbs; may be running by 18 months; throws objects at about 15 months.

    a. **Nursing interventions and coping skills**
    Allow game of tossing ball into net or bucket in bed.

2. Fine motor: uses cup proficiently; spills while using spoon; can make marks with crayon; has well-developed pincer grasp; may enjoy "plucking" or stroking the ribbon on blanket.

    a. **Critical care problems**
    Hospital food, limited desire for food.

    b. **Nursing interventions and coping skills**
    Provide a plush toy; use cup with handle; allow own blanket, especially if it has a ribbon binding.

18 to 24 Months

1. Gross motor: can walk backwards and sideways; walks upstairs holding rail but needs help walking downstairs; runs with frequent falls; may be jumping by 24 months.
2. Fine motor: scribbles spontaneously; hand dominance obvious; turns pages in a book; builds a tower of 3 to 4 blocks; uses spoon well; drinks from a glass; feeds self more neatly; removes clothes; unlaces and removes shoes; tries to put on simple garments.

a. **Critical care problems**
Hospital clothing unlike own clothing. Adult food in hospital diet.

b. **Nursing interventions and coping skills**
Provide large crayons. Nurse must prepare main dish food into small, easily scooped bites. Cut large chunks, provide bib. Let child feed self with only occasional help from nurse.

2 to 3 Years

1. Gross motor: walking is automatic; runs well; walks on tiptoe.[3] Expresses interest in different postures for urinating.[32]
2. Fine motor: builds a tower of 8 blocks; increased finger control allows child to copy straight line and circle; can feed himself but may demand that an adult do so; puts on own clothes.

   a. **Critical care problems**
   Intravenous lines, restraints, and complicated dressings.

   b. **Nursing interventions and coping skills**
   Allow to dress self entirely or partially as limitations allow.

3 to 6 Years

1. Gross motor: restless and vigorous in physical activity (1); runs; hops; skips; jumps; climbs; stands and bounces on one foot; bounces and catches ball; rides tricycle; walks downstairs alternating feet.

   a. **Critical care problems**
   May feel exhausted or too ill to be active. Fatigued. Nutritionally depressed.

   b. **Nursing interventions and coping skills**
   Ambulate or do bed exercises as soon as feasible.

2. Fine motor: likes to draw, write, cut out shapes; shows increased coordination of small muscle movements; dresses and undresses self; may tie own shoes; washes and dries hands; can assist in simple household chores.

   a. **Critical care problems**
   Immobilized by monitoring wires, lines, restraints.

   b. **Nursing interventions and coping skills**
   Allow to dress self or allow unlimited time to put on one item of clothing, e.g., socks. Encourage to help tidy surroundings as nurse does so.

6 to 7 Years

1. Demonstrates abundant energy and high activity level.

   a. **Critical care problems**
   Confined to bed. May show low energy levels with severe illness or multiple injury.

    b. ***Nursing interventions and coping skills***
    Caution about sitting or dangling without nurse supervision.

  2. Balance and coordination improving; may be able to ride bicycle.

7 to 8 Years

  1. Improved muscular skills (e.g., can tie shoes).

    a. ***Critical care problems***
    Traction, immobilization of body or parts of body.

    b. ***Nursing interventions and coping skills***
    Hand, leg, arm exercises as allowed. Overhead swing to assist in repositioning self.

  2. More serious and cautious; becoming quieter.

8 to 9 Years

  1. Active and gregarious; wants to do everything.
  2. Posture may be poor; spindly bodies tend to droop.

    a. ***Critical care problems***
    Equipment is often made for either younger child or adult.

    b. ***Nursing interventions and coping skills***
    Reposition with bedboards and footboards to make beds fit patient. Maintain correct body alignment.

  3. Hand-eye coordination continues to improve.
  4. Rhythmic sense is improved; muscle movements become smooth.

    a. ***Nursing interventions and coping skills***
    All personal objects that patient can use without help must be placed on side where it is easier to maneuver.

9 to 10 Years

  1. Hand-eye coordination fully developed.

    a. ***Critical care problems***
    Medications may cause loss of or disproportionate hand-eye coordination.

    b. ***Nursing interventions and coping skills***
    Caution about exact location of objects. Do not allow patient to reach for fear of losing balance.

10 to 11 Years

  1. Agility and mastery of motor coordination are evident.

11 to 12 Years

  1. Demonstrates good muscular control. If adolescent growth spurt begins, lack of coordination may ensue as body framework and muscle development grow disproportionately.

    a. ***Critical care problems***
    Embarrassment about teenage awkwardness is heightened by severe illness or immobilization of injured part.

   b. *Nursing interventions and coping skills*
       Acknowledge the awkwardness as fact; dwell on what child can
       do well. Be honest and help set realistic goals.

12 to 18 Years

1. Awkwardness ends as muscular development progresses. Posture
   improves. Control and grace are displayed.

   a. *Critical care problems*
       Cumbersome dressings, numerous lines and drains, physical
       limitations from pain, fractures, and so on.

   b. *Nursing interventions and coping skills*
       Continue bed exercises, passive or active, as condition allows.
       Keep good body alignment as position is changed. Place
       personal items within reach and set up environment to assist
       patient in carrying through smooth movements.

LANGUAGE DEVELOPMENT

1 to 3 Months

1. Throaty sounds, vowel sounds, squeals. Vocalizes in response to
   social stimulation.

   a. *Critical care problems*
       Intubated, unable to make sounds.

   b. *Nursing interventions and coping skills*
       Talk to baby, let him see your face while talking.

2. Cries when cold, wet, hungry.

   a. *Critical care problems*
       Drainage, urinary receptacles. Often kept naked for
       treatments.

   b. *Nursing interventions and coping skills*
       Constant vigilance to maintain comfort.

3 to 6 Months

1. Coos, chuckles, laughs, smiles, babbles. Long vowel sounds
   predominate.

   a. *Nursing interventions and coping skills*
       Be responsive to baby's communication; mimic baby's sounds.

6 to 9 Months

1. Vocalizes with people and toys. Crows with pleasure.

   a. *Critical care problems*
       Sedation, pain, limited contact with people.

   b. *Nursing interventions and coping skills*
       Special effort to encourage making sounds of pleasure.

2. Imitates speech sounds, babbles.[21]

   a. ***Critical care problem***
   Impersonality of procedures and treatments.

   b. ***Nursing interventions and coping skills***
   Have specific play times as energy permits.

3. Spends more time making babbling noises. Can grunt, growl, and gurgle. May say "mama" and "dada." Combines vowels and consonants to make syllables.

   a. ***Critical care problem***
   Time constraints of diagnostic tests, therapy, and other procedures.

   b. ***Nursing interventions and coping skills***
   Encourage parents to speak often, so their voices will become familiar.

9 to 12 Months

1. Imitates adult inflection of a specific word.

   a. ***Critical care problem***
   Multiple caregivers with different voice inflections.

   b. ***Nursing interventions and coping skills***
   Try to assign same nurse to patient for consecutive days.

2. Says "mama," "dada," and two other words.
3. Child can understand but not produce language (e.g., "no").

   a. ***Critical care problem***
   Complex communications during procedures and therapy.

   b. ***Nursing interventions and coping skills***
   Speak to child in loving, simple terms.

4. Recognizes own name.
5. Vowel sound predominate.
6. Uses the same sound to refer to the same person or collection of things (single or multiple meanings for one sound).

   a. ***Critical care problem***
   Masks may muffle speech of caregivers.

   b. ***Nursing interventions and coping skills***
   Have all staff use the same terminology, using simple terms. Use care plan to indicate each child's vocabulary of specific words, e.g., bottle, nipple, nickname, and other items as noted by parent.

7. Frequent use of holophrases in which a whole sentence is contained in a single word (e.g., "milk" means "I want milk.")[3]

12 to 18 Months

1. Uses own jargon, which develops into sentences. Has 2- to 6-word vocabulary.

a. *Critical care problems*
Intubation, complex language of adult world.

b. *Nursing interventions and coping skills*
Obtain details from parents about familiar terms and pet phrases.

2. Begins to name objects he has studied.[16]

a. *Critical care problem*
Unfamiliar staff who come and go for specific therapy.

b. *Nursing interventions and coping skills*
Post child's vocabulary on wall by head of bed.

3. Use of holophrases continues.[3]
4. Points to own body parts or objects named in picture book.

a. *Nursing interventions and coping skills*
Play "body parts" game. Help child locate body parts and associate them with comfort or pleasure; do not associate with pain or restraint.

18 to 24 Months

1. Uses 2- to 3-word phrases or sentences (telegraphic speech).[3]
2. Begins to use pronouns; "me" and "mine" predominate.
3. Gives name when asked.

a. *Nursing interventions and coping skills*
Associate name with child as person.

4. Language is disconnected; everything is taken literally.[4]

a. *Critical care problem*
Unfamiliar objects with unknown purposes.

5. Language is a blocker; toddler acts instead of talking about. Understands only simple directions.

a. *Critical care problems*
Restraints, physical limitations of illness, and trauma limit ways to act.

b. *Nursing interventions and coping skills*
Explanations should come from someone who knows child well.

6. Approximately 25% of conversation is intelligible to strangers.

a. *Critical care problem*
Many different caregivers.

b. *Nursing interventions and coping skills*
Have each caregiver utilize care plan with child's phonetically described vocabulary, to avoid frustration.

7. Actively exercises power of yes and no. Sometimes mixes them; "yes" may mean "no".

2 to 3 Years
1. Uses many simple phrases and short (4-word) sentences.
2. Hesitancy and uncertainty (normal developmental stuttering) are common in speech.

    a. Nursing interventions and coping skills
    Speak slowly and articulate plainly to give clear sounds to words.

3. Uses pronouns readily.
4. Vocabulary increases from 300 to 900 words during this period.

    a. Critical care problem
    Illness or trauma may introduce new words associated with pain and unpleasantness.

    b. Nursing interventions and coping skills
    Use books with large pictures to teach about food, clothes, and outdoors to expand child's experience beyond immediate environment.

5. Laughter is a frequent form of communication.

    a. Nursing interventions and coping skills
    Make "fun times" with laughter and pleasurable sounds.

6. By age 2, 66% of conversation is intelligible to strangers; by age 3, 90%.[3]

3 to 4 Years
1. Has vocabulary of 900 words by 3 years; 1500 words by 4 years.[3] Can use words that refer to past, present, and future.

    a. Critical care problem
    Tendency of adults to talk down to children with severe illness.

    b. Nursing interventions and coping skills
    Maintain vocabulary level of child through careful plan of communication during each stage of illness.

2. Uses plurals.
3. Lip sounds (m, p, b, w, h) intelligible.[3]

    a. Critical care problem
    Masked personnel.

4. Poor communication through speech may hinder child's development of close relationships with other children.[3]

    a. Critical care problem
    Other severely limited children in same area.

    b. Nursing interventions and coping skills
    Encourage verbalization between roommates; encourage siblings to visit (they must be prepared).

4 to 6 Years
1. Has vocabulary of approximately 2500 words by age 6.

a. *Nursing interventions and coping skills*
Repeat complex words or phrases to allow child to master them.

2. Uses 5-word sentences.
3. Tongue contact sounds added (n, t, d, k, g, x, -ing).[3]
4. Speech is completely intelligible by 4 years, with exception of difficult consonant sounds (r, l, s, th, z, sh, ch).
5. Talks constantly; highly inquisitive. Speech is a weapon; child boasts, exaggerates, threatens, verbally communicates anger.[16]

a. *Critical care problems*
Limited energy levels, limited environment, sterile cubicle, complex technical equipment, treatments.

b. *Nursing interventions and coping skills*
Be as thorough as possible in teaching, try to anticipate questions. Incorporate answers into care as child poses questions.

6 to 12 Years
1. Difficult consonants are mastered and added to vocabulary by 7 years[3] (r, s, x, th, sh, ch).
2. Articulates all sounds by 7 1/2 years.
3. Speech is tool for reasoning and expression.[3]
a. *Nursing interventions and coping skills*
Respond to child's communication with respect for his part in interaction. Provide adequate time for expressing ideas and emotions.

12 to 18 Years
1. Reading vocabulary equals listening vocabulary by 13 years (3). Use of slang is common.

a. *Critical care problems*
Media concepts of hospital are unlike real situation. Hospital, critical care terminology.

b. *Nursing interventions and coping skills*
Nurse needs to ascertain child's comprehension of situation and care. Dispel fears, correct misinterpretations. To describe care, use terminology that is the same as child's or adolescent's concept.

COGNITIVE DEVELOPMENT

Note: The age categories in this section vary from those in previous sections for ease in theoretical presentation.

1 to 4 Months
1. Piaget's sensorimotor stage, substage 2: Infant repeats actions that have produced pleasurable outcomes, learns by visual exploration, will not search for "lost object".[3,36]

   a. Nursing interventions and coping skills
      Keep toys within visual field. Remove syringes, needles, and
      other such equipment from visual field immediately.

4 to 10 Months
   1. Piaget's sensorimotor stage, substage 3: Infant's actions demon-
      strate intent; begins to understand connection between his own
      movements and desired results; demonstrates object permanence
      by searching for missing object.[3]

      a. Critical care problem
         Changing environment.

      b. Nursing interventions and coping skills
         *Establish use of same toys, food utensils and clothes. Hang
         picture or mobile that does not change.*

10 to 12 Months
   1. Piaget's sensorimotor stage, substage 4: Infant uses old and familiar
      strategies to solve problems in new situations; he now makes events
      happen.[3]

      a. Critical care problem
         Interjection of pain or discomfort with some repeatable events.

      b. Nursing interventions and coping skills
         *Create two or three situations that allow for pleasurable
         outcomes when repeated; (e.g., swallowing medications brings
         caressing pats of approval from caregiver.*

12 to 18 Months
   1. Piaget's sensorimotor stage, substage 5: Child explores and
      experiments with different ways of manipulation; child will
      search for "lost" object in more than one place if allowed to
      follow it with eyes.[3,16]

18 to 24 Months
   1. Piaget's sensorimotor stage, substage 6: Faced with a new situation,
      the child internally analyzes it to some extent and relies only
      partially on trial-and-error experimentation.[3]
   2. Child has difficulty coping with frustration because he is incapable
      of complex problem-solving and inept at expressing feelings
      verbally; temper tantrums are frequent.[5]

      a. Critical care problem
         Loss of control in many of simple tasks thus learned.

      b. Nursing interventions and coping skills
         *Be patient with child's many frustrations. Focus on happy
         expressions and substitute simple alternatives.*

   3. Child unable to differentiate between consciousness and
      unconsciousness, reality and fantasy, reason and affect.

      a. Critical care problem
         Unfamiliar with new feelings associated with illness or trauma.

    b. Nursing interventions and coping skills
    Establish reality of some familiar objects, parents and other
    people, toys.

2 to 6 Years

1. Piaget's preoperational stage: In this transitional stage, child can represent things to himself in specific terms, but he cannot tie internal representations to complex systems.[3]

   a. Critical care problems
   Complex environment; incomplete comprehension of own situation.

2. Symbolic development: Visual images and words symbolize actions or objects at about 2 years; child knows colors, age, numbers to about 20.

   a. Critical care problem
   Sterile, colorless walls.

   b. Nursing interventions and coping skills
   Use toys to allow verbalization of inner thoughts and feelings.

3. Reasoning: 2 to 4 year old child begins reasoning ability, but it is heavily influenced by his own wants and desires; level of comprehension is limited; focuses on present state of events.[21]

   a. Critical care problem
   Time span of pain, limitations, and unfamiliar environment is exaggerated by illness.

   b. Nursing interventions and coping skills
   Do not talk about future. Keep care in the here and now.
   Relate immediate past actions to their results.

4. Transductive reasoning: Concepts of place, time, space, and causality develop (i.e., two events happening simultaneously are related).[1,3]

   a. Critical care problem
   Multiple aspects of care are confusing.

   b. Nursing interventions and coping skills
   Focus on one event as priority.

5. Egocentrism: Child unable to see others' point of view; his own ways of interacting and experiencing are the only ones that exist (gradually disappears throughout pre-operational stage).

   a. Critical care problems
   Imposed treatments, necessary actions in emergency.

6. Reversibility: Until about 5 or 6 years of age, child's reasoning moves only in forward direction; reversibility develops gradually during latter part of preoperational period.

> a. *Nursing interventions and coping skills*
> *Create comfortable environment in which child can acceptably change his mind.*

7. Classification: Child begins to form concepts by grouping objects together into classes;[6] continues to be unaware of sub-groupings.
8. Memory and attention span increasing.[3]

> a. *Critical care problem*
> Selective amnesia of trauma. Loss of time intervals associated with illness or trauma.

> b. *Nursing interventions and coping skills*
> *Talk about things in the here and now and relate to past experiences. Involve in the patient activities and stories.*

6 to 11 Years

1. Piaget's stage of concrete operations: Increased ability to use reason and logic; child thinks of situations in concrete terms; uses complex mental actions (mathematics, ordering a series); understands time sequences and can project into the future; reads the clock; increased attention span; questions show thought;[1,3] belief in Santa Claus ends.

> a. *Critical care problems*
> Treatments and procedures are serial; child's help is needed to accomplish sophisticated diagnostic testing and treatments.

> b. *Nursing interventions and coping skills*
> *Have child plan and become involved in treatments, assist in describing discomfort, pain, needs, and relationships.*

2. Conservation: Certain properties of objects remain unchanged even when space and shape are altered.

> a. *Nursing interventions and coping skills*
> *Allow child to save, hoard, have secret items.*

3. Serial ordering and transitivity: Child is able to arrange things in a certain order (e.g., can name months of year in order). Child begins to understand relationships between classes of objects (e.g., apples and oranges are fruit).

> a. *Critical care problem*
> Multiplicity of events that have no relationship to each other in child's mind.

> b. *Nursing interventions and coping skills*
> *Use serial ordering to assess level of consciousness. Make associations of events to help child sort categories.*

4. Inductive logic: Specific instances or the child's personal experiences are the basis of general rules.

    a. Critical care problems
Lack of time orientation in the hospital. One catastrophic event is unlike past experiences.

    b. Nursing interventions and coping skills
Help child focus on pleasant events of past. Talk about immediate event in relation to child's perceived social ordering of past and present situations.

11 to 18 Years

1. Piaget's stage of formal operations: All operations can be performed in child's head; child is able to systematically think through a solution to a problem; is able to understand if-then relationships; increased imagination and tendency to introspection.[3,25,29]

    a. Critical care problems
Lights and noises in environment. Deforming injuries. Severity of illness or trauma may require multiple complex treatments.

    b. Nursing interventions and coping skills
All treatment and care should be carefully explained. Clarify when patient is unsure. Give positive stroking.

2. Deductive logic: Uses reason; formulates hypotheses; moves from general to specific.

    a. Critical care problems
Changing staff, multiplicity of personnel to accomplish technical care.

    b. Nursing interventions and coping skills
Use patient's ability to handle details of care and understand more complex relationships. Nurse may give important or priority data once, but when patient is severely ill, repetition will probably be necessary.

DIVERSIONAL ACTIVITIES

Note: refer to sections on sensory, perceptive, and motor development for additional information useful in this section.

1 to 3 Months

1. Play with adults (being stroked, cuddled, or talked to) is primary mode.
2. Also interested in lights, moving objects, and appropriate toys (mobiles, music boxes, rattles).

a. *Critical care problems*
Limited space. Dim or constant lighting (because of need to assess patients frequently).

b. *Nursing interventions and coping skills*
Enhance environment with lighted mobiles, rocking chairs, soft music.

3. No knowledge of sharing.[9]

3 to 6 Months

1. Stage of solitary play may begin: Infant is able to entertain himself for brief periods without adult interaction. Responsive play with someone else ("boo" or "peek-a-boo") is possible but limited.

   a. *Critical care problems*
   Separation from parents, limited consistent involvement with same person.

   b. *Nursing interventions and coping skills*
   Have parents or same nurses caring for child, if feasible.

2. Appropriate toys: pictures on crib and walls, soothing music, stuffed animals, one-piece squeeze toys, rattles, metal mirror, playpen for short periods, cradle gym for 20 to 30 minutes.

   a. *Critical care problem*
   Numerous items of hardware may crowd out toys and mirrors.

   b. *Nursing interventions and coping skills*
   Change toys when their number is limited.

6 to 9 Months

1. Solitary play continues.
2. Begins to play with appropriate toys: 1-inch blocks, water or bath, large rubber balls, stroller, pots and pans.

   a. *Critical care problem*
   Sterile environment.

   b. *Nursing interventions and coping skills*
   Toys must be of a kind that can be sterilized frequently as child drops them on floor; use balls that have return roll.

9 to 12 Months

1. Solitary play continues. Child may play spontaneously and can play in crib for long periods.

   a. *Critical care problem*
   Interruptions of treatments.

   b. *Nursing interventions and coping skills*
   Use toys that have action mechanisms when touched.

   2. Recognizes names of toys

   3. Plays "give-and-take" games with ball or other appropriate toy (push-pull toys, cloth books, balls, bells, simple open-close boxes, floating bath toys).

     a. *Critical care problems*
   Limited area for movement; restraints.

     b. *Nursing interventions and coping skills*
   Make play time a part of regular care; provide stories from pictures, allow patient interactions with bath toys; nurse can offer small boxes from such equipment as IV tubing and medications.

12 to 18 Months

   1. Stage of parallel play begins. Child pursues his own interests alongside another child.

     a. *Critical care problem*
   Separation from others because of severity of illness or sepsis.

   2. Still unable to share.

   3. Likes motor action activities (running, push-pull toys). Other appropriate toys are toy telephone, balls, large books, phonograph records, throwing toys.

     a. *Nursing interventions and coping skills*
   Allow short intervals in play area; supervise if IV therapy or other restraints inhibit the child.

18 to 24 Months

   1. Parallel play continues.

   2. Still lacks ability to play with other children (either hugs or pushes).

   3. Hoards toys. Appropriate toys are dolls, soft clay, finger paint, soapy water, picture puzzles (2 to 4 pieces), big books, large crayons and paper, large beads with string, blocks.

     a. *Nursing interventions and coping skills*
   Allow child to have two or three of his own toys. Incorporate toys with bath. Caution: small objects may still be placed in mouth and aspirated or swallowed.

2 to 3 Years

   1. Stage of associative play: Child's activity not related to activity of another child.

   2. Continues to lack ability to play cooperatively with other children.

   3. Imaginary friends (good or bad) are frequent.

     a. *Nursing interventions and coping skills*
   Tell stories to allow for fantasy of imaginary friends.

   4. Appropriate toys are tricycle, family of dolls, puzzles (3 to 6 pieces), role dolls (doctor, dentist), nesting boxes, easel and

paintbrush, song games, crayons, blunt scissors and paper, clay, mud, sand.

   a. *Critical care problem*
     Environment is too limited for large toys.

   b. *Nursing interventions and coping skills*
     Role play with dolls representing family members and hospital personnel. Provide clean clay for "feeling" type of play.

3 to 6 Years

1. Associative play continues.
2. Stage of cooperative play may begin in later years of this period: Children play at the same game or work on the same project.
3. Fantasies common (e.g., magical words, imaginary playmates); enjoys "let's pretend" situations.

   a. *Critical care problem*
     Hospital environment may be fantasy world.

   b. *Nursing interventions and coping skills*
     Nurse must relate fantasized care and treatments to reality. Maintain a clear reality for child without minimizing enjoyment of "let's pretend."

4. Child plays with any age group but likes to be "bigger than" other children.

   a. *Critical care problem*
     Illness creates feelings of smallness.

5. Boys' and girls' interests are similar; they play together.
6. Boys more quarrelsome than girls.
7. New roles are tried (mother, doctor, teacher).

   a. *Nursing interventions and coping skills*
     Can use other children to interact in small bed games and provide peer interest.

8. Everything becomes a game.
9. Plays simple sit-down games but dislikes losing; will change rules to win.

   a. *Nursing interventions and coping skills*
     Introduce easily won games to provide positive outcome when illness and trauma are severe "negatives."

10. Both locomotor and manipulative play enjoyed.

   a. *Critical care problems*
     Loss of control; physical restraint.

   b. *Nursing interventions and coping skills*
     Lift swings on overhead frames.

11. Appropriate toys and games are checkers, simple cards, tag, hide-and-seek, dress-up, doctor and nurse kits, story-telling,

puppets, costumes, simple group games (musical chairs), paste and paper, cars and trucks.

    a. *Nursing interventions and coping skills*
       Use hospital clothing as "costumes" with decorations to help patient assume other roles and personalities.

6 to 12 Years

1. Cooperative activities continue.
2. Increasing interest in table games and hobbies.

    a. *Nursing interventions and coping skills*
       Involve child in care planning and implementation as much as possible.

3. Increasing involvement in sports.

    a. *Critical care problems*
       Illness and trauma reduce energy. Limited space and opportunity to make noise.

    b. *Nursing interventions and coping skills*
       Provide bed activities that require large muscle coordination; use bed board and overhead swings.

4. Becomes increasingly interested in how things work; eager to learn; wants to complete tasks.

    a. *Critical care problem*
       Prolonged treatments of complex nature.

    b. *Nursing interventions and coping skills*
       Provide short-term goals with attainable positive results to help patient realize a completed task.

5. Prefers to play with someone rather than alone; interested in group activities.

    a. *Critical care problem*
       Isolation.

6. Begins collections (a type of hoarding); saves everything (e.g., baseball cards).
7. Peers of same sex are important as friends.

    a. *Critical care problem*
       Social immobilization.

    b. *Nursing interventions and coping skills*
       Allow telephone privileges to a special friend.

8. Games show superstitions, teasing, and insults.

    a. *Nursing interventions and coping skills*
       Nurse may be brunt of insult; show how to be good sport.

9. Appropriate diversional materials are comics, puzzles, TV, table games, hobbies, team sports, movies, crafts, clubs, science experiments, stamp and coin collections.

   a. *Nursing interventions and coping skills*
   Provide reading material of interest, television at selected intervals. Relate patient's experiences to scientific principles to help clarify understanding of body functions and effects of treatment.

12 to 18 Years
1. Skills develop in both individual and group games and activities.
2. Outdoor activities become more interesting.

   a. *Critical care problem*
   Confinement.

3. Organized, competitive games and sports desirable.

   a. *Nursing interventions and coping skills*
   Use competition as motivation to get well. Stimulate desire to accomplish treatments and progressive self-care.

4. Activities differ for boys and girls.

   a. *Critical care problem*
   Mixed patient census.

5. Groups, clubs, and cliques are important; both sexes are included.

   a. *Critical care problem*
   Social isolation.

   b. *Nursing interventions and coping skills*
   Allow family and selected special friends to visit.

6. Diversional activities are softball, soccer, TV, telephones, darts, ping-pong, radio, stereo, more mature games, complex jigsaw puzzles, sewing, models, microscope sets.

   a. *Nursing interventions and coping skills*
   Use radio with earphones.

———————— CONSCIENCE AND VALUES ————————

Note: The age categories in this section vary from those in previous sections for ease in theoretical presentation.

1 Month to 6 Years
1. "Conscience" initially denotes the child's incorporation of parental moral values into his own personality; this occurs through the processes of imitation and identification.[3,24]

    a. Critical care problem
    Absolute control by staff over level of care, time when
    care is delivered, and need for special interventions.

    b. Nursing interventions and coping skills
    Maintain parent-family-patient relationships for stability.

2. Young child has little concept of right and wrong until standards are established; controlled entirely by external forces (mother, environment).

    a. Nursing interventions and coping skills
    Set reasonable limits that are with type of illness or trauma.

3. External controls necessary until child develops inner controls.
4. Later in this period, imaginary friends are often invented to blame for wrongs.

    a. Critical care problem
    Completely strange world of hospital.

    b. Nursing interventions and coping skills
    Accept the fact that child will blame others. Set out the reality of actual event to help child distinguish fact from fiction.

5. Rudimentary self-control evidenced by control of some of own urges, e.g., saying "no" while reaching for a forbidden object.
6. Acts are perceived as totally right or wrong.
7. Guilt arises from deviation from established "rules."

    a. Nursing interventions and coping skills
    Have child help set rules.

8. Adult is perceived as always right; punishment is deserved.[1,19]

    a. Critical care problem
    Imposition of treatments or care that may be painful or disliked.

    b. Nursing interventions and coping skills
    Show that patient is "right" and respected by nurse.

9. No understanding of rule flexibility.
10. Actions are "good" or "bad" depending upon consequences rather than intent.

    a. Nursing interventions and coping skills
    Provide comfort and some pleasurable experiences, e.g., having special visit from clown or a well-liked food (if possible).

6 to 12 Years

1. Standards established earlier in childhood serve to inhibit antagonistic impulses as they arise.
2. Still exploring and questioning own standards.

   a. Nursing interventions and coping skills
     Set realistic expectations for patient involvement in care.

3. Has regard for social laws and rules; discipline and rules contribute to sense of security.[33,37]

   a. Critical care problem
     Absolute rules for critical care delivery and emergency treatments.

   b. Nursing interventions and coping skills
     Accept periodic rebellion against standards.

4. Thinks logically about principles, rights, and justice in comparison to other individuals and community.

   a. Critical care problem
     Loss of control.

   b. Nursing interventions and coping skills
     Nurse needs to expect frequent questioning about "my rights" and "why is this happening to me." Help establish perspective of real fact versus speculation.

5. Recognizes that actions affect others; continues to think of own needs and satisfactions first.
6. Recognizes relationship between action and consequences.
7. Fixed rules and rituals of peer group influence value development; conformity to peer group principles is strong.

   a. Critical care problem
     Adult-child relationships. Authority of staff.

   b. Nursing interventions and coping skills
     Nurse needs to understand peer pressure and be flexible regarding dress, moral and spiritual codes.

8. Recognizes the effects of labels (e.g., "bad girl").

12 to 18 Years

1. Confusion over values results as complex experiences increase and horizons widen.

   a. Critical care problem
     Complexity of trauma and illness.

   b. Nursing interventions and coping skills
     May benefit from spiritual counselor: priest, minister, rabbi.

2. Child is able to make moral judgements about behavior.

   a. Critical care problems
     Pain, intense stimulation.

   b. Nursing interventions and coping skills
     Reduce sensory overload. Separate fact from value judgment.

_____ **FEARS** _____

1 to 3 Months
1. Being uncovered or held loosely.

   a. *Critical care problem*
   Child is often undressed, may have to be naked.

   b. *Nursing interventions and coping skills*
   If unable to wrap or swaddle, place rolled towel on each side of torso.

2. May dislike bathing.

   a. *Critical care problem*
   Frequent handling and cleansing are necessary.

3. Loud noises are startling.

   a. *Critical care problem*
   Equipment discharges.

   b. *Nursing interventions and coping skills*
   Play quiet lullaby music into cubicle.

3 to 6 Months
1. Loss of support.
2. Startles and cries at loud noises.

   a. *Critical care problem*
   Frequent loud and strange noises.

   b. *Nursing interventions and coping skills*
   Modify and reduce sudden noises as much as possible. Alert all professional and support staff to need for modification of noise.

6 to 9 Months
1. Anxiety about strangers.

   a. *Critical care problem*
   Various personnel entering and leaving unit.

2. May spontaneously fear something previously enjoyed (e.g., bathtub), fears reflect momentary need for more dependency and usually precede spurts of independence.[6]

   a. *Nursing interventions and coping skills*
   Go slowly, allow child to regress without reprimanding comments or actions.

3. Separation anxiety; doesn't like parents to leave, no others can care for him; controls disappearance and reappearance to overcome anxiety.[5,16]

   a. *Critical care problem*
   Parent separation for long intervals during procedures or when other siblings require parent.

4. Begins to play out fears with toys.

   a. *Nursing interventions and coping skills*
       Allow the child to bring anxieties to the surface where
       they can be controlled better. For example, the child
       may wish to control his fear of falling by letting a toy
       fall from a chair and then comforting the toy.

9 to 12 Months

1. Separation anxiety continues.

12 to 18 Months

1. Separation anxiety continues.
2. Wakens at night and may need reassurance (e.g., a quick little pat).[16]

   a. *Critical care problems*
       Unfamiliar surroundings. Often dim lighting for 24 hours. No differentiation between night and day.

   b. *Nursing interventions and coping skills*
       Child may need to be picked up and held when awakened
       (increased reassurance).

3. Dreams are real; child needs much reassurance; dreams may repeat bad experience (e.g., stranger); takes long time for even parents to console; dreams may recur until child can control and overcome anxiety.

   a. *Critical care problem*
       Many frightening experiences and procedures.

   b. *Nursing interventions and coping skills*
       Games like peek-a-boo during day may help alleviate recurrent
       dreams during night.

18 to 24 Months

1. Other fears may appear (e.g., bathtub, thunder, dogs, darkness).

   a. *Critical care problem*
       Noisy equipment.

   b. *Nursing interventions and coping skills*
       Employ familiar sounds: bells, music boxes, children's voices.

2. May be unable to function in strange bathroom.

   a. *Critical care problem*
       Urinary bladder catheterization.

2 to 3 Years

1. Mutilation fears, especially when boys and girls discover girls don't have a penis.[16]

   a. *Critical care problems*
       Eyes patched. Co-ed rooms.

b. *Nursing interventions and coping skills*
Avoid abrupt action. Describe body parts being washed. If bath time is observed by both sexes in same room, identify girls with mothers, boys with fathers.

2. Concerned about scratches, cuts, and wounds of any kind; body perceived as a shell.[16] Archaic fears merge with real dangers.

a. *Critical care problems*
Unfamiliar procedures, dressing changes, pain.

b. *Nursing interventions and coping skills*
Give child as honest and complete a picture as possible of illness or injury.

3 to 6 Years

1. Afraid of pain and bodily injury; worries over real or imagined physical threats.

a. *Critical care problems*
Pain; invasive procedures.

b. *Nursing interventions and coping skills*
Have parent stay at bedside as much as possible.

2. Nightmares and fear of dark or night occur periodically.

a. *Critical care problems*
Shadows and noises of strange equipment.

b. *Nursing interventions and coping skills.*
Nurse must provide assurance of her presence and be quickly available when called. Provide a call device; leave night light on.

3. Castration fears: one part of body (usually genitals) symbolizes another.

6 to 12 Years

1. Superstitious.
2. Denies fear; display bravado when feeling fear of helplessness.[1]

a. *Critical care problems*
Grotesque dressings, equipment, traction, and so on.

b. *Nursing interventions and coping skills*
Play game: have patient point out equipment while nurse explains what it does. "Show and tell" all procedures or changes in care before implementing change.

3. Fears displacement of former role in family or peer group.[21]

a. *Critical care problems*
Child is alone, in pain, away from known environment.

4. Fears mutilation and death.

a. *Critical care problems*
Invasive procedures and monitoring. Death of others in unit.

b. *Nursing interventions and coping skills*
Emphasize usefulness of equipment.
Note all positive change.

12 to 18 Years

1. Fears failure in school, career, or friendship.

   a. *Critical care problem*
   Visiting limited to immediate relatives.

   b. *Nursing interventions and coping skills*
   Allow for messages from classmates, work colleagues.

2. Fears loss of identity (bodily or emotionally).
   a. *Critical care problems*
   Dismemberment, catastrophic multiple injuries.

   b. *Nursing interventions and coping skills*
   Use greeting cards as room or cubicle decorations. Refer to specific body parts as part of a whole.

————— HOSPITALIZATION AND DEATH —————

There are three phases of behavior possible during hospitalization, as described by Robertson.[30]

Protest Phase

1. Crying, rejecting attitude. Watches and calls for mother unceasingly; this decreases tension.

   a. *Critical care problems*
   Many children who are ill and crying. Limited view of hall and other adults.

   b. *Nursing interventions and coping skills*
   Stay close and accept child, do not reject. Speak gently and touch child. Seeing mother and nurse together may help child. Mother should stay with child if possible.

2. Expressing agression and hostility gives child greater ability to respond favorably when mother comes.

   a. *Critical care problem*
   Crying, hostile, aggressive behavior disturbs other children.

3. This phase may last several hours to several days, depending on energy and level of illness.[30]

Despair Phase

1. Increasing hopelessness; child is passive and suspicious.

   a. *Critical care problem*
   Changing caregivers.

   b. *Nursing interventions and coping skills*
       Stay close and accept child; speak gently and touch child.
       Seeing mother and nurse together may help child. Mother
       should stay with child if possible.

2. Activities may include thumb sucking, masturbation, head
   banging, rocking, fingering locks of hair, sitting quietly,
   clutching toy.
3. Deepened depression and withdrawal.
4. Continues to watch for mother.[30]

   a. *Critical care problem*
       Limited view.

Denial Phase

1. Seems to improve; doesn't call for mother, eats better, etc. Much
   psychic energy is used to block unbearable facts. When visited by
   mother, child may appear indifferent.[30]

   a. *Critical care problem*
       Withdrawal may be reinforced by kindness and soft words of
       personnel busy with more critically ill patient.

   b. *Nursing interventions and coping skills*
       Prevention, using interventions just described. Keep mother
       with child as much as possible. Have a consistent caregiver
       to develop trust. Much parent teaching is necessary during
       this phase; which is very painful for parents. Much explanation
       may be needed to prevent further estrangement. Open visiting
       is very important. [14]

2. When discharged, child may show lack of affect or resist closeness.
   Regression to infantile behavior or resistance to even momentary
   separation may be evidenced.[5]

   a. *Nursing interventions and coping skills*
       Parent teaching is essential. Child may need extra "babying"
       for a while to restore trust and security.

CONCEPT OF DEATH

Under 4 Years of Age

1. Vague; death is associated with that observed in plants, which
   disappear and then come up again.

   a. *Nursing interventions and coping skills*
       A dying child or infant will make people around him tense;
       the child will sense this and become anxious and may even
       withdraw or become apathetic. [14]

2. A dead object is "asleep."[33]

> *a. Critical care problem*
> May fear bedtime because of association of death with sleep.
>
> *b. Nursing interventions and coping skills*
> *Hold or touch child at bedtime.*

3. Denial of death as final. As with sleeping and waking up again, going away but coming back again, one may die but come alive again.[34]

   > *a. Critical care problem*
   > Sleep deprivation due to multiple and frequent treatments and care.
   >
   > *b. Nursing interventions and coping skills*
   > *Child usually has little trouble sleeping if allowed. Nightmares may begin at 4 years of age.*

4. At this age child does not have enough "I" concept to understand a "not I" situation Death of self is not questioned.[35]

   > *a. Critical care problem*
   > In an accident, parents of hospitalized child may die.
   >
   > *b. Nursing interventions and coping skills*
   > *Honesty is necessary with regard to death of others (especially a parent). If told that mother or father "went away," his or her return is expected, and child will feel abandoned when they don't return.*

4 to 6 Years

1. Death is still a difficult concept for the child. Denial of death, especially in those most frightened of illness, is frequent.[29] Death is perceived as something that happens to others or as punishment for "bad" thoughts".[32]

   > *a. Critical care problems*
   > Many frightening sounds and experiences; pain; discomfort of illness or treatments.
   >
   > *b. Nursing interventions and coping skills*
   > *Children's books dealing with the concept of death may facilitate the child's expression of thoughts and anxieties. Be honest and supportive. Assure the child that his actions or wishes will not cause death.*

6 to 12 Years

1. In this period the child realizes the irreversibility of death, identifies death as personal event.

   > *a. Critical care problem*
   > Child sees or knows that other die in environment he is now in.
   >
   > *b. Nursing interventions and coping skills*
   > *Adult (whom child trusts) needs to present reality. Allow verbalization and acting out of fears. Never try to prepare*

*child for death, but allow expression of thoughts and
anxieties.* [29]

2. In the early school age years, death is perceived as being caused by
an external agent; feelings of guilt are evident.

3. In late childhood the universality, permanence, and inevitability of
death are perceived.[32]

   a. *Critical care problem*
   Sees or knows other in unit who have died.

   b. *Nursing interventions and coping skills.*
   Assist child to know about his personal faith or religion.
   Provide comfort during the dying process.

4. The older child perceives the non-verbal messages of family and
staff easily.[32] It is very difficult to hide the diagnosis of a fatal
illness.

   a. *Critical care problems*
   Progressive physical decline; increased discomfort and
   weakness.

   b. *Nursing interventions and coping skills*
   *Support child as family and staff learn to be honest about
   their feelings.*

12 to 18 Years

1. Adult-level concept of death and its universality and permanence.

   a. *Critical care problem*
   Death is frequent occurence in hospital environment.

2. Although inevitability of death is recognized, thoughts of one's own
death cause much turmoil ("death before fulfillment" concept).[32]

   a. *Critical care problem*
   Multiplicity of injuries.

   b. *Nursing interventions and coping skills*
   *Support religious desires of patient. Consistent and honest
   answers from all—family, nurses, doctors.*

BIBLIOGRAPHY

1. Anthony, S.: The Discovery of Death in Childhood and After. New York, Basic Books, 1972.

2. Babcock, D. and Keepers, T.: Raising Kids O.K.. New York, Grove Press, 1976.

3. Bee, H.: The Developing Child. New York, Harper & Row, 1975.

4. Bergmann, T. and Freud, A.: Children in the Hospital. New York, International Universities Press, 1965.

5. Blake, F., et al.; Nursing Care of Children, 8th ed. Philadelphia, J. B. Lippincott Co., 1970.

6. Brazelton, T.; Infants and Mothers. New York, Dell Publishing Co., 1969.

7. Brazelton, T.: Toddlers and Parents. New York, Dell Publishing Co., 1974.

8. Breckenridge, M., and Murphy, M.; Growth and Development of the Young Child, 8th ed. Philadelphia, W. B. Saunders Co., 1969.

9. Brown, M., and Murphy, M.: A child grows: How the child grows and develops psychologically, socially and culturally. Pediatric Nursing, 1:4, 1975.

10. Brown, M., and Murphy, M.: A child grows: the child's cognitive development. Pediatric Nursing, 1:7, 1975.

11. Brown, M., and Murphy, M.: A child grows: The child's perceptual and linguistic development. Pediatric Nursing, 2:19, 1975.

12. Chapman, J., and Chapman, H.: Behavior and Health Care. St. Louis, C. V. Mosby Co., 1975.

13. Chinn, P.: Child Health Maintenance. St. Louis, C. V. Mosby Co., 1974.

14. Easson, W.; The Dying Child. Springfield, Ill., Charles C Thomas, 1970.

15. Erikson, E.: Childhood and Society. New York; W. W. Norton & Co., 1950.

16. Fraiberg, S.; The Magic Years. New York, Charles Scribner's Sons, 1959.

17. Ginott, H.: Between Parent and Child. New York; Avon Books, 1965.

18. Ginott, H.: Betweeen Parent and Teenager. New York; Avon Books, 1969.

19. Grollman, E.; Concerning Death. Boston, Beacon Press, 1974.

20. Haller, J.; The Hospitalized Child and His Family. Baltimore, Johns Hopkins Press, 1967.

21. Kempe, C., et al.: Current Pediatric Diagnosis and Treatment, 5th ed. Los Altos, Cal., Lange Medical Publications, 1978.

22. Lewis, M.: Clinical Aspects of Child Development. Philadelphia; Lea & Febiger, 1971.

23. Lindheim, R., et al.: Changing Hospital Environments for Children. Cambridge, Mass., Harvard University Press, 1972.

23a. Lowrey, G., M.D.: Growth and Development of Children, 6th Ed. Chicago, Yearbook Medical Publishers, Inc., 1973, p. 233.

24. Maier, H.: Three Theories of Child Development. New York, Harper & Row, 1969.

25. Marlow, D.: Textbook of Pediatric Nursing, 5th ed. Philadelphia; W. B. Saunders Co., 1977.

26. Millar, H.: Approaches to Adolescent Health Care in the 1970's. Washington, D.C., U.S. Department of Health, Education, and Welfare Publication No. (HSA)76-5014, 1975.

27. Mussen, P., et al.: Child Development and Personality. New York; Harper & Row, 1963.

28. Petrillo, M., and Sanger, S.: Emotional Care of the Hospitalized Child. Philadelphia, J. B. Lippincott Co., 1972.

29. Plank, E.: Working with Children in Hospitals. Chicago; Year Book Medical Publishers, 1971.

30. Robertson, J.: Young Children In Hospitals. London, Tavistock Publications, 1970.

31. Rybicki, L.: Preparing Parents to Teach Their Children About Human Sexuality. American Journal of Maternal Child Nursing, 1:3, 1976.

32. Scripien, G., et al.: Comprehensive Pediatric Nursing. St. Louis; C. V. Mosby Co., 1975.

33. Shore, M.: Red is the Color of Hurting. Bethesda, Md., National Institute for Mental Health, 1967.

34. Silver, H., et al.: Handbook of Pediatrics. Los Altos, Cal. Lange Medical Publications, 1975.

35. Stone, L., and Church, J.: Childhood and Adolescence. New York, Random House, 1968.

36. Suen, M., and Solnit, A.: Common Problems in Child Development and Behavior. Philadelphia; Lea & Febiger, 1968.

37. Sutterly, D., and Donnelly, G.: Perspectives in Human Development. Philadelphia; J. B. Lippincott Co., 1973.

38. Vaughan, V., and McKay, R. (eds.): Nelson Textbook of Pediatrics, 11th ed. Philadelphia, W. B. Saunders Co., 1979.

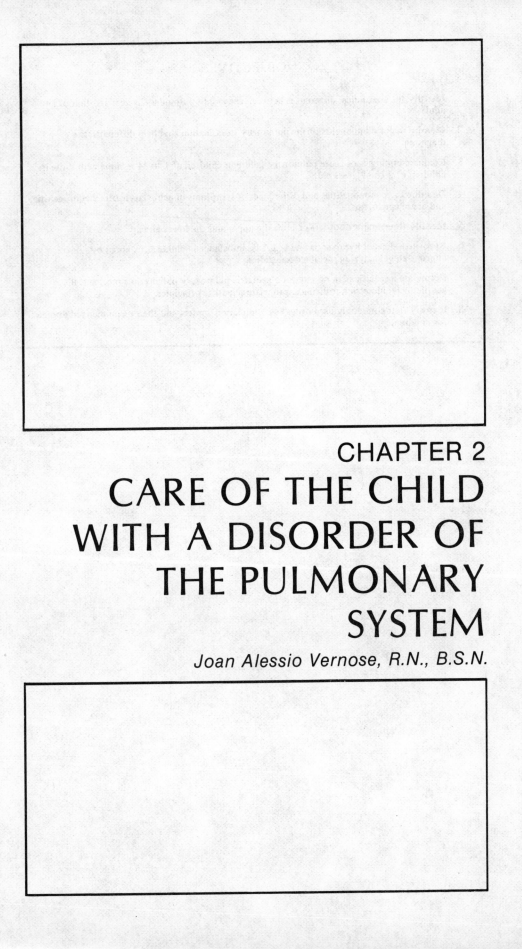

CHAPTER 2
CARE OF THE CHILD WITH A DISORDER OF THE PULMONARY SYSTEM

Joan Alessio Vernose, R.N., B.S.N.

OBJECTIVES

1. Identify the anatomical differences between the child's pulmonary system and that of an adult.

2. Identify major components of the pulmonary examination that help differentiate a diagnosis.

3. Compare etiologies of acute pulmonary failure in children of 1 to 24 months with those in children of 2 to 12 years old.

4. Describe the commonalities and differences of symptoms of acute laryngotracheobronchitis and acute epiglottitis.

5. Identify three major disorders of both the upper and the lower airway.

6. Recognize signs of hypoxemia and acid-base imbalance in children, as noted by appropriately analyzing specific case studies.

7. Formulate a specific plan of care for a pediatric pulmonary patient on a mechanical ventilator (volumetric), utilizing appropriate scientific principles.

8. Identify four commonly used drugs in pulmonary disorders and their recommended dosages for children.

Characteristics of the Lung

1. At birth the lung is underdeveloped.
2. At 23 weeks gestation, exchange of oxygen and carbon dioxide becomes possible.
3. The shape of the lung is cylindrical. The anteroposterior diameter is equal to or greater than the transverse diameter.
4. By the age of 3 1/2, the adult chest wall configuration is attained.
5. Growth of the lung continues until approximately 8 years of age, with increased dimensions of air space and alveoli.
6. Proportion of total lung weight to body weight is constant from infancy to adulthood.
7. With normal breathing the thorax of the infant is much more compliant than that of the adult. The thorax stiffens with age.
8. There is a smaller functional residual capacity (FRC) in infants, resulting in a smaller amount of "buffer gas". This makes it more difficult to balance sudden changes of gas concentrations, thus increasing the chances of atelectasis.

Characteristics of Alveoli

1. Alveolar growth patterns
   a. There are 20 million alveoli at birth, 200 million alveoli by one year of age, and 300 million alveoli, the same as the adult, by eight years of age. Thereafter, only the size of the alveoli increases to further lung growth.
   b. Pulmonary surface area in relation to body weight almost doubles by 18 months and triples by 3 years of age. Therefore, the younger child has smaller reserve surface of gas exchange than the older child. Normally there is no need for reserve because of the lack of heavy exercise at this age. However, if the infant develops a pulmonary ailment he increases his workload, which leads to danger.
   c. The young child has fewer communications between adjacent alveoli, alveolar ducts, alveolar bronchioles, and segments of the lung. Some of these channels are called "old pores of Kohn." These communications serve a purpose in decreased functional states in which collateral ventilation blocks the normal air conducting system so that the alveoli can be bypassed. Therefore, the child has less capacity for collateral ventilation.
2. Alveolar walls
   a. Thickness of the walls is increased in the newborn, thus affecting the diffusion of gases across the alveolar capillary barrier.
   b. Interstitial edema and other pathologic factors impair transfer of gas from alveoli to capillary blood.
   c. Muscular arteries accompanying the airways do not extend into the periphery in children as they do in adults. This factor ordinarily aids in adaptation to regional hypoxia.

Characteristics of Airway
1. Airway growth patterns
    a. Bronchial tree in children has the same number of branches as in adults.
    b. Diameter of parts of the air conducting system grows on different scales from birth to adult age.
        1) Tracheal diameter increases threefold.
        2) Bronchioles increase twofold. Peripheral bronchioles have increased resistance in children less than 5 years of age. Therefore, peripheral airway disease, e.g. bronchiolitis, is severe in the young child.
2. Nasal passages
    a. In infants, resistance of nasal passages to airflow is 40% of total air conducting system (as compared with 60% in adults).
    b. Larynx is high, uvula nearly touches soft palate, the tongue is large.
        1) Infant breathes through nose except when crying.
        2) Any obstruction to nasal passages is extremely dangerous.

Characteristics of Bronchi
1. Bronchi at any age are lined with ciliated columnar epithelium.
2. The cells are shorter and wider in infants and more slender in the older child.
3. Airways have different internal diameters; with congestion or edema these cells or tissues decrease the size of functioning bronchi, increasing the airway resistance.
4. In the child, there is less muscle in the small bronchi than in the adult. They are, therefore, more collapsible.
5. There is lower static recoil pressure in children. This accounts for less pull on bronchi, which allows airway closure or air trapping at a larger lung volume. Such conditions cause the severe consequences of an airway obstruction.

Characteristics of Mucous Glands
1. There are more mucus-producing structures in children than in adults.
2. Conditions that result in overproduction of mucus will exaggerate the obstruction in the child.

CLINICAL ASSESSMENT OF PULMONARY STATUS _____

History
1. Clinical presentation
2. Previous medical history
3. Family medical history
4. Growth and developmental stage
5. Immunization status
6. Medication history

7. Allergies
8. Evaluation of present illness

Physical Examination[2,4,5,10,14,19]

1. Inspection
   a. Cyanosis: distribution, degree, duration, response to oxygen therapy (suspect right-to-left shunt if cyanosis persists).
   b. Respirations.
      1) Rate: varies with age and whether the child is awake or asleep. Record when the child is at rest.
      2) Depth: difficult to assess except in these extremes.
         a) Hyperpnea occurs with fever, severe anemia, salicylism, metabolic acidosis, respiratory alkalosis, and those disorders associated with increased physiologic dead space.
         b) Hypopnea occurs with metabolic alkalosis (e.g., pyloric stenosis), and respiratory acidosis (e.g., central nervous system depression).
      3) Quality.
         a) Labored respirations: note the time of onset, duration, predisposing factors, any retractions or nasal flaring.
         b) Noisy breathing: describe sound heard to differentiate the snore of nasal obstruction from stridor of laryngeal or tracheal origin.
         c) Wheezing: prolonged and high-pitched musical sound of varying degrees of intensity. May be heard without a stethoscope. Timing suggests diagnosis.
            (1) Inspiratory: upper airway obstruction (e.g., croup, cord paralysis, epiglottitis).
            (2) Inspiratory and expiratory: midtracheal lesions or progressive bronchospasm.
            (3) Expiratory: early phase of bronchospasm; intra-thoracic airway obstruction.
         d) Labored breathing and wheezing together: suggest either a single high obstruction (trachea or main stem bronchus) or multiple lower obstruction (lobar, segmental, or subsegmental bronchi).
         e) Paroxysmal: suggests impairment of diaphragm function.
   c. Cough.
      1) Nonproductive: suggests allergy or virus.
      2) Productive: suggests bronchorrhea, chronic bronchitis, or bronchiectasis.
      3) Paroxysmal: suggests foreign body or pertussis.
      4) Recurrent with wheeze: suggests tracheobronchial obstruction, cystic fibrosis, asthma, or foreign body.
      5) Croupy (sounds like the bark of a seal or dog): denotes subglottal involvement.

6) Cough associated with swallowing: suggests aspiration into tracheobronchial tree, anomaly or mass in hypopharyngeal area, achalasia of esophagus, or tracheoesophageal fistula.

7) Cough with aphonia or dysphonia: indicates hypopharyngeal or laryngeal foreign body, papilloma of larynx, croup, or psychoneurosis.

d. Sputum.

1) Most secretions formed by infants are swallowed and therefore compose some of the material in vomitus and stools.

2) Assess volume, color, viscosity, and odor of sputum if the child is able to cooperate.

e. Clubbing (progressive changes in nail curvature and shape of terminal phalanges).

1) Suggests chronicity of disorder.

2) Caused by

a) Pulmonary disorders (bronchiectasis, empyema, chronic pneumonia, cystic fibrosis, neoplasms, pulmonary abscess).

b) Cardiac disorders (cyanotic heart disease).

f. Halitosis: suggests bronchiectasis, lung abscess, paranasal sinusitis, nasal foreign body, adenoidal infection, allergic rhinitis.

g. Nutritional status: failure to thrive may be manifestation of severe or chronic respiratory disorder.

h. Grunting: suggests respiratory distress syndrome (RDS), chest pain, acute pneumonic process with pleural involvement, pulmonary edema, congestive heart failure.

i. Thoracic disfiguration (e.g., "barrel chest," pectus excavatum).

2. Palpation

a. Note tenderness, masses, and defects of bony structures.

b. Note any enlargements of the chondrocostal junctions, which may suggest rickets.

c. Palpate for fremitus and friction rubs.

d. Note the extent and symmetry of lateral movements of the chest.

3. Percussion

a. Chest wall of the infant is more resonant than that of the adult, so percussion should be light so as to better indicate the variations of sounds.

b. Direct percussion on the chest wall is sometimes a better method to indicate dullness or other changes.

4. Auscultation

a. Cooperation from the child is necessary for adequate assessment of breath sounds.

b. The stethoscope head should be relatively small to localize sounds. The bell type is preferred to the diaphragm, since it does not make a tight seal with the skin of the chest wall. Pediatric sizes are available.

c. Breath sounds of an infant and young child are relatively louder than those of the adult.

d. Auscultate in both upright and supine positions if possible.

e. Vocal resonances may be detected during crying or during conversation.

f. Hold the stethoscope to the infant's mouth to determine relative air exchange and evidence of hyperpnea. Rhonchi can also be heard by this method.

5. Vital signs (pediatric norms)
   a. Systemic blood pressure.
      1) Use flush technique or preferably a Doppler device to determine blood pressure in the infant.
      2) In the older infant and child, pediatric cuffs measuring two thirds of the upper arm should be used.
   b. Pulse, respiration, temperature (see Normal Physical and Physiologic Development, pp. 3–10).
   c. Pulmonary wedge pressure (5–10 cm H_2O pressure). Pressures vary with disorders. Need for stretching above norms to improve cardiac output and myocardial function.

Laboratory Studies

1. Blood.
   a. CBC.
   b. Hemoglobin.
   c. Hematocrit.
   d. Electrolytes.
   e. Arterial blood gases.
2. Urine.
   a. Routine.
   b. Specific gravity.
   c. Osmolality.
3. Pulmonary function tests.
   a. Young infant and child.
      1) Arterial blood gases.
      2) Acid-base studies.
      3) Measurements of intrapulmonary shunting.
   b. Older cooperative child.
      1) Vital capacity.
      2) Tidal volume.
      3) Forced expiratory volume.
      4) Dead space/tidal volume (VD/VT ratio).
      5) Peak mid-expiratory flow rates.
   c. Indications for study.
      1) Assessment of degree of respiratory failure.
      2) Determination of type of respiratory insufficiency.
      3) In anticipation of a major thoracic procedure and/or major anesthesia.

4) To evaluate treatment regimen.

5) To establish prognosis.

Diagnostic Studies

1. Chest x-ray film.
2. Bronchography.
   a. Indications.
      1) Chronic productive, purulent cough with persistent localized rales on auscultation in a child who does not have cystic fibrosis.
      2) Follow-up care of a child with bronchiectasis whose disease has not responded to medical management.
      3) Recurrent focal pneumonia of unknown origin.
      4) Severe or recurrent hemoptysis of unknown origin.
      5) Segmental localization of asymptomatic intrapulmonary masses.
   b. Study may aid in delineating congenital abnormalities of the bronchi.
   c. Performed under general anesthesia with an endotracheal tube in place to permit controlled or assisted ventilation and rapid aspiration of secretions and contrast medium.

HYPOXEMIA AND OXYGEN THERAPY _____

Assessment

Since hypoxemia is manifested early in many pediatric pulmonary disorders, oxygen therapy is frequently necessary. Early recognition is important.

1. Hypoxemia
   a. Detected by cyanosis, PaO_2 level, oxyhemoglobin saturation, hemoglobin concentration, cardiac output, distribution of blood flow, or any unusual displacement of the oxyhemoglobin dissociation curve.
   b. Tissue hypoxemia may occur at normal PaO_2 levels in the presence of severe anemia, decreased cardiac output, shock, or an extreme shift of the oxyhemoglobin dissociation curve to the left.
2. True right-to-left shunt (oxygen therapy is usually unsuccessful in increasing the PaO_2 significantly).
3. Upper airway disorders.
4. Lower airway disorders.

Therapeutic Principles

1. Administer lowest concentrations of oxygen necessary to achieve desired PaO_2 (60 to 80 mm Hg) not exceeding 100 mm Hg.
2. Record concentration and duration.

Administration

1. Gas must be humidified.

2. Nasal catheters are not well tolerated by children.
3. Nasal cannulas are preferred but are only as valuable as the child is cooperative. This method allows freedom of movement.
4. Oxygen tents are usually well accepted by children. They allow some movement, especially to the younger child. Care must be taken to keep the tent tightly tucked in place to insure adequate oxygen concentrations.
5. Oxygen hoods provide easier access to neonates and infants and insure greater oxygen concentration.
6. Simple rebreathing masks may also be used. They should be pediatric size and be made of soft vinyl. Protect the top of the child's ears by placing cotton under the head strap of the mask. Wipe inside of mask dry occasionally to prevent skin breakdown.
7. Artificial airways should be accompanied by heating nebulizer and use of short insulated tubing to maintain the temperature of gas near normal body temperature at the tubing outlet.
8. Method of administration depends on disorder, age, acceptance by the child, location of the child with reference to nurse surveillance.

Hazards
1. Oxygen toxicity may involve:
   a. The retina, leading to retrolental fibroplasia, especially in the newborn.
   b. The lung, leading to pulmonary oxygen toxicity, which is dependent on alveolar oxygen tension level, alveolar hemorrhage.
   c. The brain, leading to cerebral vasoconstriction.
   d. The erythrocytes, leading to a mild hemolytic tendency.
2. Indirect risk of oxygen administration is the possibility of inducing alveolar hypoventilation in a chronically hypercapnic patient whose respiratory center may be insensitive to the $PaCO_2$, e.g., the child with cystic fibrosis.

ACID-BASE IMBALANCE AND SODIUM BICARBONATE THERAPY

Assessment
Metabolic acidosis may be seen in a variety of pulmonary disorders.
1. Metabolic acidosis: pH less than 7.25.
2. Evaluating metabolic acidosis.
   a. Acid-base status of blood in relation to clinical history and knowledge of antecedent therapy the patient has received.
   b. Plasma bicarbonate concentration is 20 to 22 mEq/liter in first two years of life.
   c. Whole blood base excess is 1.0 to 3.0 mEq/liter.

Therapeutic Principles

1. Estimate dose of sodium bicarbonate to correct a measured degree of metabolic acidosis. Factors to be considered:
   a. The magnitude of the metabolic acidosis.
   b. Any correction to above data to take into account the "distribution" effect resulting from buffering carbonic acid in states of CO_2 retention.
   c. Anticipated clinical course over the period of sodium bicarbonate administration.
   d, Expected result of concomitant therapy.
   e. Estimated bicarbonate space (30 to 50% of body weight); higher value pertains to newborns and premature infants.

Administration

1. Required dose is usually 1 mEq/kg, not exceeding 2 mEq/kg/min.
2. Blood acid-base data are required to monitor and evaluate therapy.

Hazards

1. Overcorrection can lead to metabolic alkalosis.
2. Osmolar poisoning due to too rapid administration (should Not exceed 6 mOsm/kg/hour).
3. Local toxicity at site of infusion.

Collection of Blood Samples for Oxygen and Acid-Base Determination

1. Direct puncture: the femoral artery should be the last resort owing to the increased risk of infection.
2. Arterialized capillary blood sampling: safe, convenient, and relatively accurate for acid-base status of blood. Its role in oxygen measurement is less secure owing to greater effect of incomplete "arterialization" of blood on oxygen tension than on carbon dioxide tension.
3. Indwelling arterial lines: insertion of a plastic catheter into an artery, preferably the radial. It is used for both sampling of blood and monitoring systemic arterial pressure. Both can be accomplished by using the "Sorenson Intraflow," which allows the line to be flushed continually and to be monitored at the same time. Before radial artery cannulation, precaution should be taken to establish the existence of the ulnar arterial supply to the hand by manually compressing the radial artery (Allen test). Failure of the palm to blanch confirms the presence of adequate collateral perfusion.

Interpretation of Arterial Blood Gases

1. Normal values for the pediatric age group:
   a. PaO_2: 60 to 80 mm Hg in first few days of life, 90 to 100 mm Hg thereafter.
   b. $PaCO_2$: 34 mm Hg in first two years of life, 40 mm Hg in older children.
   c. pH: 7.35 to 7.45

PATHOLOGIC CONDITIONS

According to a survey conducted by the United States Government, one of every ten children is handicapped by asthma, bronchitis, bronchiectasis, cystic fibrosis, or some other pulmonary disorder. In addition, 42% of hospitalized children have a respiratory disorder.

ACUTE RESPIRATORY FAILURE

Acute respiratory failure is a condition in which the impairment of gas exchange in the lungs poses an immediate threat to life.

Etiology.
1. Infants (1 to 24 months of age).
   a. Bronchopneumonia.
      1) Bacterial.
      2) Viral.
      3) Aspiration.
   b. Upper airway obstruction.
   c. Congenital heart disease.
   d. Status asthmaticus.
   e. Septicemia.
   f. Foreign body aspiration.
   g. Intrathoracic anomalies.
      1) Diaphragmatic lesions.
      2) Vascular ring.
      3) Lobar emphysema.
   h. Encephalitis.
   i. Poisoning.
   j. Cystic fibrosis.
2. Children (2 to 12 years of age).
   a. Status asthmaticus.
   b. Congenital heart disease.
   c. Bronchopneumonia.
   d. Encephalitis.
   e. Peripheral polyneuritis.
   f. Septicemia.
   g. Poisoning.
   h. Trauma.
      1) Thoracic injury.
      2) Head injury.
      3) Traumatic shock.
   i. Near-drowning.
   j. Burns.
   k. Renal failure.

Pathophysiologic Description.
1. Primary pulmonary disorder.
   a. Obstruction of lower airways: edema, thick secretions, smooth muscle spasm of bronchial wall leading to trapping of gas distal to obstructed airways.
   b. Increased airway resistance in a child less than 5 years old.
   c. With many disorders the basic pulmonary defect is "wasted perfusion," pulmonary capillary flow through unventilated or poorly ventilated alveoli resulting in a venoarterial shunt with consequent fall in systemic PaO_2.
2. Primary cardiovascular disease.
   a. Effect of pulmonary capillary blood flow:
      1) Decreased, e.g., tetralogy of Fallot, severe pulmonic stenosis.
      2) Increased, e.g., ventricular septal defect.
   b. Pulmonary venous hypertension results in pulmonary vascular obstruction, which in turn leads to alveolar capillary congestion and increased bronchial secretions. This leads to atelectasis with venoarterial shunting and further hypoxemia.
3. Primary nervous system disease.
   a. Due to loss of central control of ventilation (e.g., cerebral edema, cerebral vascular accidents, central nervous system depression associated with drug overdose or poisoning) culminates in the loss of protective upper airway reflexes, thus predisposing the patient to aspiration.
   b. Diseases of peripheral nervous system, e.g., Guillain-Barré syndrome.
   c. Abnormalities associated with prolonged convulsive seizures, e.g., status epilepticus.
4. Primary skeletal muscle disorder.
   a. Severe muscle weakness.
   b. Intense muscular spasma.
   c. Neuromuscular diseases.

Clinical Presentation
1. Signs and symptoms.
   a. Clinical criteria:
      1) Decreased or absent inspiratory breath sounds.
      2) Severe inspiratory retractions and use of accessory muscles.
      3) Cyanosis in 40% ambient oxygen.
      4) Depressed level of consciousness and response to pain.
      5) Poor skeletal muscle tone.
   b. Physiologic criteria:
      1) $PaCO_2$ equal to or more than 60 mm Hg.
      2) PaO_2 equal to or less than 100 mm Hg in 100% oxygen.
   c. Clinical and one physiologic equals acute respiratory failure.
2. Criteria for infants and children with congenital heart disease.
   a. Clinical criteria:
      1) Severe retractions.

2) Apnea or gasping in 100% oxygen.
3) Decreased to absent inspiratory breath sounds.
4) Expiratory grunting.
5) Tachypnea (rate equal to or more than 20% above normal range).
6) Arterial hypotension and/or bradycardia (equal to or more than 20% under normal range).
b. Physiologic criteria:
1) PaO_2 equal to or less than 30 mm Hg in 100% oxygen (cyanotic lesion).
2) PaO_2 equal to or less than 60 mm Hg in 100% oxygen (acyanotic lesion).
3) $PaCO_2$ equal to or more than 50 mm Hg.

Objective of Therapy
1. Establish airway patency.
2. Promote effective respiration, spontaneous or ventilator-assisted.
3. Reduce complications.
4. Prevent sequelae.

Therapeutic Management
Assess presence of hypoxemia and need for oxygen therapy (for details see p. 66-67).
Administer humidified oxygen. Methods depend on disease, age, acceptance, and location of child with reference to nurse surveillance (see also p. 67 for detailed description and hazards of therapy).
Assess presence of acid-base imbalance and need for sodium bicarbonate therapy (for details see p. 67-68).
Administer sodium bicarbonate according to this general rule: 2 mEq/kg/ minute, not to exceed 8 mEq/kg/day (see also p. 68 for details and hazards of therapy).
Based on arterial blood analysis, administer $NaHCO_3$ (sodium bicarbonate) according to this formula: 0.03 × body weight × base deficit in mEq/liter.
Assess possible respiratory acidosis.
a. Evaluate arterial blood gas data.
b. Correction depends on clinical disorder and method of treatment in progress.
Obtain, monitor, and interpret arterial blood gases (for details see p. 68).
Drain excess secretions from tracheobronchial tree.
a. Postural drainage: side-back-side is most frequently used position. If condition allows, have patient assume other positions for postural drainage.
b. Mechanical vibration: Usually tolerated very well by children. It is quite effective in moving secretions along and is less painful than percussion, especially when there is a chest incision. (A mechanical toothbrush can be used for the newborn).
c. Breathing exercises (same as for adult): Use of incentive spirometry for the child who is not intubated is recommended, since the child views this exercise as a game.

    d. Percussion (same as for adult): Remember to stop every 30 seconds to allow the child to fully expand his chest. They tend to splint during the entire procedure and decrease their inspiratory volume.

Suction secretions from tracheobronchial tree.
    a. Nasopharyngeal.
    b. Tracheal.

Establish and maintain artificial airway.
    a. Oral airway.
    b. Endotracheal tubes.
        1) Equipment:
            a) Pediatric tube (size 2.0 mm to 8.0 mm), clear with radiopaque markings. It should be implant tested and have circle markers displayed at 2 cm and 4 cm. The internal diameter should be noted proximally for quick identification. The tube should fit so that there is a leak, to prevent necrosis and stenosis. Because the cricoid diameter in small children is narrow and insures an adequate seal, cuffed tubes are not used.
            b) Larynogoscope and blade of appropriate size.
            c) Introducing forceps.
            d) Tube of appropriate size and several tubes of assorted sizes in case of difficulty.
            e) Stethoscope.
            f) X-ray apparatus ready to take film as soon as possible after intubation. Keep child's head in neutral position while film is taken, since tube changes position when neck is either extended or flexed and may give false information.
            g) Oxygen apparatus.
            h) Suction equipment.
            i) Waterproof tape.
            j) Benzoin and applicators.
        2) Selection process:
            a) Oral tracheal tubes are used for emergency airway management and for patients who have nasal obstruction.
            b) Nasotracheal tubes are preferred and should replace an oral tracheal tube as soon as possible. Nasotracheal tubes may be more easily stabilized.
        3) Complications:
            a) Post-intubation croup due to mucosal swelling at sub-glottic level. Treatment consists of oxygen therapy and mist. Racemic epinephrine (0.25 ml to 0.5 ml of 0.25%) with 3 to 4 ml of sterile water delivered by aerosol is sometimes used, although this treatment is controversial. Steroid therapy may also be used, although it too is controversial.

b) Stenosis, primarily at subglottic level. Treatment consists of:
  (1) Tracheostomy for children aged 1 to 5 years until larynx and trachea enlarge; tracheostomy with multiple tracheal dilatations; dilatation and direct injection of adrenocortical steroids; resection of subglottal scar; stent; granulation tissue removal by microlaryngoscopy or laser beam excision.
  (2) An adult sleeve resection of trachea with end-to-end anastomosis is not used, since trauma occurs at cricoid level where resection presents risk of irreparable damage to vocal cords.

c. Tracheostomy should be performed in an operating room under controlled conditions and after prior establishment of an airway and adequate ventilation.
  1) Indications:
    a) Congenital or acquired disease of the upper airway. Facilitation of long-term mechanical ventilation or suctioning because of chronic lung disease.
    b) Congenital webs, stenosis, polyps, lymphangiomas, laryngomalacia, papillomas, postinfectious states, post-traumatic stenosis, direct trauma to larynx.
  2) Complications:
    a) Mechanical.
      (1) Accidental decannulation: restrain patient if necessary.
      (2) Occlusion: position head to maintain patent airway.
    b) Infection.
      (1) Routine culture and sensitivity tests should be performed.
      (2) Use sterile technique.
    c) Stenosis.
    d) Tracheal bleeding.
    e) Tracheomalacia.
    f) Tracheal erosion.
  3) Considerations for care of the child with a tracheostomy:
    a) Explain thoroughly, especially to the toddler who has just mastered verbalization, the reason why he can no longer talk.
    b) Keep small toys, dry cereal, etc. out of the reach of the child to avoid accidental aspiration.
    c) Because of short, stubby neck of young children, it is necessary to place a roll or pad under the shoulders to prevent occlusion of the tube.
    d) Tie tracheostomy tape with neck flexed; make a knot, not a bow, to secure tube.

When testing for security, only one finger should fit between tape and neck.

   e) Be sure end flaps of tape are not over tracheostomy opening.

   f) Drain water from condensation traps frequently to avoid accidental drowning and allow gas flow; secure water trap to bed.

   g) Skin care:

      (1) Clean around tracheostomy site with one-half strength hydrogen peroxide frequently. Dry site, and avoid dusting powders.

      (2) Change tracheostomy strings every day after the first 4 to 5 days postoperatively.

   h) Emergency equipment should be at the bedside at all times. This includes:

      (1) Extra tracheostomy tube.

      (2) Kelly clamp.

      (3) Suction equipment and apparatus.

      (4) Extra caps for use when hyperventilating and when closed system is needed.

      (5) Extra double swivel connector to allow free movement at site; the axes of free rotatory movements are at right angles to each other (Pediatric swivel, National Catheter, Argyle, New York).

      (6) If the tube should become dislodged in the first few days postoperatively, one can place traction on the sutures, pulling the stoma into the skin incision; replacement of the tube is then possible.

  4) Decannulation:

   a) Criteria include that the disease be under control, that there be no acute respiratory infection, and that the coughing mechanism be intact.

   b) Procedure: Emergency reintubation equipment should be readily available. Dexamethasone may be given 24 hours prior to decannulation. The child should be sedated and placed in an oxygen tent for removal of the tracheostomy tube. Older children may be weaned with progressively smaller tubes.

   c) Careful observation for signs of airway obstruction is important.

   d) Vigorous chest physiotherapy to compensate for ineffective cough is likely to be necessary.

Maintain adequate ventilation.

  a. Indications for mechanical ventilation include acute respiratory failure and reserve of ventilatory effort, e.g., neuromuscular disease.

  b. Types of mechanical ventilation (positive pressure) include:

    1) Volume pre-set, time-cycled ventilator is preferred. Large internal compliance (compression volume) may require ventilator tidal volume to be 50 to 150% greater than patient tidal volume.

    2) Pressure-cycled assister-controllor. The assist mode is generally of less value in small children, owing to wide range of sensitivities and response times.

  c. Complications of mechanical ventilation may include:

    1) Airway: extubation, occlusion, edema, stenosis, granuloma.

    2) Pulmonary.

      a) Secretions due to dry gas (do not use ultrasonic nebulizers with mechanical ventilation, owing to excess volume of water with unpredictable volume of water in lungs).

      b) Atelectasis.

      c) Pneumonitis.

      d) Oxygen toxicity.

      e) Hyperinflation (trapped gas).

      f) Interstitial emphysema.

      g) Pneumothorax: increased hazard when peak airway pressure is more than 40 cm water pressure or when CPAP is more than 10 cm water pressure. Thoracotomy tube should be inserted and attached to an underwater seal system.

      h) Pneumomediastinum.

      i) Decrease in urinary output and retention, with or without interstitial pulmonary edema. Fluid restrictions and diuretics may be necessary.

    3) Mechanical.

      a) Disconnection.

      b) Kinked tubing.

      c) Valve malfunction.

      d) Power failure.

      e) Leaks.

      f) Humidifier water level either too high or too low.

      g) Condensation of water in tubing.

    4) Infection.

      a) Tracheitis.

      b) Bronchopneumonia.

      c) Septicemia.

      d) Sources: hands, nonsterile airway care, vascular lines, connections, patient's skin, humidifiers, nebulizer, ambient air, any equipment tubing not changed every 24 hours.

  d. Intermittent mandatory ventilation (IMV). IMV is a method of operating a ventilator to provide for both spontaneous breathing (bypassing the ventilator) and delivery of machine breaths. A circuit connected to a fresh gas source enables the patient to take unrestricted, unassisted, spontaneous breaths supplemented by mechanical breaths.

   1) Indications for use:

      a) Weaning patients from mechanical ventilation. IMV permits a gradual reduction of ventilator support, minimizing out-of-phase breathing.

      b) IMV allows development of negative intrapleural pressure and regular contraction of respiratory muscles.

  e. Positive end-expiratory pressure (PEEP). PEEP is a method of maintaining higher than atmospheric pressure in the lungs at the end of expiration.

   1) It maintains the lungs in a state of slight hyperinflation.

   2) It increases functional residual capacity (FRC) to combat the tendency of small airways and alveoli to collapse when deprived of surfactant.

   3) It increases intrathoracic pressure.

   4) The amount of PEEP depends on the needs and response of patient.

   5) End-expiratory pressure may be used on patients who are breathing spontaneously or receiving mechanical ventilation.

   6) The terms constant positive pressure breathing (CPPB), constant positive airway pressure (CPAP), and continuous positive pressure ventilation (CPPV) may also be used, the precise nomenclature varying with the authority consulted.

   7) The physiologic responses to PEEP include:

      a) Increased FRC.

      b) Increased lung compliance.

      c) Decreased work of respiratory effort.

      d) Decreased venous admixture.

   8) Complications of PEEP may be:

      a) Pneumothorax.

      b) Mediastinal and subcutaneous emphysema.

      c) Decreased cardiac output.

      d) Increased lung water.

    Maximal upper limits of PEEP are not known at the present time.

  f. A dual system of monitoring with alarm systems may be necessary to detect the absence of respiratory circuit pressure.

   1) Keep a flow sheet at the bedside to indicate various parameters relating to machine function and physiologic monitoring for immediate correlation between machine adjustments and the patient's response.

   2) Coordination of the patient with the mechanical ventilator can often be achieved merely by providing adequate alveolar ventilation and oxygenation. The child, however, is more apt to "fight" the system. The restless infant or

child may require sedation and slight depression of the respiratory drive.

  g. Weaning from respiratory assist devices (mechanical ventilation) is generally accomplished with use of IMV device.

    1) The indications for weaning are:

      a) Control of underlying disease.

      b) Improvement, as evidenced by chest film.

      c) Vital capacity greater than 15 ml/kg.

      d) Improved blood gas and pH data.

      e) Stable cardiac status.

      f) Control of infections.

      g) Positive psychological response.

      h) Thin secretions.

      i) Inspiratory pressure equal to or greater than 20 cm H_2O.

Nursing Skills

1. Pulmonary history and physical exam.
2. Assessment parameters for oxygen therapy.
3. Administration of oxygen therapy.
   a. Communication with patient and family regarding need for therapy and type of equipment to be used.
   b. Monitoring and recording oxygen concentrations every 15 minutes until patient is stable, then every 2 hours.
   c. Recording of inflating pressures, amount of CPAP, IMV hourly or in conjunction with vital signs.
4. Comfort and protection of patient receiving oxygen therapy.
   a. Cotton or sponge on top of ears if head strap is used.
   b. Wipe inside of mask occasionally to prevent skin breakdown.
   c. Oxygen hood should be kept close to the neck, but friction and pressure on the neck should be avoided.
   d. Use cleansing soap on inside of hood to reduce clouding from condensation.
5. Chest physiotherapy, including postural drainage, mechanical vibration, breathing exercises, percussion, airway suctioning.
6. Sterile tracheostomy care.
7. Skin and eye care.
8. Pressure monitoring.
9. Psychological and communication approaches necessary for therapeutics.
10. Play therapy.
11. Emergency life support.

CARE OF THE CHILD WITH UPPER AIRWAY OBSTRUCTION

Significant signs and symptoms vary with the site and cause of obstruction. Inspiratory stridor occurs with lesions near the entrance to the larynx, where the airway tends to become narrower during inspiration. Stridor may have a vibrating or crowing character and tends to be reduced by placing the child in the prone position. Inspiratory and expiratory stridor occur with obstruction at sites between the pharynx and the carina. Change in the quality of the voice occurs when the vocal cords are involved.

Infections
1.   Acute laryngotracheobronchitis: This is a common infection of infants and young children in which the larynx, trachea, and bronchi are inflamed. Obstruction to the airway tends to be severe. Inflammation causes swelling of the mucosal lining of these structures. Thick, viscous, purulent secretions are present and further obstruct the airway.
   a.   Etiology and predisposing factors.
      1)   Most common causative agent: parainfluenza viruses, especially types 1 and 2.
      2)   Bacterial cultures may show streptococci, pneumococci, staphylococci, and *Haemophilus influenzae.*
      3)   Peak incidence: 6 months to 3 years.
      4)   Winter months.
      5)   Preceded by upper respiratory infection.
   b.   Pathophysiologic description.
      1)   Inflammation and edema of larynx, trachea, and bronchi.
      2)   Severe airway obstruction complicated by purulent secretions.
      3)   Asphyxia and exhaustion of respiratory muscles.
   c.   Clinical presentation.
      1)   "Croupy" cough (like bark of a seal).
      2)   Stridorous respirations.
      3)   Hoarseness.
      4)   Attack commonly occurs in middle of night.
      5)   Restlessness due to hypoxia and hypercapnia.
      6)   Retractions of intercostal muscles and accessory muscles.
      7)   Tachypnea.
      8)   Prolonged inspiratory phase.
      9)   Temperature elevation.
   d.   Objective of therapy.
      1)   Prevention of acute respiratory failure.
   e.   Therapeutic Management.
      1)   Establish and maintain a patent airway and adequate ventilation.
         a)   Provide cool, humidified oxygen therapy (40 to 60% initially) (see also p. 67–68).
         b)   Allow child to assume position of comfort.
         c)   Administer medications, e.g., racemic epinephrine delivered with face mask IPPB. May cause further obstruction if child resists.

2) Prevent further obstruction to airway.
   a) Handle child minimally.
   b) Sometimes small amounts of Nembutal or morphine and Nembutal are used intermittently. If morphine and Nembutal are used, monitor closely for respiratory depression.
3) Decrease external stimuli; provide quiet environment.
4) Parental teaching to help decrease stimulation.
5) Observe, monitor, and record:
   a) Level of fatigue.
   b) Vital signs.
   c) Type and degree of retractions.
   d) Degree of stridor.
   e) *Changes in heart rate, decreased respiratory rate, and decreased stridor indicate acute obstruction requiring immediate attention.*
6) Maintain hydration through intravenous therapy and strict intake and output.
7) Obtain diagnostic studies as ordered:
   a) Chest x-ray.
   b) Arterial blood gases.
   c) Nasopharyngeal and blood cultures and sensitivities.
8) Begin antibiotic therapy as ordered, e.g., ampicillin 100 to 150 mg/kg/24 hours, every 6 hours parenterally.
9) Identify need for tracheostomy. Indications include:
   a) Failure of medical regimen.
   b) Maximum respiratory effort with tight fitting translaryngeal artificial airway.

f. Complications.
   1) Hypoxic CNS damage.
   2) Asphyxia.
   3) Subglottic stenosis.
g. Nursing skills are the same as in acute respiratory failure (p. 77).

2. Acute epiglottitis (acute supraglottitis).[1,2,5,12,14,17,20,43]
   a. Etiology and predisposing factors.
      1) Commonly *Haemophilus influenzae,* type B.
      2) May be pneumococci, group A streptococci.
      3) Victims are most commonly aged 3 to 6 years.
      4) Infection is more common in the winter months.
      5) Antecedent upper respiratory tract infection, sore throat, dysphagia.
   b. Pathophysiologic description.
      1) Severe, rapid, progressive infection of epiglottis and surrounding area.
      2) Vocal cords are not involved.

    c. Clinical presentation.
        1) Rapid onset.
        2) Drooling resulting from painful inflammatory swelling of supraglottic tissue.
        3) Minimal cough.
        4) Child usually assumes upright position, with chin forward and tongue protruding to facilitate breathing.
        5) Appears anxious and frightened.
        6) Stridor.
        7) Retractions of intercostal and accessory muscles.
        8) Temperature elevation.
        9) Large, edematous, fiery-red epiglottis is a classical sign.
      10) Will not eat or drink.
      11) Elevated white cell count, bacterial infection.
    d. Objective of therapy: Prevention of acute respiratory failure.
    e. Therapeutic management:
        1) Since the tongue must be depressed for visualization, repeated examinations are most dangerous. Physicians should examine the child together to minimize the number of examinations.
        2) Patients are usually intubated in the operating room, using anesthesia and oxygen.
        3) This procedure may be immediately followed by a tracheostomy. Present practice, however, favors leaving the tube in place and reevaluating the patient's condition under light anesthesia and laryngoscopy every 24 hours to consider extubation.
    f. Complication: sudden occlusion of airway.
    g. Nursing skills are the same as for acute respiratory failure (p. 77). Special attention should be given to the danger of accidental extubation or decannulation.

Aspiration of Foreign Body[2, 5,12,14]
  1. Etiology and precipitating factors.
    a. Nature of foreign body.
        1) Size and structure.
        2) Composition.
            a) Metallic.
            b) Vegetal.
                (1) Irritating quality causes mucosal swelling.
                (2) Some foreign bodies (beans, seeds, peanuts) may swell and cause further obstruction.
    b. Age of patient is usually 1 to 4 years.
    c. Level of consciousness.
    d. State of health.
    e. Right lung is more frequently invaded, owing to sharper angulation of left main stem bronchus.
  2. Pathophysiologic description.

    a. A foreign body lodging in pharynx, larynx, trachea, or bronchi.

    b. If initially without symptoms, localized inflammation, swelling, and necrosis may occur.

3. Clinical presentation.

    a. Sudden onset of dyspnea and/or paroxysmal cough.

    b. Sudden onset of aphonia or dysphonia.

    c. Choking, gagging, wheezing, cough.

    d. Symptomless period commonly occurs, which may last from hours to weeks.

    e. Symptoms may vary depending on the location of the foreign object.

        1) If in the larynx, the patient may present with:

            a) Hoarseness.

            b) Croupy cough.

            c) Dysphonia.

            d) Inspiratory stridor.

        2) If in the trachea:

            a) Audible slap and palpable thud due to momentary expiratory impaction at the subglottic level.

            b) Expiratory stridor.

        3) If in the bronchus:

            a) Limited expansion of chest wall.

            b) Decreased vocal fremitus.

            c) Diminished breath sounds distal to foreign body.

            d) Atelectasis.

            e) Lobar emphysema.

            f) Recurrent cough.

            g) Dyspnea.

            h) Cyanosis, if large bronchus is involved.

            i) Infectious process at site: fever, cough, malaise, tachypnea.

            j) If foreign body is a lipid, the symptoms may be confused with those of cystic fibrosis.

            k) Recurrent pneumonia, especially if there is incomplete clearing between attacks.

4. Diagnostic studies:

    a. Lateral and anterior-posterior chest films.

    b. Laryngoscopy.

    c. Contributing factors to diagnosis.

        1) Mediastinal shift.

        2) Atelectasis.

        3) Emphysema.

5. Objectives of therapy.

    a. Remove foreign body.

    b. Prevent acute respiratory failure.

6. Therapeutic management.
   a. Prevention.
   b. Removal of foreign object.
      1) By direct laryngoscopy.
      2) By bronchoscopy.
      3) Instruct and elicit cough if possible.
   c. Administration of drug therapy if warranted by secondary infection.
   d. If airway is totally obstructed, use American Heart Association procedure for clearing airway.
      1) Chest "squeeze" and sweeping foreign contents from mouth.
      2) Attempt to ventilate with four quick breaths.
   e. Do not make rash attempts at foreign body removal, e.g., inverting child or injecting finger down airway, as this may cause it to relocate and compound a difficult removal.
   f. Administer oxygen if there is respiratory distress.
   g. In asphyxia, insert 14 gauge needle through cricothyroid membrane for temporary airway.
   h. Have tracheostomy set ready for emergency procedure.
7. Complications.
   a. Dislocation of object to a more critical part of the airway.
   b. Asphyxia.
   c. Bronchiectasis.
   d. Parenchymal infection.
   e. Stenosis.
8. Nursing skills.
   a. Establishing emergency airway.
   b. Chest "squeeze" method of removing foreign body in airway.
   c. Teaching prevention.
      1) Remind parents and personnel of the risk factors that predispose children to aspirate foreign bodies.

Anomalies (Vascular Rings) [10,35,40,54,56]

1. Etiology.
   a. Congenital malformations.
2. Pathophysiologic description.
   a. Double aortic arch.
   b. Right aortic arch with left ligamentum arteriosum or patent ductus arteriosus.
   c. Retroesophageal subclavian artery.
   d. Anomalous origin of innominate artery.
   e. Anomalous origin of left common carotid artery.
3. Clinical presentation.
   a. Raucous respirations.
   b. Intercostal retractions.
   c. Dyspnea.
   d. Tachypnea.

      e. Feeding problems that lead to coughing and cyanosis, resulting in decreased nutritional status and, possibly, anemia.

      f. Prolonged expiration and impeded air exchange.

      g. Stridor.

      h. Recurrent pneumonia in older infant.

      i. Flexion of neck causes severe dyspnea and cyanosis.

      j. Resultant features of vascular ring are compression and narrowing of tracheoesophageal complex.

      k. Hacking cough.

      l. Increased secretions of respiratory tract.

      m. Dysphagia.

      n. Aspiration.

      o. Expiratory wheeze and diffuse rhonchi on auscultation.

4. Diagnostic studies.

      a. Barium swallow.

      b. Chest x-ray.

      c. Tracheogram.

      d. Cardiac catheterization.

5. Objectives of therapy.

      a. Repair anomaly.

      b. Prevention of acute respiratory failure.

6. Therapeutic management.

      a. Establish and maintain adequate airway and ventilation.

         1) Oxygen therapy.

         2) Intubation as necessary.

         3) Frequent suctioning, usually pharyngeal.

      b. Provide adequate nutrition.

         1) Intravenous therapy.

         2) Nasogastric feedings.

      c. Surgical correction is usually performed through a left thoracotomy.

      d. Provide antibiotic therapy as necessary.

      e. Continue airway surveillance for several weeks. Vascular rings may continue to partially obstruct the airway at the previous site of constriction for some weeks or even months after surgery.

7. Complication: tracheal malacia.

8. Nursing skills are the same as for acute respiratory failure (p. 77). Observe for signs of tracheal edema.

CARE OF THE CHILD WITH LOWER AIRWAY DISORDER

The general signs and symptoms indicating a lower airway disorder are prolonged expiratory phase with forced expirations, some increase in inspiratory effort and retractions of soft tissue, increased antero-posterior diameter, and increased workload of breathing.

Cystic Fibrosis [2,5,12,14]
1. Etiology.
   a. Of obscure origin.
   b. Hereditary disorder, autosomal recessive trait.
   c. Multisystem disorder involving widespread dysfunction of exocrine glands.
   d. Occurs in 1:2000 live births, predominately in Caucasians.
2. Pathophysiologic description: Cystic fibrosis (CF) affects many of the systems and organs of the body.
   a. The pancreas is smaller, thinner, and firmer than normal. The lesions are progressive, resulting in atrophy with fibrosis or replacement by fat. There is also a reduction or absence of pancreatic enzymes from the duodenal fluid.
   b. The intestine is obstructed around the region of the terminal ileum because of the viscous nature of the meconium. Not all patients with CF have meconium ileus. If they do not, the symptoms of malnutrition appear between 4 weeks and 6 months of age. There is abdominal distention and emaciation, and excretion of fat in the stools (steatorrhea). The stools are large, clay colored, and frothy.
   c. The liver shows cell atrophy, fatty metamorphosis, periportal fibrosis, proliferation of bile ducts, and focal obstructive lesions.
   d. The cardiovascular system may demonstrate right ventricular hypertrophy, related to obstructive pulmonary disease and pulmonary hypertension.
   e. The initial respiratory system signs and symptoms are chronic or paroxysmal cough, possibly leading to vomiting; thick secretions; wheezing; increased respiratory rate; and easy fatigue. The initial lesion in the lung is bronchial obstruction due to sticky sputum or mucopurulent secretions followed by overdistension of alveoli. Infection often occurs and may give rise to an abscess. Later complications include hemoptysis, pneumothorax, cor pulmonale, or nasal polyps.
3. Clinical presentation.
   a. Varies greatly with state of illness. It is important to incorporate pathophysiology of disease in the individual assessment. Patient may have manifestations of all affected organs and systems or may have only a few at any one time.
   b. Assessment.
      1) Note general activity.
      2) Note physical findings.
      3) Note nutritional status.
      4) Assess laboratory data and chest x-ray report.

4. Diagnostic studies.
   a. Cystic fibrosis analyzer is available to show the increase in electrolyte concentration in sweat. A positive result is more than 60 mEq/liter of chloride. The study is not done prior to 3 to 4 weeks of age, since sweat glands do not function until that time.
   b. Pancreatic function tests.
   c. Family history.
   d. Chest radiograph reveals irregular aeration with scattered areas of atelectasis.
   e. Diagnostic studies are performed on any child who has symptoms of pancreatic insufficiency or malabsorption, e.g., failure to thrive, large appetite, large foul-smelling stools, protuberant abdomen, rectal prolapse, intestinal obstruction in the newborn, fecal impaction in an older child, and milk allergy in an infant.
   f. CF is suspected in any child with chronic pulmonary disorders.
5. Objectives of therapy.
   a. To enable the child to lead as normal a life as possible.
   b. Combating, slowing, or preventing secondary effects or complications.
   c. Protection from respiratory infection.
   d. Using the team approach to the child's care, because of the magnitude of this chronic disease and its psychosocial problems.
6. Therapeutic management.
   a. Establish and maintain adequate airway and ventilation (See p. 71–80 for details). Administration of bronchodilators and expectorants.
   b. Administration of antibiotic therapy based on culture and sensitivity tests at the time of exacerbations.
   c. Prevent diaphoresis; keep child away from extreme temperatures.
   d. Provide dietetic and pancreatic therapy.
      1) Restrict fat.
      2) Increase protein and caloric intake.
      3) Replace pancreatic enzymes by using preparations with meals and cold foods, e.g., Viokase powder.
      4) Administer vitamin supplements (water soluble), especially A, B complex, and K.
   e. Digoxin and diuretics may be given if there is evidence of cardiac failure.
   f. Provide measles vaccine and protect from respiratory infections.
   g. Arrange for team conferences, including medicine, nursing, clinical psychologist, and social or mental health workers.
   h. Select sites for injections most carefully; avoid wasted muscle.
   i. Observe stools carefully and record findings to assist in evaluating dietary regimen.

      j. Administer meticulous skin care, since skin is unusually susceptible to breakdown, which increases the risk of infection.

      k. Note signs of rectal prolapse.

      l. Weigh daily.

      m. Participate in home care regimen.

      n. Remember that these parents may feel especially guilty about their child's illness.

7. Complications.
   a. Sepsis.
   b. Irreversible destruction of lung tissue.
8. Nursing skills are the same as those for respiratory failure (p. 77).
   a. Family teaching to prepare for patient's activity levels, which regress.

Pneumonia

1. Incidence and etiology: Interstitial plasma cell pneumonia is frequently seen in pediatric patients undergoing critical care.
2. Pathophysiologic description.
   a. *Pneumocystis carinii* is an organism whose taxonomic classification is controversial. It is believed to be a protozoan, since it responds to Pentamidine.
   b. Typically affects immune-compromised infants and children.
   c. Most of these patients are receving adrenocorticosteroids and/or antimetabolites.
3. Clinical presentation.
   a. May be contagious.
      1) Incubation period of 40 days.
      2) Insidious onset.
   b. Signs and symptoms include poor feeding, pain in anterior part of chest or substernal region, vomiting, diarrhea, tachycardia, flaring of alae nasi, irritability, tachypnea, cyanosis, and cough.
   c. Physical findings include little or no resonance. On auscultation there may be good air exchange, with occasional scattered rales and rhonchi.
   d. Course of disease may be rapid; child may expire within a few days from respiratory failure.
4. Diagnostic studies.
   a. Trans-bronchial lung biopsy, using a flexible bronchoscope, is now preferred over the needle and open lung biopsy techniques.
   b. Chest x-ray reveals extensive patchy interstitial infiltrates, with areas of emphysema.
   c. The organism is demonstrated in hypopharyngeal and tracheal secretions.
5. Objectives of therapy.
   a. Supportive therapy.
   b. Combat causative organism.
6. Therapeutic management.
   a. Establish and maintain adequate airway and ventilation (See p. 71–80 for details).

    b. Maintain isolation.
    c. Provide adequate hydration through intravenous therapy.
    d. Give oxygen and humidity as indicated by clinical course.
    e. Administer medications.
       1) Bactrim (trimethoprim and sulfamethoxazole), 20 mg/Kg
          trimethoprim and 100 mg/Kg sulfamethoxazole every
          6 hrs orally for 14 days.
          a) Maintain adequate fluid intake during therapy to
             prevent crystalluria and stone formation.
          b) Complete blood count should be done frequently so
             that any blood dyscrasia can be noted.
       2) Pentamidine Isethionate, 100 to 150 mg/m^2 body
          surface area, parenterally, daily for 10 days.
          a) Store Pentamidine in refrigerator.
          b) Adverse reactions to Pentamidine.
             (1) Decrease in systemic blood pressure.
             (2) Increase in heart rate.
             (3) Increase in BUN.
             (4) Hypoglycemia.
             (5) Nausea.
             (6) Vomiting.
7. Complications
    a. Acute respiratory failure.
    b. Anaphylaxis due to Bactrim and/or Pentamidine.
8. Nursing skills are the same as for acute respiratory failure (p. 77).
    a. Rapid assessment of ensuing shock.

Aspiration (Near Drowning)
1. Definitions.
    a. Drowning without aspiration is death from respiratory
       obstruction and asphyxia while submerged in fluid medium.
    b. Drowning with aspiration is death from the combined effects
       of asphyxia and changes secondary to aspiration of fluid while
       submerged.
    c. Near drowning without aspiration is survival, at least temporary,
       following asphyxia due to submersion in fluid.
    d. Near drowning with aspiration is survival, at least temporary,
       following aspiration of fluid while submerged.
2. Incidence and etiology.
    a. 6000 to 8000 deaths yearly.
    b. Highest incidence of death occurs in persons between 10 and
       19 years of age.
    c. Second most common cause of death in persons under 24 years
       of age.
3. Pathophysiologic changes depend on fluid types.
    a. Fresh water (lake, canal, bathtub).
       1) Fluid rapidly enters circulation, leading to hemodilution,
          hemolysis of red blood cells, hemoglobinemia, and
          hyperkalemia.

     2) Increased circulating blood volume leads to circulatory overload, congestive heart failure, and pulmonary edema, aggravating the perfusion-diffusion defect (this hypervolemia is transient).

     3) Decreased pulmonary compliance results from washing out of surfactant.

     4) Protein, sodium, and chloride are drawn into alveolar spaces, increasing the hemodilution.

     5) Asphyxia with hypoxia and hyperkalemia predisposes to ventricular fibrillation.

  b. Salt water.

     1) Increased concentration of electrolytes.

     2) Fluids leave the intravascular spaces, resulting in hemoconcentration and hyperelectrolytemia.

     3) Increased electrolyte concentrations act as chemical irritants, resulting in inflammation and pulmonary edema with patchy areas of atelectasis and emphysema.

     4) Shift of fluid into pulmonary spaces leads to hemoconcentration, decreased circulating blood volume, and shock.

4. Clinical presentation (depends on age, previous state of health, duration of submersion, amount aspirated, and type of fluid aspirated).

  a. Physiologic effects: hypoxia, hypercapnia, and acidosis.

  b. Bronchospasm.

  c. Distended abdomen, usually from large amounts of swallowed water.

  e. Cardiac dysrhythmias.

  f. Neurological changes and loss of consciousness.

5. Objectives of therapy.

  a. Prevention of central nervous system hypoxia.

  b. Restoration of effective ventilation.

  c. Maintenance of adequate circulation.

6. Therapeutic management.

  a. Establish and maintain adequate ventilation.

     1) Clear airway.

     2) Administer oxygen.

     3) Ventilate if necessary by intubation.

     4) Chest physiotherapy every hour.

     5) CPAP.

     6) Sedation to coordinate patient with ventilator.

  b. Correct circulatory status.

     1) Blood transfusions, especially of packed cells, are commonly administered to counter hemolysis and hemodilution (particularly with fresh water drowning).

     2) Plasma is administered to reduce shock and restore intracellular fluids in cases of salt water drowning.

     3) Provide 2/3 to 3/4 maintenance fluids; dextrose 5% in 1/4 normal saline or dextrose 5% in 1/2 normal saline to avoid hyponatremia and to minimize cerebral edema.

    c. Administer medications.
       1) Steroids to reduce cerebral edema.
       2) Sodium bicarbonate to correct acidosis.
       3) Diuretic therapy to treat hemodilution or cardiac failure.
       4) Consider broad-spectrum antibiotics for aspiration pneumonitis.
       5) Consider bronchodilating agents.
    d. Monitor vital signs.
       1) Temperature may be labile.
       2) If patient appears to be obtunded, hypothermia to 32°C may be indicated.
    e. Central venous pressure line to assess right heart function.
    f. Indwelling arterial line.
    g. Strict intake and output.
    h. Careful neurological assessment.
    i. Frequent arterial blood gas measurement to direct therapy.
  7. Complications.
    a. Acute respiratory failure.
    b. Infection.
    c. Neurologic deficit.
  8. Nursing skills are the same as those for acute respiratory failure (p. 77).

Inhalation Burns[2,12,37]

  1. Etiology: see Care of the Burned Child (Chap. 11).
  2. Pathophysiologic description.
    a. Thermal burn, caused by excessive heat, may produce injury to respiratory mucosa, especially above the trachea.
    b. Inhalation of heated air alone does not damage the lung because it cools by the time it reaches the level of the carina.
    c. Steam at 100°C produces more serious damage at all levels of the respiratory tract.
    d. Respiratory burn is actually a chemical burn induced by inhalation of suspended particles (smoke) and the toxic products of incomplete combustion.
    e. Alveolar capillary disruption.
    f. Pulmonary hemorrhage.
    g. Mucosal edema and slough.
  3. Clinical presentation.
    a. Neurological status.
       1) Assess brain stem reflexes for hyper- and hypoactivity.
       2) Regular evaluation of supratentorial function or depressed level of consciousness.
       3) Intracranial pressure monitoring for increases in pressure.
    b. Cardiovascular and circulatory status.
       1) Tachycardia or bradycardia.
       2) Increased systemic blood pressure.
       3) Hemodilution or hemoconcentration.
       4) Hypoxemia.
       5) Decreased or increased cardiac output.

    c. Pulmonary status.
       1) Hypoxia.
       2) Infiltrates noted in lung fields on chest x-ray.
       3) Rales, rhonchi, wheezes, decreased breath sounds.
       4) Atelectasis.
       5) Hypercarbia or hypocarbia.
    d. Urinary status.
       1) Increased specific gravity, showing urine concentration.
       2) Oliguria.

4. Objectives of therapy.
    a. Maintain CNS integrity through respiratory, cardiovascular, and renal homeostasis.
    b. Regulate fluids to achieve solute-solvent balance and red blood cell homeostasis.

5. Therapeutic management.
    a. Establish and maintain adequate airway and ventilation. Tracheostomy is usually contraindicated, owing to the increased risk of infection.
    b. Monitor vital signs and neurologic signs.
       1) Pulmonary wedge pressure in severe cases.
       2) Central venous line.
       3) Arterial line.
       4) Levels of consciousness and abstract thought.
       5) Careful observations of temperature.
    c. Maintain fluid and electrolyte balance.
       1) Obtain osmolality studies.
       2) Hemoglobin and hematocrit as needed.
       3) Supplement losses or shifts with intravenous therapy.
    d. Strict output calculations for assessment of renal status.
    e. Obtain arterial blood gases and respiratory compliance measurements.
    f. Prevent infection by careful control of patient and environment.
       1) Regular culture and sensitivity tests on tracheal secretions.
       2) Antiobiotic therapy.
       3) Sterile suctioning technique.
       4) Good mouth care.
    g. Additional management is like that employed for acute respiratory failure.

6. Complications.
    a. Sepsis.
    b. Neurological deficit.

7. Nursing skills.
    a. Same as for acute respiratory failure
    b. Scrupulous aseptic technique.

Status Asthmaticus [5-12,23,26,34,41,47,53,54]

Definition: bilateral intense wheezing that is unresponsive to 2 subcutaneous injections of epinephrine (0.0/mg/kg) given within 30 minutes, thoracic hyperinflation, and allergic history.

1. Etiology and predisposing factors.
   a. Biochemical abnormalities.
   b. Immunological factors.
   c. Infections.
   d. Endocrine factors.
   e. Psychological factors.
2. Pathophysiologic description.
   a. Characterized by spasms of bronchial smooth muscle, edematous mucosa, and tenacious secretions that obstruct air flow through bronchi and bronchioles.[13]
   b. Results in increased work load of respiratory muscles, lungs, and surrounding thoracic structures.
   c. Decreased efficiency of breathing.
   d. May progress to hypoventilation and respiratory failure.
3. Clinical presentation.
   a. History.
      1) Known allergy history.
      2) Family history.
   b. Signs of upper respiratory infection for a few hours prior to attack.
   c. Peak times of the year are fall and winter.
   d. Paroxysmal hacking cough in the older child.
   e. Infant appears restless and unable to suck or sustain feeding; skin may seem sallow.
   f. Signs and symptoms: violent respiratory effort, hyperventilation leading to minimal or limited respiratory movements and accompanied by see-saw undulation of abdomen, grunting with gaping mouth, supraclavicular and intercostal retractions, respiratory rate more than 70/min, pulse rate more than 140/min.
   g. Pulsus paradoxus: a sign of impending respiratory failure.[13]
   h. Papilledema: associated with presence of $PaCO_2$ greater than 75 mm Hg.
   i. Associated symptoms: otitis media, pharyngitis, fever, pneumonia.
   j. Sudden disappearance of precardiac dullness may indicate the development of pneumomediastinum.[13]
   k. Dehydration signs.
4. Objectives of therapy.
   a. Establish adequate ventilation to alleviate hypoxemia.
   b. Remove secretions from bronchial tree.

    c.   Avoid acute respiratory failure.

    d.   Remove causative agent.

5. Therapeutic management is generally the same as for acute respiratory failure.

    a.   Establish and maintain adequate airway and ventilation.

        1) Note danger if wheezing suddenly stops; this may indicate sharp rise in $PaCO_2$ and accompanying hypoxemia.

    b.   Administer medications.

        1) Aminophylline infusion of 10 to 20 mcg/ml. Achieve this therapeutic level by rapid infusion (15 minutes) followed by constant infusion.[13]

        2) Monitor serum theophylline levels to define optimal amounts.

        3) Be alert to theophylline toxicity as indicated by CNS irritability, headache, nausea, vomiting, and abdominal cramps. Slow infusion until emergency level can be obtained.[13]

        4) Steroid therapy: hydrocortisone or its equivalents should be administered; 4 mg/kg every 2 hours for 6 doses; then 10 mg/kg/day given in three divided doses per day.

        5) Bronchodilator inhalant.

        6) Isoproterenol intravenous infusion: begin with 0.1 mcg/kg/min and progress to effective dose.

        7) Mechanical ventilation: consider neuromuscular blockade to prevent pulmonary barometric trauma. Also, consider sedation with 0.1 mg/kg of Morphine or diazepam (Valium) every 4 to 6 hours.

        8) Obtain laboratory studies.

           a) Arterial blood gases or arterialized capillary blood gases.

           b) Complete blood count.

           c) Electrolytes.

           d) Urinalysis.

        9) Provide intravenous fluids at maintenance rate until the child stabilizes.

     10) Monitor vital signs frequently.

     11) Monitor vital signs frequently.

          a) Keep indwelling arterial line for frequent evaluation of blood gases and acid-base balance.

6. Complications are the same as those of acute respiratory failure, with the added problem of chronicity of disease after critical attack.

7. Nursing skills are the same as for acute respiratory failure (p. 77).

    a.   Special attention to the following is needed:

        1) Psychological measures: avoid teaching during acute attack.

        2) Assess causative factors of attack.

        3) Evaluate parent-child relationship.

        4) Psychiatric consultation as needed.

BIBLIOGRAPHY

Books

1. Avery, M., and Fletcher, B.: The Lung and Its Disorders in the Newborn Infant, 3rd ed. Philadelphia, W. B. Saunders Co., 1974.
2. Doerchuk, C.: Development of the lung. Respiratory physiology and pathophysiology. *In* Vaughan, V., and McKay, J. (eds.): Nelson Textbook of Pediatrics, 11th ed. Philadelphia, W. B. Saunders Co., 1979.
3. Egan, D.: Fundamentals of Respiratory Therapy. St. Louis, C. V. Mosby Co., 1973.
4. Jones, R., and Owen-Thomas, J.: Care of the Critically Ill Child. Baltimore, Williams & Wilkins, 1971.
5. Kendig, E. (ed.): Disorders of the Respiratory Tract in Children. Vol. I: Pulmonary Disorders, 2nd ed. Philadelphia, W. B. Saunders Co., 1972.
6. Leifer, G.: Principles and Techniques in Pediatric Nursing, 3rd ed. Philadelphia, W. B. Saunders Co., 1977.
7. Lightwood, R., et al: Paterson's Sick Children. Philadelphia, J. B. Lippincott Co., 1971.
8. Lough, M., et al.: Pediatric Respiratory Therapy. Chicago, Year Book Medical Publishers, 1974.
9. Modell, J.: The Pathophysiology and Treatment of Drowning and Near-Drowning. Springfield, Ill., Charles C Thomas, 1972.
10. Prior, J., and Silberstein, J.: Physical Diagnosis. St. Louis, C. V. Mosby Co., 1968.
11. Schwartz, S. (ed.): Principles of Surgery. New York, McGraw-Hill Book Co., 1969.
12. Scipien, G., et al.: Comprehensive Pediatric Nursing. New York, McGraw-Hill Book Co., 1975.
13. Smith, C. (ed.): The Critically Ill Child, 2nd ed. Philadelphia, W. B. Saunders Co., 1977.
14. Tooley, W.: Respiratory Function and Pulmonary Disease in Older Infants and Children. *In* Barnett, H. (ed.): Pediatrics, 15th ed. New York, Appleton-Century-Crofts, 1972.
15. Varga, C.: Handbook of Pediatric Medical Emergencies. St. Louis, C. V. Mosby Co., 1973.
16. Wasserman, E., and Slobody, L.: Survey of Clinical Pediatrics. New York, McGraw-Hill Book Co., 1974.
17. Zschoche, D. (ed.): Mosby's Comprehensive Review of Critical Care. St. Louis, C. V. Mosby Co., 1976.

Articles

18. Aberdeen, E., and Downes, J.: Artificial Airways in Children. Surg. Clin. North Am., *54*:1155, 1974.
19. Alexander, M., and Brown, M.: Physical Examination Part 12: Chest and Lungs. Nursing '75, *5*:44, 1975.
20. Bass, J. et al.: Acute epiglottitis, a surgical emergency. J.A.M.A. *229*: 671, 1974.
21. Belenky, W., et al.: Treatment of acquired subglottic stenosis. Ann. Otol. Rhinol. Laryngol., *82*:822, 1973.
22. Civetta, J., et al.: "Optimal PEEP" and intermittent mandatory ventilation in the treatment of acute respiratory failure. Respir. Care, *20*:551, 1975.
23. Cotton, E., and Parry, W.: Treatment of status asthmaticus and respiratory failure. Pediatr. Clin. North Am., *22*:162, 1975.
24. Downes, J., et al.: Acute respiratory failure in infants and children. Pediatr. Clin. North Am., *19*:423, 1972.
25. Downes, J., and Raphaely, R.: Pediatric intensive care. Anesthesiology, *43*:238, 1975.
26. Franklin, W.: Current concepts — treatment of severe asthma. N. Engl. J. Med., *290*:1469, 1974.
27. Gardner, H., et al.: The evaluation of racemic epinephrine in the treatment of infectious croup. Pediatrics, *52*:52, 1973.

28. Geffin, B., et al.: Stenosis following tracheostomy for respiratory care. J.A.M.A., *216*:1984, 1971.

29. Glegen, W., and Denny, F.: Epidemiology of acute lower respiratory disease in children. N. Engl. J. Med., *288*:498, 1973.

30. Kirby, R.: Is intermittent mandatory ventilation a satisfactory alternative to assisted and controlled ventilation? Annual Refresher Course Lectures, American Society of Anethesiologists, Annual meeting, Chicago, Illinois, 1975.

31. Johnson, D., and Jones, R.: Surgical aspects of airway mangement in infants and children. Surg. Clin. North Am., *56*:263, 1976.

32. Johnson, D., and Stewart, D.: Management of acquired tracheal obstructions in infancy. J. Pediatr. Surg., *10*:709, 1975.

33. Jordan, W., et al.: New therapy for postintubation laryngeal edema and tracheitis in children. J.A.M.A., *212*:585, 1970.

34. Lecks, H.: Explosive asthma in the infant and young child under two years. Clin. Pediatr., *15*:135, 1976.

35. Lincoln, J., et al.: Vascular anomalies: simplified classification. Chest, *62*:39, 1972.

36. Mellins, R., et al.: Committee report: Respiratory care in infants and children. The scientific assembly on pediatrics of the American Thoracic Society, National Tuberculosis and Respiratory Disease Association, New York, 1971.

37. Mellins, R., and Park, S.: Respiratory complications of smoke inhalation in victims of fire. J. Pediatr., *87*:1, 1975.

38. Meyasaka, K., et al.: Complications of radial artery lines in the pediatric patient. Canad. Anaesth. Soc. J., *23*:9, 1976.

39. Newth, C., et al.: The respiratory status of children with croup. J. Pediatr., *81*:1068, 1972.

40. Park, C., et al.: Tracheal compression by the great arteries in the mediastinum. Arch. Surg., *103*: 626, 1971.

41. Parry, W., et al.: Management of life-threatening asthma with intravenous isoproterenol infusions. Am. J. Dis. Child, *130*:39, 1976.

42. Polgar, G.: Pediatric lung diseases: can they be explained by age related properties of the respiratory system? Pediatr. Portfolio, *2*:5, 1973.

43. Raphin, R.: Tracheostomy in epiglottitis. Pediatrics, *52*:426, 1973.

44. Redding, J.: Saving victims of near drowning. Med. Opin., *5*:32, 1976.

45. Repsher, L., et al.: Diagnosis of *Pneumocystis carinii* pneumonitis by means of endobronchial brush biopsy. N. Engl. J. Med., *287*:340, 1972.

46. Shin, H., et al.: Pulmonary diseases in childhood. Clin. Notes Respir. Dis., *14*:3, 1975.

47. Soleymani, Y., et al.: Management of life-threatening asthma in children. Am. J. Dis. Child, *123*:533, 1972.

48. Stockes, J.: The management of respiratory failure in infancy. Anes. and Int. Care, *1*:486, 1973.

49. Taussig, L. et al.: Treatment of laryngotracheobronchitis (croup). Am. J. Dis. Child, *129*:790, 1975.

50. Todres, I., et al.: Endotracheal tube displacement in the newborn infant. J. Pediatr., *89*:126, 1976.

51. Wolfsdorf, J.: The acute care of respiratory problems in the neonate, infant and child. (Source unknown.)

52. Wood, D., et al.: A clinical scoring system for the diagnosis of respiratory failure. Am. J. Dis. Child, *123*:227, 1972.

53. Wood, D., et al.: The management of respiratory failure in childhood status asthmaticus. J. Allergy Clin. Immunol., *50*:75, 1972.

54. Wood, D., and Downes, J.: Intravenous isoproterenol in the treatment of respiratory failure in childhood status asthmaticus. Ann. Allergy, *31*:607, 1973.

55. Wychulis, A., et al.: Congenital vascular ring: surgical considerations and results of operation. Mayo Clin. Proc., 46:182, 1971.

56. Vedne, B., et al.: Aortic arch anomalies: simplified classification. Chest, 62:39, 1972.

CHAPTER 3
CARE OF THE CHILD WITH A DISORDER OF THE CARDIOVASCULAR SYSTEM

Judy Huntington, R.N., B.S.

OBJECTIVES

1. Identify the differences between fetal circulation and normal circulation after birth.

2. Recognize the differences in heart rate and conduction patterns between adults, infants, and children.

3. Identify priority components which constitute the complete cardiovascular physical exam of a child.

4. Recognize murmurs according to grade.

5. Describe six major acyanotic and major cyanotic congenital heart defects by pathophysiology, treatment, complications, and nursing intervention.

6. Formulate a plan of care for a post-operative pediatric cardiovascular surgical patient.

7. Identify three arrhythmias common in children.

8. Describe five major causes of congestive heart disease in children.

9. Identify the essential actions of effective cardiopulmonary resuscitation for infants and children.

10. Identify basic settings for defibrillation according to age of child.

11. Identify four commonly used drugs in resuscitation and their recommended doses for pediatric use.

Normal Circulation

1. Fetal Circulation
   Very small blood flow to liver and lungs.
   a. Special umbilical vessels allow blood to flow into and out of the placenta.
      1) Ductus venosus.
         a) Allows oxygenated blood returning from the placenta through the umbilical veins to enter fetal circulation.
         b) Allows blood from portal veins to bypass the liver and empty into general venous system.
   b. Fetal blood bypasses nonaerated lungs by two routes.
      1) Foramen Ovale.
         a) Opening in atrial septum allowing blood to flow from right atrium into left atrium.
         b) Oxygenated blood from umbilical vein flows through inferior vena cava to right atrium, through foramen ovale to left atrium and left ventricle, through aorta to brain and systemic circulation.
      2) Ductus Arteriosus.
         a) Blood that does not bypass right ventricle is pumped into the pulmonary artery and then through this vessel directly into the aorta.
         b) Unoxygenated blood from the superior vena cava flows into right atrium and right ventricle through main pulmonary artery, ductus arteriosus, and descending aorta back to placenta.
2. Normal Child Circulation. All three fetal circulation openings close shortly after birth, and blood flows through liver and lungs as in adult.
   a. Ductus Venosus.
      1) Closes in first few weeks of life.
      2) Decreased blood flow from umbilical veins is not sufficient to maintain opening.
   b. Ductus Arteriosus.
      1) Closes in first few weeks of life.
      2) Closes because of backward blood flow from aorta into pulmonary artery—possibly oxygen related.
   c. Foramen Ovale.
      1) Maintains opening as long as pressure in right atrium is greater than in left atrium.
      2) After lungs expand, right heart pumps blood easily and right atrial pressure falls about 3 mm Hg less than in left atrium.
      3) Backward pressure causes valve of foramen ovale to close and blood flow through it to stop.

Heart Rates in Infants and Children[21,22,31]

Age	Heart Rate (Beats/Minute)		
	Average	Minimum	Maximum
0 to 24 hours	125	88	166
1 day to 1 week	138	100	188
1 week to 1 month	162	125	188
1 to 3 months	161	115	215
3 to 6 months	147	125	215
6 to 12 months	147	115	188
1 to 3 years	130	100	188
3 to 5 years	105	68	150
5 to 8 years	102	75	150
8 to 12 years	88	51	125
12 to 16 years	83	38	125

Conduction System[21,22,31]

1. Duration EKG intervals in children (values in seconds).

Age	P–R Interval		QRS Duration	
	Lower Limit	Upper Limit	Lower Limit	Upper Limit
Birth to 1 day	.08	.12	.04	.10
1 day to 1 week	.08	.12	.04	.08
1 week to 1 month	.08	.12	.04	.07
1 to 3 months	.08	.16	.05	.08
3 to 6 months	.08	.12	.05	.08
6 to 12 months	.08	.14	.04	.08
1 to 3 years	.08	.16	.04	.08
3 to 5 years	.10	.16	.04	.09
5 to 8 years	.10	.18	.04	.09
8 to 12 years	.10	.20	.05	.10
12 to 16 years	.10	.20	.04	.10

———————— CLINICAL ASSESSMENT ————————

Medical History
1. Symptoms and course.
2. Estimations of limitations.
3. Etiologic factors and family history.

Physical Examination
1. Growth patterns.
   a. May be normal in minor defects and some obstructive anomalies.
   b. Markedly altered with large left-to-right shunts.
2. Extracardiac anomalies.
   a. Children with multiple congenital anomalies often have some form of heart defect.

3. Face.
   a. Edema of eyelids (especially on awakening) often associated with congestive heart failure.
   b. Hypertelorism of eyes (wide-set eyes) often associated with pulmonic stenosis.
4. Neck.
   a. Size of thyroid: to rule out hyperthyroidism as cause for tachycardia, cardiomegaly, and flow murmurs.
   b. Thrills in neck associated with (alone or in combination):
      1) Patent ductus arteriosus (PDA).
      2) Coarctation of the aorta.
      3) Pulmonic stenosis.
      4) Aortic stenosis.
      5) Truncus arteriosus.
   c. Neck veins.
      1) Difficult to evaluate in infant.
      2) In child, engorged neck veins suggest right heart failure.
5. Peripheral Pulses.
   a. Bounding arterial pulses (wide pulse pressure):
      1) Aortic run-off lesion.
      2) PDA.
   b. Narrow pulse pressures:
      1) Low cardiac output.
      2) Congestive heart failure (CHF).
      3) Shock.
   c. Weak pulses:
      1) In early infancy, characteristic of hypoplastic left heart lesions.
   d. Difference in upper and lower extremity pulses:
      1) Coarctation of aorta—decreased, delayed, or absent in lower extremities.
   e. Absence of peripheral pulses:
      1) Vascular anomaly.
      2) Percutaneous arteriotomy at cardiac catheterization with thrombus and/or spasm.
      3) Sacrifice of vessel after palliative repair (Blalock-Taussig operation).
      4) Thrombosis or embolism in cyanotic heart disease.
6. Digits.
   a. Abnormal number of digits is often associated with defect in atrial septum.
      1) Ellis-van Creveld syndrome (polydactylism): single atrium.
      2) Holt-Oram syndrome (missing digits): atrial septal defect (ASD), sometimes ventricular septal defect (VSD).
7. Desaturation and Cyanosis.
   a. Color of mucous membranes and nail beds.
   b. Reddening of the lips.
   c. Polycythemia.

d. Clubbing of digits.

e. Paroxysmal hyperpneic spells (tet spells)

8. Chest and respirations.

    a. Character of respirations.

    b. Murmurs.

    c. Precordial pulsations.

    d. Chest deformities.

       1) Left chest prominence with cardiac enlargement.

       2) Harrison's grooves (marked scalloping or scooping of lower chest bilaterally) associated with long-term, large left-to-right shunt.

       3) Kyphoscoliosis.

    e. Cor pulmonale.

9. Dextrocardia: cardiac impulse on right side.

    a. Mirror-image dextrocardia (situs inversus): low incidence of congenital heart disease.

    b. Dextroversion developmental (rotational anomaly): high incidence of associated congenital heart disease.

    c. Dextroposition (cardiac shift secondary to chest cage or lung pathology): usually no associated congenital heart disease.

10. Abdomen.

    a. Palpation of liver and spleen: asplenia associated with high incidence of transpositions.

    b. Ascites rare in infants and children, but does occur with constrictive pericarditis.

11. Legs.

    a. Dependent edema from CHF is usually in sacral area or face rather than legs.

       1) Present in child after he starts walking.

       2) Most severe with endocardial fibroelastosis.

12. Palpation of precordium.

    a. Infants: difficult to differentiate left ventricular from right ventricular activity.

    b. Children: analysis of ventricular activity is feasible.

13. Auscultation.

    a. As many as 3/4 of normal children have heart murmurs.

    b. Difficult to differentiate innocent from organic murmurs by auscultation alone.

    c. Grading of murmurs[21]

       1) Faintest murmur that is audible on careful auscultation; generally not heard at all during the first few seconds of auscultation.

       2) Somewhat louder murmur that can be heard immediately.

       3) Moderately loud murmur unaccompanied by a thrill.

       4) Loud murmur with thrill.

       5) Loud murmur that cannot be heard if entire stethoscope is removed from the chest but is audible if one edge of stethoscope is in contact with the chest.

6) Loudest possible murmur, (rare): can be heard with stethoscope 1 cm or more from chest wall.

d. Children often have murmurs with fever.

1) Usually are functional systolic murmurs due to increase in cardiac output.

2) Should be reevaluated after recovery from fever.

e. Evaluation of heart sounds.

1) Evaluation of both components:
   a) Movement with respiration.
   b) Intensity.
   c) Whether both components can be heard.

2) Single S_2 may mean:
   a) Aortic and pulmonary valves closing simultaneously.
   b) One valve absent or atretic.
   c) One valve closing inaudibly.

3) Increased second (pulmonic) component of the second sound may indicate:
   a) Pulmonary hypertension.
   b) Increased pulmonary flow.

4) Third heart sound (S_3)
   a) Very prominent in older children

5) Fourth heart sound (S_4)
   a) Difficult to hear.
   b) Immediately preceeds S_1.

6) When S_3 and S_4 are more prominent than S_1 and S_2:
   a) Always suspect myocardial disease.

f. Functional (innocent) murmurs.

1) Vibratory murmur ("twanging string" or "groaning" murmur).
   a) Early- to mid-systolic musical murmur.
   b) Grade 3 or less.
   c) Heard best over mid-precordial area.
   d) Increases in intensity with exercise and varies with respirations.

2) Pulmonic ejection murmur.
   a) Early- to mid-systolic murmur.
   b) Grade 3 or less.
   c) Loudest in second and third left intercostal spaces parasternally.
   d) Increased cardiac output: increased intensity of murmur.
   e) Common in preadolescents.
   f) Pulmonary artery crunch (sounds like crunching paper).

3) Venous hum.
   a) Low to medium pitched hum.
   b) Heard best in neck and second right intercostal space parasternally.
   c) Rarely associated with thrill.

          d) Maximal intensity occurs at diastole.
     4) Early- and mid-systolic murmur.
          a) Most common in first and second year of life.
          b) Maximal along the left lower sternal border.
  g. Ejection clicks.
     1) Sound like two coins striking together.
     2) Pulmonary ejection clicks.
          a) Can be normal.
          b) Also found with valvular pulmonic stenosis.
          c) Heard maximally in second left intercostal space and not transmitted to the apex.
     3) Aortic ejection clicks.
          a) Usually pathologic in origin; aortic stenosis

Radiologic Examination
1. Abdomen.
2. Chest cage.
  a. Distortion of normal rib cage pattern associated with congenital anomalies.
     1) Generalized rib notching with coarctation associated with increased collateral circulation.
3. Lungs.
  a. Patients with heart disease often have associated pulmonary disease, such as:
     1) Pneumonitis.
     2) Pleural fluid.
     3) Atelectasis.
     4) CHF.
4. Pulmonary vasculature.
  a. Vasculature prominence may be increased or decreased.
     1) If increased, may be due to left-to-right shunt lesion or pulmonary venous obstruction.
5. Cardiac positions, size, and shape.
  a. Boot shape.
  b. Globular, cushion defects.
  c. Snowman: total anomalous pulmonary venous return (TAPVR).
  d. Others.
6. Analysis of great vessels.
  a. Pulmonary artery.
     1) Enlargement of pulmonary trunk and left main pulmonary artery; may be present in:
          a) Normal children.
          b) Idiopathic dilatation of the pulmonary artery.
          c) Pulmonic valve stenosis.
          d) Increased pulmonary blood flow (left-to-right shunts).
          e) Pulmonary artery hypertension.
     2) Absence of the pulmonary knob may indicate:
          a) Pulmonary artery smaller than normal.
          b) Pulmonary artery in abnormal position.

b. Thoracic aorta.
   1) Most common congenital cardiac lesions of thoracic aorta:
      a) Localized dilatation of ascending aorta.
         (1) Aorta valvular stenosis.
      b) Prominence of ascending aorta and aortic knob.
         (1) PDA.
         (2) Coarctation of aorta.
         (3) Truncus arteriosus.
      c) Abnormal great vessels arising from aortic arch.
         (1) Tetralogy of Fallot.
         (2) Coarctation of aorta.
      d) Congenital heart disease with right aortic arch.
         (1) Increased vascular markings: truncus.
         (2) Decreased vascular markings: tetralogy.

7. Right atrium.
8. Left atrium.
   a. Left atrial enlargement caused by:
      1) Excessive blood flow into atrium.
      2) Obstruction to outflow from atrium.
9. Ventricles.
   a. Evaluate for:
      1) Enlargement due to dilatation, hypertrophy, or
         pericardial lesions.
      2) Dilatation: increase in chamber lumen or vessel lumen size.
      3) Hypertrophy: increase in chamber of vessel wall
         thickness.

Electrocardiography (ECG)
Procedure is essentially the same as in the adult.

Vectorcardiography
1. Newborn
   a. Initial QRS vector.
      1) Anterior, inferior, usually rightward.
   b. Mean QRS forces.
      1) Rightward and anterior.
   c. Terminal QRS forces.
      1) Rightward and either anterior or posterior.
   d. All three planes.
      1) Direction usually clockwise.
      2) Rarely, figure eight or counterclockwise.
2. Childhood
   a. Initial QRS forces.
      1) Rightward, anterior, and superior.
      2) Leftward forces are abnormal; may indicate right
         ventricular hypertrophy or defects associated with the
         conduction system.
   b. QRS loop starts changing from clockwise to counterclockwise
      almost immediately after birth.

1) 1 month: only 18% of horizontal QRS loops are inscribed completely clockwise.
2) 2 to 3 months: 5% clockwise.
3) After 3 months: clockwise rotation of QRS loop is abnormal, associated with right ventricular hypertrophy.

Echocardiography

This is a noninvasive ultrasonic method of evaluating:

1. Position, function, and size of semilunar and atrioventricular valves.
2. Relationships of great vessels to each other and to ventricular origins.
3. Cardiac chamber size and ventricular function.
4. Establishes the diagnosis of effusion and quantitates its amount.

Cardiac catheterization

Procedure is essentially the same as in the adult. Use a catheter size commensurate with child's anatomic maturation. The child may be given a general anesthetic, thus causing potential complications during the immediate post-procedure period.

PATHOLOGIC CONDITIONS

CONGENITAL HEART DEFECTS

Although congenital heart defects can occur in numerous combinations, the following defects will be presented as individual entities.[5,6,8,10,14,16,21,22,24,27]

ACYANOTIC HEART DEFECTS

These are heart defects that do not result in cyanosis.

Patent Ductus Arteriosus (PDA)

1. Incidence: second most common congenital heart defect, approximately 12% of all cases.
2. Pathophysiology.
   a. Fetal connection between thoracic aorta and pulmonary artery.
   b. Normally closes in first eight weeks of life.
   c. Causes increased blood flow to lungs (left-to-right shunt), pulmonary edema, increased volume of work in left ventricle, and left ventricular hypertrophy (if not corrected).
3. Surgical treatment.
   a. Definitive (closed) either by ligation or by division and closure of the two ends. (Always by division unless risk of surgery is too great to allow time for more than ligation).
      1) Premature infants with PDA and associated pulmonary disease require immediate closure of PDA, usually by ligation.
   b. Operative mortality: less than 1%. Closure decreases pulmonary flow and increases systemic flow and pressure.

4. Specific nursing interventions.
    a. Intensive pulmonary care.
    b. Pain control to allow for good inspiratory effort.
        1) Incisional pain is greater than with median sternotomies.
5. Complications.
    a. Usually rare except in cases associated with other defects.
    b. Bleeding.
    c. Atelectasis.

Coarctation of the Aorta:
1. Incidence: sixth most common congenital heart defect, approximately 6% of all cases.
2. Pathophysiology.
    a. Constriction or narrowing of thoracic aorta, usually just distal to left subclavian artery, but found anywhere along aorta.
        1) Preductal: proximal to the ductus arteriosus.
            a) Usually presents in infancy.
            b) Often associated with more serious cardiac anomalies (71%).
        2) Postductal: distal to ductus or ligamentum.
            a) Usually found in asymptomatic older children.
            b) Associated with better collateral circulation and low incidence (4%) of other related defects.
        3) Ductal ligamentum joins aorta at site of coarctation.
    b. All types cause increased pressure work for left ventricle and left ventricular hypertrophy.
    c. Signs and symptoms include:
        1) Dyspnea and frank CHF in newborns.
        2) Hypertension of upper extremities, with hypotension or diminished or absent pulses in lower extremities.
        3) Infants: CHF, tachypnia, failure to thrive.
        4) Older children: often asymptomatic or with intermittent claudication following exercise.
        5) Systolic murmur over left upper chest anteriorly or near the angle of the left scapula posteriorly.
3. Surgical treatment.
    a. Definitive (closed): by resection of the coarctation and anastomosis of the ends or by insertion of a graft (usually only necessary after age 15).
    b. Operative mortality: less than 1% in children, higher in adults (5 to 15%).
4. Specific nursing interventions.
    a. Monitor blood pressure closely.
    b. Watch for abdominal pain, tenderness, fever, leukocytosis.
    c. Watch chest drainage closely for amount and type of drainage.
5. Complications.
    a. Hemothorax (most common): due to bleeding from chest wall collateral network.

    b. Abdominal pain: bruising and clots in mesentery, probably due
to increased flow into thin-walled arterioles. Can cause
infarction of bowel.

    c. Chylothorax: from injury to thoracic duct during surgery.

    d. Paradoxial hypertension: due to response of blood pressure
receptors in carotid arteries to sudden decrease in previous
hypertension.

      1) Usually corrects itself within six months to a year.

      2) May need to be treated with antihypertensive agent, such
as reserpine.

    e. Recurrence of coarctation: a late complication caused by
stricture formation at the anastamosis.

    f. Vomiting intestinal contents owing to increased circulation
to the GI tract.

Aortic Stenosis

1. Incidence: 4% of all cases.
2. Pathophysiology.

    a. Obstruction of left ventricular flow causing increased pressure
work for left ventricle—left ventricular hypertrophy.
Obstruction may be at the valvular, subvalvular, or
supravalvular level.

      1) Valvular: most common; caused by fusion of valvular
cusps; may also be due to bicuspid valve.

      2) Subvalvular: second most common; usually due to a fibrous
diaphram located just below normal valve leaflets; can be
caused by muscular hypertrophy of intraventricular septum
(idiopathic hypertrophic subaortic stenosis).

      3) Supravalvular: least common; similar to coarctation in that
aorta is constricted just above coronary ostia; valve
leaflets may be normal or thickened.

    b. Signs and symptoms.

      1) Systolic murmur over second interspace to right of
sternum (may be absent).

      2) Syncope may be noted in childhood or in later life.

      3) Severe aortic stenosis; CHF in neonate.

      4) Mild aortic stenosis may be asymptomatic except for
murmur.

3. Surgical treatment.

    a. Indications for surgery.

      1) Gradient across left ventricular outflow tract of 50 mm Hg
or greater.

      2) Progressive left ventricular strain, as indicated by
electrocardiogram.

    b. Definitive (open heart) procedures.

      1) Valvular: fused commissures are incised to free the leaves,
usually producing a bicuspid valve; if secondary fibrosis
and calcification make valvotomy and reconstruction
impossible, replacement with an artificial valve is necessary.

    2) Subvalvular: excision of any fibrous diaphragms or hypertrophy; care must be taken not to cause irreversible damage to the conduction system.

    3) Supravalvular: if constriction is well localized and aorta not thickened above and below, the defect may be totally resected. Most commonly, a patch graft (Dacron) and endarterectomy are necessary for repair.

  c. Operative mortality: 7 to 9%.

4. Specific nursing interventions
   a. Monitor blood pressure closely; watch for diastolic pressure under 60 mm Hg (indication of aortic insufficiency).
   b. Check for large or increasing pulse pressures.
   c. Watch for arrhythmias; patients with high right atrial or left atrial pressures prior to surgery may have tendency to fibrillate.
   d. Pacemaker required for heart block.

5. Complications.
   a. Hemorrhage.
   b. Congestive heart failure: carryover from process leading to surgery, should respond to medical therapy if valvotomy adequate.
   c. Aortic insufficiency: rarely a problem in early postoperative period; results from valvotomy.
   d. Heart block (after subaortic stenosis): most common if left ventricular approach was used.

Congenital Mitral Stenosis

1. Incidence: rare, less than 1% of cases.
2. Pathophysiology.
   a. Fusion of commissures of mitral valve.
   b. Presents in early infancy with passive congestion of the lungs and pulmonary hypertension.
   c. Very rare; most mitral stenosis results from rheumatic fever.
   d. Associated endocardial fibroelastosis usually found in patients with severe congenital mitral stenosis.
   e. Symptoms in infancy include:
      1) Pulmonary vascular obstruction.
      2) Large left atrium.
      3) Mitral diastolic murmur.
      4) Pulmonary arterial hypertension and increased pulmonary venous wdge pressures at cardiac catheterization (right heart).
3. Surgical treatment.
   a. High risk because of associated anomalies.
   b. Definitive (open heart): open mitral commissurotomy—fused commissures incised under direct vision.
   c. Mitral valve replacement when child is of sufficient size.
4. Specific nursing interventions.
   a. Routine postoperative cardiovascular nursing care.

5. Complications.
  a. Hemorrhage.
  b. Mitral regurgitation.

Cor Triatriatum

1. Incidence: very rare, 0.1% of cases.
2. Pathophysiology.
   a. Pulmonary veins empty into a separate receptacle but communicate through one or several small openings across a membrane with the "true" left atrium.
   b. Causes passive congestion of the lungs and pulmonary hypertension.
   c. Signs and symptoms:
      1) Very similar to those of congenital mitral stenosis and TAPVR.
      2) Murmur may or may not be present.
      3) Pulmonary arterial wedge pressure appreciably higher than left arterial pressure.
   d. Without adequate communication between third chamber and left atrium, most infants die of pulmonary edema, pneumonia, or chronic left-sided and right-sided failure, but patients have survived to teens.
3. Surgical Treatment.
   a. Definitive (open heart): creation of an adequate opening between the posterior chamber and left atrium (difficult in infants because of small structure, size, and posterior position of the third chamber).
4. Nursing interventions.
   a. Routine postoperative cardiovascular nursing care.
5. Complications.
   a. Heart block.
      1) atrial pacing usually sufficient.

Pulmonary Stenosis

1. Incidence: 7 to 9% of all cases.
2. Pathophysiology.
   a. Narrowing of right ventricular outflow resulting in increased pressure work for the right ventricle without producing cyanosis. May be of three types.
      1) Valvular: most common; due to fusion of all three valve cusps of small valve ring.
      2) Infundibular: due to muscular ring or fibrous obstruction 1 to 3 cm below the valve; may occur alone or with valvular stenosis.
      3) Supravalvular or peripheral: not common; due to narrowing of main or peripheral pulmonary arteries.
   b. Signs and symptoms:
      1) Systolic ejection murmur: loudest in left second intercostal space near sternum.
      2) Exertional dyspnea in older children.

      3) Frank CHF in infants.

      4) Mild or absent if right ventricular pressure is under 100 mm Hg.

3. Surgical treatment.
   a. Indications for surgery.
      1) Right ventricular pressures higher than systemic pressure in infants or a pressure gradient greater than 70 mm in a child older than 5 years.
      2) Progressive right ventricular hypertrophy.
   b. Definitive (open heart): type of procedure depends on pathology.
      1) Valvular: valvotomy by incising along the fusion to free the valve cusps.
      2) Infundibular: excision of infundibular obstruction or widening of the outflow tract and valve ring with a patch (results in some pulmonary regurgitation.)
      3) Peripheral: surgical repair not possible unless stenosis is close to the heart.
   c. Operative mortality: 1 to 2%.
4. Specific nursing intervention.
   a. Routine postoperative cardiovascular nursing care.
5. Complications.
   a. Hemorrhage.
   b. Pulmonary valve regurgitation: frequently occurs, but not a problem if pulmonary artery pressure is normal and no other defects are present.

Aorticopulmonary Window (AP Window)

1. Incidence: rare.
2. Pathophysiology.
   a. Characterized by a large defect between the ascending aorta and the pulmonary trunk just above the semilunar valves.
   b. Causes increased left ventricular volume of work (much like PDA).
   c. Diagnosis: Made by cardiac catheterization and selective aortography.
3. Surgical treatment.
   a. Definitive (open heart) primary closure of defect.
   b. Mortality rate: high, up to 30% because of frequent preexisting pulmonary hypertension; also varies according to size of defect.
4. Specific nursing interventions.
   a. Routine postoperative cardiovascular nursing care.
   b. Good pulmonary therapy.

Ventricular Septal Defect (VSD)

1. Incidence: most common congenital heart defect, 30% of all cases.
2. Pathophysiology.
   a. Hole in the interventricular septum causing left-to-right shunt and increased volume of work for left ventricle.

    b. A large VSD will create increased volume of work for both left and right ventricles, because pulmonary venous blood entering the left ventricle during diastole will flow through the septal defect into the right ventricle.

    c. Classified as to most common types by position of defect.

       1) Supracristal (Type I): situated between the crista supraventricularis and the pulmonary valve.

       2) Membranous (Type II): just caudal to crista supraventricularis.

       3) Atrioventricular (Type III): posteriorly beneath septal leaflet of the tricuspid valve.

          a) This is an area where AV conduction bundle is especially susceptable to injury.

          b) Left ventricular outflow tract involvement can occur.

       4) Muscular (Type IV): found in muscular septum near its caudal and anterior portion; tendency is to multiple swiss-cheese type; difficult to find all defects.

    d. Often associated with other defects such as ASD, pulmonary stenosis, PDA transposition, coarctations, and tricuspid atresia.

    e. Symptoms depend on size of defect and degree of pulmonary vascular resistance.

       1) Small VSDs: Children are usually asymptomatic; heart size may be normal or slightly enlarged. May have loud murmur, with or without thrill.

       2) Moderate sized VSDs: Children are usually asymptomatic, may tire more easily, may have frequent bouts of pneumonia, usually do not develop CHF.

       3) Large VSDs: Patients often present in CHF at an early age; frequent bouts of pneumonia and failure to thrive; murmur may be softer than in smaller defects because large size produces less of a jet through the septum.

  3. Surgical treatment.

    a. Indications for surgery.

       1) Infants with large left-to-right shunts resulting in CHF, when medical therapy does not relieve symptoms (usually under 1 year of age).

       2) Children with elevated pulmonary vascular resistance, to prevent pulmonary vascular disease.

    b. Palliative repair (closed): pulmonary artery banding.

       1) Some surgeons prefer to do a pulmonary artery banding and postpone complete repair until child is older.

       2) A fabric band is placed around the pulmonary artery and narrowed until the pulmonary artery pressure is decreased to about one third, thus decreasing the volume of the left-to-right shunt and relieving heart failure.

       3) Contraindicated where pulmonary pressure is equal to systemic pressure and a right-to-left shunt is present.

    c. Definitive repair (open heart): closure of VSD.
        1) Accomplished either by direct suture or with the aid of a Dacron or pericardial patch. This may be performed through a ventriculotomy or via the right atrium and tricuspid valve.
        2) If the patient was previously banded, the band is cut and removed at the time of VSD repair. If the pulmonary artery lumen is insufficient, it is made larger by a longitudinal incision with transverse closure, by a pericardial patch, or by resection and anastomosis.
        3) Mortality rate: About 5% higher in infants and patients with pulmonary hypertension than in any other patient group.

4. Specific nursing interventions.
    a. Routine postoperative cardiovascular nursing care.
    b. Intensive pulmonary therapy.
    c. Monitor volume status closely.
    d. Monitor cardiac output.
    e. Watch for arrhythmias.
    f. Watch for CHF and pulmonary edema.
    g. With pulmonary artery banding, have atropine available at bedside.

5. Complications.
    a. Hemorrhage: from chest wall, ventriculotomy, or periphery of pulmonary artery patch.
    b. Pulmonary edema: associated with pulmonary artery banding that is too tight or associated with other defects; in patients with high pulmonary vascular resistance.
    c. Heart block and arrhythmias: due to swelling; usually temporary, but may require pressor support and pacing. (May also be due to damage to conduction circuits.)
    d. Bradycardia in first 12 hours post banding is usually indicative of a tight pulmonary artery band.
        1) Responds to atropine.
        2) If persistent, may require surgical loosening of band.
    e. Cyanosis, dyspnea, and hypotension due to low cardiac output may be observed 24 to 48 hours after surgery.

Atrial Septal Defect (ASD)

1. Incidence: fourth most common congenital heart defect, 9 to 10% of cases.
2. Pathophysiology.
    a. Hole in the interatrial septum; may occur in various locations; classified accordingly.
        1) Ostium secundum: a defect occurring at the site of the foramen ovale and separated from the coronary sinus and tricuspid valve by a large strip of septal tissue.
        2) Sinus venosus: occurs high in the septum near the orifice of the superior vena cava.

   a) Frequently associated with anomalous drainage of the right pulmonary veins into the right atrium at this point.

  3) Ostium primum (simple): a defect occuring very low in the septum, with its inferior margin formed by the fused septal leaflets of the mitral and tricuspid valves.

   a) When associated with clefts in the mitral or tricuspid valves, this defect or VSD becomes an AV canal.

 b. Produces increased volume of work for the right ventricle.

 c. Symptoms.

  1) Ostium secundum and sinus venosus are asymptomatic.

   a) Asymptomatic.

   b) Electrocardiogram shows right ventricular hypertrophy.

   c) May have some exertional dyspnea.

  2) Ostium primum often associated with CHF.

3. Surgical treatment.

 a. Indications for surgery.

  1) Usually done around 2 to 6 years of age unless severe failure unrelieved by medication is present earlier.

  2) Older children should be operated on as soon as diagnosis is established.

   a) Advancing years bring increased pulmonary artery pressure and higher operative risk (PVD).

 b. Definitive procedure (open heart): closure of ASD by direct suture or by means of a patch.

  1) Ostium secundum: primary closure is usual; large defect is closed by patch.
  Mortality rate: 1 to 2%.

  2) Sinus venosus.

   a) Simple sinus venosus is usually closed by patch to minimize atrial arrhythmias caused by strain on the sinus node.

   b) If it is associated with anamalous drainage, the patch is usually required to act as a baffle.

  3) Ostium primum (simple): patch closure often associated with arrhythmias because AV bundle runs in close proximity to site of trpair. Mortality rate: 3 to 5%.

4. Specific nursing interventions.

 a. Routine postoperative cardiovascular nursing care.

 b. Monitor of volume status closely.

 c. Monitor closely for arrhythmias.

5. Complications.

 a. Pulmonary edema: Occurs most commonly after ostium secundum repair; usually transient; occurs most frequently in patients with severe pulmonary hypertension.

 b. Heart block: due to swelling; associated with ostium primum repairs; usually transitional; may require pressors or pacing.

Endocardial cushion defects (AV canal)
1. Incidence: about 3% of all cases.
2. Pathophysiology.
   a. Partial AV canal: ostium primum defect of the atrial septum and a cleft of the anterior leaflet of the mitral valve.
   b. Transitional AV canal: Ostium primum with cleft in mitral valve and septal leaflet of the tricuspid valve.
   c. Complete AV canal or atrioventricular canal: hole in the middle of heart due to ostium primum; both mitral and tricuspid clefts, and communicating VSD.
   d. Defect results in increased volume of work for both the left and right ventricules owing to large left-to-right shunt, mitral regurgitation, and pulmonary artery hypertension (secondary to increased left atrial and pulmonary venous pressures).
   e. Often associated with Down's syndrome, up to 30% of cases in some studies.
   f. Signs and symptoms vary greatly depending on type of defect.
      1) Complete AV canal results in early CHF and death in first three years if not treated.
      2) Partial AV canal with minimum initial regurgitation may remain asymptomatic for many years.
      3) CHF or susceptability to respiratory infections is common.
      4) X-ray film increased heart size of all four chambers.
      5) P-R interval is prolonged.
3. Surgical treatment.
   a. Indications for surgery.
      1) Massive congestive heart failure.
   b. Palliative repair (closed): Pulmonary artery banding.
      1) Occasionally used in severely compensated infants to allow them to grow before complete repair.
   c. Definitive repair (open heart): involves careful repair or replacement of the mitral valve, patch repair of the ostium primum, repair of the tricuspid cleft, and closure of the VSD if present.
      1) Mortality rate depends on degree of mitral regurgitation, preexisting CHF, and increased pulmonary resistance. Approximately 7 to 8%.
4. Specific nursing interventions.
   a. Routine postoperative cardiovascular care.
   b. Close observation for arrhythmias.
   c. Close monitoring of volume status.
   d. Intensive pulmonary therapy.
5. Complications.
   a. Pulmonary edema: especially in patients whose mitral regurgitation has not been alleviated by surgery but whose ASD has been closed.

1) Cause: Blood regurgitating through mitral valve results in increased left atrial pressure and increased pulmonary resistance.
   b. Heart block: see complications of ostium primum (simple).
   c. Residual mitral or tricuspid insufficiency.

CYANOTIC HEART DEFECTS

These are heart defects that result in some degree of cyanosis.

Tetralogy of Fallot

1. Incidence: Approximately 11% of all cardiac disease in children. Most common cause of cyanotic heart disease in older children (after the age of 4, 75% of children with cyanotic heart disease have tetralogy of Fallot.)
2. Pathophysiology.
   a. Defect consists of a large high VSD and pulmonary stenosis (valvular, infundibular, or a combination) associated with right ventricular hypertrophy and dextroposition of the aorta.
   b. In severe cases with pulmonary valvular atresia, the defect is sometimes referred to as pseudotruncus.
   c. Consists of large right-to-left shunt (because of pulmonary stenosis, blood flows from right ventricle through VSD to aorta). Degree of cyanosis and right ventricular hypertrophy (from increased pressure of work) depends on degree of pulmonary stenosis.
      1) Patients with very little pulmonary stenosis may have balanced interventricular shunts or even left-to-right shunts.
         a) These are termed atypical of "pink tets" because they are not cyanotic.
   d. Signs and symptoms:
      1) Cyanosis: rarely present at birth, but progressive once it is present. Clubbing of fingers and toes common in older children.
      2) Exertional dyspnea and squatting, very poor exercise tolerance. Squatting common in patients with infundibular stenosis (increases venous return from lower extremities and arterial oxygenation of the remaining circulating blood).
      3) Tet spells – Approximately half of these infants have hypoxic spells characterized by paroxysmal hyperpnea and cyanosis, often accompanied by limpness and rolling back of eyes.
         a) These are common but dangerous (as many as 10% may have a cerebral vascular accident or die following a tet spell).

(1) documented tet spell is indication for immediate surgery.
b) Murmuring diminishes with spell.
c) Treatment of tet spells.
(1) Placement of infant in knee-chest position to mimics squatting.
(2) Sedate with morphine sulfate.
(3) Some centers advocate use of O_2
4) Electrocardiogram shows right axis deviation and right ventricular hypertrophy.
5) A loud harsh systolic murmur.
6) Because a portion of the normal right heart volume has gone through the VSD directly to the aorta, the volume going to the lungs and ultimately to the left heart may be proportionately smaller, leaving the left heart's normal volume less than the right heart.
a) These patients have smaller than normal left ventricles and may need to be shunted before complete repair to allow the left ventricle time to grow its normal size.
3. Surgical treatment.
a. Indications for surgery.
1) Pink tets: repair should be done at about the age of 6 (best time both physically and psychologically).
2) Asymptomatic or minimally cyanotic children should be repaired between the ages of 6 and 8.
3) Symptomatic cyanotic children should be repaired when symptoms appear.
a) Infants can be repaired primarily or palliated with a shunt, depending on their individual anatomy and size.
b. Palliative (closed heart) procedures (most commonly referred to as shunts): increase blood flow to the lungs (decreased cyanosis) and increase the volume going to the left ventricle, allowing it to increase to its normal size before complete repair.
1) Potts anastomosis: side-to-side anastomosis between the descending thoracic aorta and the left pulmonary artery.
a) Done less frequently now because it is difficult to remove when doing a full repair.
2) Waterston anastomosis: side-to-side anastomosis between ascending aorta and right pulmonary artery. Usually done on infants too young for a Blalock shunt (less than 6 months); has generally replaced the Potts procedure.
a) Too large a shunt will rapidly lead to CHF, pulmonary hypertension, and hypercirculation to right lung.
b) Mortality rate: 10%
3) Blalock-Taussig anastomosis: end-to-side anastomosis between the subclavian artery and the pulmonary artery on the side opposite the aortic arch.

a) Infant: can be done as long as subclavian artery and pulmonary artery are of sufficient size.
b) Mortality rate: 1 to 2%.
c) Definitive (open heart) repair: removal of shunt (if previously done), repair of the pulmonary artery (may require patch grafting if closure is due to hypoplastic pulmonary artery, and reapir of the VSD with a patch.
   (1) Severely hypoplastic right ventricular outflow tract of atresia requires a conduit bypass (Rastelli procedure).

4. Specific nursing interventions. Note: Patients with tetralogy of Fallot, transposition of the great vessels, and total anomalous pulmonary venous return have similar postoperative complications and needs for nursing intervention.
   a. Maintenance of correct volume status (See Table 3–1).

Table 3–1. VOLUME OVERLOAD AND VOLUME DEPLETION

Signs and Symptoms	
Volume Overload	*Volume Depletion*
"Cardiac asthma"	Decreased urine output
Wheezy, congested respirations not relieved by suctioning.	Less than 1 cc/kg/hr with 3/4 maintenance; less than 0.5 cc/kg/hr if on less that 1/2 maintenance.
Pulmonary edema	
Severe pulmonary congestion with excessive, pink, frothy secretions.	Cold, cool extremities
	Particularly of feet and lower legs
Increasing $PaCO_2$	Decreased or absent pedal pulses
Indicative of increasing pulmonary congestion.	Low dichrotic notch on arterial tracing
Low serum Na and Cl	Low CVP, BP, PA, wedge pressures
Indicative of free water overload.	Not always present. Infants and children can be severely volume depleted before showing change in BP or CVP.
Increased heart size of haziness of lung fields on x-ray	By shutting down peripherally they will maintain their central pressure and BP.
Increase or rising BP, CVP, PA, wedge pressures, LA pressures	Dichrotic notch and warmth of extremities are of key importance.
	Increased pulse rate
Treatment	
Volume Overload	*Volume Depletion*
Fluid restriction	Replace chest loss
Less than maintenance fluids.	As it occurs (at least hourly). cc/cc depending on Hct.
Diuretics	
Digitalize	Fluid given
If CHF is severe	Usually colloid, which tends to stay in vascular space more than crystalloid.

    1) Left atrial central venous pressure and blood pressure must be high enough to perfuse bodily tissues and at the same time low enough to prevent CHF and pulmonary edema. May necessitate cardiotonic agents or pacemaker.

    2) Arrhythmias: from swelling, irritability of the myocardium, or drugs.

      a) Treatment depends on frequency and type of arrhythmias.

  b. Close obervation for hemorrhage and tamponade—frank bleeders, leakage from suture lines, or diffuse oozing from surrounding areas.

    1) Diffuse oozing: check clotting and platelet levels and treat accordingly.

    2) Frank bleeders: may require further surgery. With heavy bleeding, strip chest tubes frequently to avoid pooling of blood.

    3) Tamponade must be treated immediately.

      a) Muffled heart sounds, tachycardia, narrowing pulse pressure, increased CVP, decreased blood pressure, increase in size of mediastinum as shown by x-ray film; any combination of these is cause for immediate alarm.

      b) Continuous stripping of chest tubes to keep blood and clots from pooling around heart; surgical intervention usually necessary.

      c) Be prepared to open lower edge of suture line (midline sternotomies). A gloved finger slid under the sternum will release clots and provide an outlet for trapped blood.

  c. Maintenance of adequate cardiac output.

    1) Patients who have marginal cardiac output may need support of pressor agents.

      a) Watch for consistently low blood pressure, faint pulses, CVP in abnormal range in spite of adequate volume and supportive measures.

      b) Pressor agents such as Isuprel, dopamine, or Levophed/Regitine may be used.

5. Complications.

  a. After shunts.

    1) Pleural effusion: occurs occasionally; responds to thoracentesis.

    2) Cerebral embolism or thrombosis.

    3) Congestive heart failure: usually occurs only if shunt is too large; may necessitate further corrective surgery.

    4) Hemothorax.

    5) Early occlusion of shunt: requires another operation later; closures are managed by total repair.

  b. After total repair.

    1) Hemorrhage: rare.

2) Heart block: rare.
3) Pulmonary edema: common.
4) Low cardiac output: most common cause of death.

Transposition of the Great Vessels
1. Incidence: seventh most common cardiac anomaly, approximately 8%.
2. Pathophysiology.
   a. Aorta arises from the right ventricle; pulmonary artery arises from the left ventricle.
      1) Always accompanied by some intercommunication between the two sides of the heart (e.g., ASD, PDA, VSD) or it is not compatible with life. May have associated pulmonary stenosis.
      2) ASD is the most desirable defect; palliative treatment is aimed at creating one.
   b. Causes severe hypoxia, owing to systemic circulation arising from right ventricle, and increased volume of work of the left ventricle, owing to recirculation of large volume of blood through pulmonary circuit.
   c. Infants usually die from CHF and hypoxia unless treated in the first few months of life.
   d. Signs and symptoms:
      1) Severe hypoxemia: cyanosis at birth, occasional anoxic unconsciousness.
      2) If patent ductus is present, cyanosis may be less in trunk and lower extremities than in head and upper extremities
      3) Pulmonary congestion: tachypnea, irritability, and difficulty in feeding.
      4) X-ray film shows "egg-shaped" heart with a narrow vascular pedicle.
      5) Electrocardiogram shows right axis deviation and right ventricular hypertrophy.
3. Surgical treatment.
   a. Palliative procedures: creation of larger ASD to improve mixing of pulmonary and systemic circulation, thereby decreasing cyanosis.
      1) Balloon Atrial Septostomy (Rashkind procedure): nonoperative; done at time of cardiac catheterization.
         a) Balloon septostomy accomplished by passing a balloon-tipped catheter from the femoral vein through the foramen ovale into the left atrium, inflating the balloon, and pulling it forcibly back through the foramen ovale, tearing the margin and increasing its size.
            (1) Creates common mixing chamber and increases the average oxygen concentration.
      2) Blalock-Hanlon procedure: closed operative method of enlarging the ASD. Usually done only when attempts at balloon septostomy are unsuccessful.
         a) Operative mortality rate: approximately 10%.

    3) Patients with transposition of the great vessels associated with pulmonary stenosis.
       a) Pulmonary stenosis is usually of a very complex subvalvular type and difficult to correct.
       b) These patients usually also require a Blalock-Taussig shunt to increase blood flow to the lungs.
       c) Definitive repair for this type of defect with VSD requires a Rastelli procedure (see truncus arteriosus).
       d) These patients have a high operative mortality.
  b. Definitive procedures: Open Heart.
    1) Retransposition of the great arteries: Efforts at this used to fail because coronary arteries could not be retransplanted. Currently, however, efforts have been more successful and results are encouraging.
    2) Mustard Procedure (interatrial venous transposition): Interatrial septum is excised and an internal baffle of pericardium or fabric is placed so that blood from vena cava is directed into the left ventricle and pulmonary venous return is directed into the right ventricle, in essence, creating a transposition of the veins to compensate for that of the arteries.
       a) Usually done at about 1 year of age.
       b) Operative mortality: approximately 10%.
    3) Rastelli procedure (done for patients who have transposition with VSD and severe pulmonary stenosis): closure of VSD with a baffle that directs flow from the left ventricle through the VSD into the aorta. The pulmonary artery is removed from the left ventricle and attached by anastomosis end to end with a valve conduit. The remaining end is then attached to the right ventricle, reestablishing normal flow patterns.
4. Complications.
  a. Pulmonary edema: most common complication after creation of the ASD.
  b. Hemorrhage: most common complication after total correction.
    1) Most often caused by diffuse oozing.
5. Specific nursing interventions.
  a. See section on tetralogy of Fallot.
  b. Care should be taken when turning patients, particularly to the left side.
    1) Watch for arrhythmias, decreased cardiac output, and sudden cardiac arrest.

Total Anomalous Pulmonary Venous Return (TAPVR)
1. Incidence: approximately 2% of cases.
2. Pathophysiology.
  a. All pulmonary venous blood drains into the right atrium either directly or via the coronary sinus, superior vena cava, or inferior vena cava. A patent foramen ovale or ASD provides a

right-to-left shunt and thus mixed oxygenated blood to the left ventricle.

    b. Anomaly divided into four basic groups.

        1) Cardiac type: pulmonary veins connect directly or via coronary sinus with the right atrium.

        2) Supracardiac type: Pulmonary veins connect with superior vena cava via a common pulmonary vessel and an anomalous left ascending vessel into the left innominate vein.

        3) Infracardiac type: pulmonary blood drains from a common vessel into a descending vein that traverses the diaphram to enter the inferior vena cava, portal vein, or ductus venosus.

        4) Mixed type: pulmonary blood enters the right atrium by a different route from each lung.

    c. Degree of obstruction and pathway directly affects prognosis.

        1) Defects occuring below the diaphragm where blood empties into the inferior vena cava, portal vein, or ductus venosus are immediately life-threatening and must be repaired as soon as possible. These infants have a poor prognosis.

        2) In defects occuring above the diaphragm, a balloon septostomy is usually sufficient to allow the infant to grow until he can tolerate a complete repair.

    d. Causes increased volume of work for right ventricle and increased pulmonary blood flow.

    e. Structural changes:

        1) Hypertrophy and dilatation of right atrium, right ventricle, and pulmonary artery.

        2) Small left atrium.

    f. Signs and symptoms:

        1) Pulmonary congestion and cardiac failure.

           a) Usually symptomatic at birth.

           b) Frank failure occurs before 6 to 12 weeks of age.

        2) Tachypnea on exertion and often at rest.

        3) Failure to thrive.

        4) Variable cyanosis.

        5) Pulmonary systolic ejection murmur frequently present.

        6) "Snowman" contour on x-ray film (in children over 1 year).

        7) Electrocardiogram shows right axis deviation and right ventricular hypertrophy. P waves are unusually tall and peaked. Presence of Q wave in right precordial leads.

        8) Infants with TAPVR and obstruction have small heart and pulmonary venous congestion on x-ray film, without obstruction, have increased heart size and increased flow (CHF).

  3. Surgical treatment.

    a. Indications for surgery.

        1) Most patients will die in first six months if not treated.

2) Poor response to medical treatment or recurrent cardiac failure.
  b. Palliative repairs: Done when ASD is too small to allow for adequate mixing.
    1) Balloon septostomy: see transposition.
      a) Temporarily effective for patients with defects above the diaphragm and with minimal obstruction.
  c. Definitive (open heart).
    1) Pulmonary venous blood is rerouted to left atrium by means of anastomosis grafts and baffles.
    2) If the left atrium is small, the ASD is frequently left open.
      a) Allows left-to-right shunt to operate until left atrium is able to handle a full load.
      b) ASD is closed in a separate operation.
    3) Operative mortality: 10%
4. Specific nursing interventions.
  a. Essentially the same as for tetralogies and transpositions.
5. Complications.
  a. Pulmonary edema: most common complication after total repair.
  b. Hemorrhage.
  c. Heart block: most common with cardiac type or TAPVR.
  d. Pulmonary hypertension: if left atrium small and ASD is closed.

Hypoplastic Left Heart Syndrome

1. Incidence: most common congenital defect causing CHF in the newborn and during the first week of life.
2. Pathophysiology.
  a. Mitral valve, left ventricle aortic valve, and ascending aorta are markedly hypoplastic, with the valves severely stenotic or atretic.
  b. Causes passive congestion of lungs owing to inadequate left ventricular output.
  c. Symptoms.
    1) Cyanosis, mainly in lower half of body.
    2) Frank congestive heart failure.
  d. Usually diagnosed by echocardiography; catheterization not usually necessary.
3. Treatment.
  a. No effective treatment.
  b. Death occurs as ductus closes.

Tricuspid Atresia

1. Incidence: approximately 3% of cases.
2. Pathophysiology.
  a. Tricuspid valve is atretic; right ventricle is hypoplastic.
  b. Systemic blood reaches left ventricle through ASD.
  c. Blood reaches the lungs via a PDA or VSD.

      d. Defect causes three main problems.
         1) Systemic venous congestion due to obstruction of flow out of right atrium.
         2) Cyanosis due to right-to-left shunt through ASD.
         3) Inadequate flow through lungs.
      e. Signs and symptoms.
         1) Cyanosis or CHF, depending on type.
         2) Electrocardiogram shows left axis deviation.

3. Surgical treatment.
    a. Palliative repairs.
        1) Fontan procedure.
           a) Glenn takedown.
           b) Close ASD.
           c) Valve in.
           d) Conduit with valve from right atrium to left pulmonary artery.
        2) Aortic-pulmonary shunts (Potts, Waterston, Blalock-Taussig).
           a) Usually the first step.
           b) Establishes arterial shunt and allows patient to grow until vessels are large enough for Glenn procedure.
        3) Glenn procedure: direct end-to-end anastomosis of the superior vena cava to the right pulmonary artery.
           a) Palliates all three physiologic problems but requires adequate pulmonary artery size and no pulmonary hypertension.
           b) Operative mortality: 20%.
    b. Definitive repairs.

4. Specific nursing interventions.
    a. Routine postoperative cardiovascular nursing care.
    b. Watch closely for atrial arrhythmias.

5. Complications.
    a. Hemorrhage.
    b. Intractable CHF.
    c. Left ventricular hypertrophy.
    d. Operative mortality for the Fontan procedure is very high. Most common complications:
        1) Heart block.
        2) Atrial arrhythmias; Complete loss of cardiac output will occur; requires atrial pacing.

Truncus Arteriosus

1. Incidence: approximately 1% of all cases.
2. Pathophysiology.
    a. Consists of high VSD and a single vessel, the truncus, arising from the base of the heart. The pulmonary arteries arise from the truncus and do not have a separate valve.
    b. Symptoms:
        1) Early onset of CHF.

    2) Cyanosis may or may not be present.

    3) Harsh systolic murmur.

    4) Pulse pressure often widened; bounding peripheral pulses.

    5) X-ray film shows presence of right aortic arch.

3. Surgical treatment.
   a. Indications for surgery.
      1) Most patients will die from CHF in first six months.
   b. Palliative repair.
      1) Pulmonary banding may be of temporary help for infants with severe CHF.
   c. Definitive repair.
      1) Rastelli Procedure: VSD is closed with Dacron patch; segment with pulmonary arteries is cut out of truncus and resulting defect is closed; woven Dacron graft with prosthetic valve is attached to pulmonary arteries; then anastomosis is performed between proximal end of graft and edges of ventriculotomy.
         a) Mortality: 30 to 50%.

4. Specific nursing interventions.
   a. Much the same as for VSD.

5. Complications.
   a. Hemorrhage.
   b. Pulmonary edema.
   c. Heart block.
   d. Low cardiac output.

Other Cyanotic Congenital Heart Defects of Rare Incidence

Pulmonary Atresia With Intact Septum, With ASD or PDA

1. Incidence: rare (probably less than 1% of all cases).
2. Pathophysiology.
   a. Defect consists of intact ventricular septum and small hypertrophic right ventricle with complete obstruction of the outflow tract at the pulmonary valve or the muscle just below it.
   b. Main pulmonary artery is almost always patent.
   c. Blood reaches the lungs via the ductus and bronchial arteries.
   d. Signs and symptoms:
      1) Marked cyanosis.
      2) Murmur usually is absent.
      3) Electrocardiogram shows left ventricular hypertrophy with (perhaps) right ventricular hypertrophy.
         a) Degree of right ventricular hypertrophy has no relationship to size of right ventricular chamber.
      4) Reduced pulmonary vascular markings on x-ray film.
      5) Cardiac catheterization shows:
         a) Complete obstruction of pulmonary valve.

b) Increased pressure in right ventricle.
c) Right-to-left atrial shunt.
3. Surgical treatment
   a. Surgery is necessary, or death occurs when PDA closes.
   b. Palliative: emergent—protect against closure of PDA.
      1) Balloon atrial septostomy.
      2) Blalock-Taussig or Waterston shunt.
      3) Injection of PDA with formalin to prevent closure.
      4) Closed valvotomy (Brock procedure).
   c. Definitive: open.
      1) Valve conduit from right atrium to main pulmonary artery.
      2) ASD closure.
      3) PDA ligation.
4. Specific nursing interventions.
   a. Routine postoperative cardiovascular nursing care.

Double Outlet Right Ventricle With Pulmonary Stenosis (Taussig-Bing Syndrome)

1. Incidence: less than 1% of all cases.
2. Pathophysiology.
   a. Clinically difficult to distinguish from tetralogy of Fallot.
   b. Defect consists of aorta and pulmonary artery that arise from right ventricle, and left-to-right shunt through VSD.
   c. Causes decreased blood flow to lungs because of pulmonary stenosis.
   d. Aortic valve sits just above the right ventricle and is medial to the pulmonary valve in the frontal plane.
   e. VSD usually present; may be:
      1) Subcristal, or
      2) Supracristal.
   f. Pulmonary stenosis is due to:
      1) Large pulmonary artery with pulmonary valvular obstruction, or
      2) Subpulmonic infundibular stenosis.
   g. Depending on status of pulmonary outflow tract, may resemble tetralogy with large VSD.
3. Surgical treatment.
   a. Palliative repair: arterial shunt such as Blalock-Taussig or Potts.
   b. Definitive (open heart): very difficult.
      1) Combination of repairs.
         a) Rastelli procedure: closure of VSD, establishment of continuity between left ventricle and pulmonary artery.
         b) Venous baffle.
         c) Operative mortality: too few cases to report, but very high.
4. Specific nursing interventions.
   a. Routine postoperative cardiovascular nursing care.
   b. See transposition nursing care.

5. Complications.
   a. Similar to those of truncus and transposition repairs.

Ebstein's Anomaly With ASD.
1. Incidence: rare.
2. Pathophysiology.
   a. Defective structures: tricuspid valve is deviated toward the apex of the right ventricle, and the septal and posterior cusps of the valve are shortened and are attached to the ventricular wall near the apex.
   b. Results in decreased size of the right ventricle.
      1) Actual pumping portion of right ventricle is on the right atrial side of the tricuspid valve orifice.
   c. Tricuspid valve is seldom stenotic.
   d. Right-to-left shunt.
   e. Decreased pulmonary blood flow.
   f. Signs and symptoms:
      1) Cyanosis.
      2) Massive cardiomegaly.
      3) Profound congestive heart failure.
      4) Electrocardiogram may show:
         a) Wolff-Parkinson-White syndrome (WPW).
         b) 1 degree AV block.
         c) Right bundle branch block (RBBB).
         d) Right ventricular hypertrophy (RVH) very rare.
3. Surgical treatment.
   a. Palliative repair (closed): Glenn procedure.
      See tricuspid atresia repair.
   b. Definitive repair: Relocation or replacement of tricuspid valve.
4. Specific nursing interventions: same as for tricuspid atresia.
5. Complications: see tricuspid atresia.

Single Chambered Atrium
1. Incidence: rare.
2. Pathophysiology.
   a. Absence of atrial septum results in common mixing chamber for all pulmonary venous and systemic blood.
   b. Often associated with Ellis-van Creveld syndrome.
   c. Usually tolerated well in infancy.
3. Surgical treatment.
   a. Usually done at preschool age, 4 to 5 years.
   b. Definitive repair (open heart): atrium is partitioned with a polyvinyl graft.
   c. Mortality: estimated at 50%.
4. Specific nursing interventions: same as for ASD repair.
5. Complications.
   a. Inappropriate ADH (antidiuretic hormone).

Single Chambered Ventricle
1. Incidence: rare.

2. Pathophysiology.
   a. Absence of ventricular septum; mixing of all systemic and venous blood in a common ventricular cavity results in increased ventricular volume of work.
   b. Pulmonary flow is increased.
   c. Symptoms.
      1) Cyanosis in infancy, particularly when associated with pulmonary stenosis.
         a) Dyspnea.
         b) Congestive heart failure.
   d. Defect is tolerated poorly because of ventricular failure.
3. Surgical treatment.
   a. Palliative (closed): pulmonary artery banding (see VSD); geared toward associated anomalies.
      1) Systemic to pulmonary artery shunt.
         a) With severe pulmonary stenosis.
   b. Definitive (open).
      1) Creation of a ventricular septum.
         a) Exceedingly difficult, poor risk.
4. Specific nursing interventions.
   a. Same as for VSD repair.
5. Complications.
   a. Complete heart block.

POSTOPERATIVE NURSING MANAGEMENT OF THE PEDIATRIC CARDIOVASCULAR SURGERY PATIENT

Objectives of Postoperative Care
1. Prevent complications.
2. Attain normal physiological and psychological homeostasis.

Monitor Physiologic Parameters Closely
1. Vital Signs.
   a. Temperature: Control with antipyretics and warming or cooling blankets as needed; especially important in infants.
      1) Elevated temps add stress to myocardial function.
      2) Low temps increase acidosis and decrease cardiac output.
      3) Measure hourly.
   b. Pulse rate, respiratory rate, blood pressure, central venous pressure, left atrial pressure, and pulmonary artery pressure. (Not all pressures always monitored.)
      1) Indicators of hemodynamic and pulmonary status.
      2) Values will vary with age and defect; find out base line parameters.
         a) Report any deviations.
         b) Maintain pressures within limits using drugs, pacemakers, respirators according to patient needs.
      3) Measure every one-half to one hour.

      c.   Neurological status.

          1)   Pupil checks (microaggregates, clots, air embolism, or anoxia can cause cerebral vascular accident or increased intracranial pressure).

2. Electrocardiogram status.

    a.   Monitor electrocardiogram continuously.

    b.   Watch for arrhythmias and treat accordingly.

        1)   Drugs (See drug section).

        2)   Pacemaker.

    c.   Often disrupted because of site of defect and swelling along suture line; disruption may be transitory or permanent.

    d.   **Caution:** In paced patients, electrocardiogram does not indicate adequacy of cardiac output; monitor blood pressure closely.

3. Urine output and kidney function.

    a.   At least 0.5 to 1 cc/kg/hr excreted and collected by pediatric urimeter.

    b.   Measure hourly.

    c.   Check specific gravity every 4 hours.

    d.   Check for sugar and acetone every 4 to 6 hours if patient is on high dextrose concentration 10% dextrose, 20% dextrose, or hyperalimentation.

    e.   Check urine electrolytes, blood urea nitrogen (BUN).

    f.   Give adequate fluids for kidney perfusion.

    g.   Give drugs as necessary to increase urine output.

    h.   Peritoneal dialysis sometimes necessary.

        1)   Acute tubular necrosis due to low cardiac output or prolonged hypovolemia.

        2)   Peritoneal catheter is also occasionally used as a means of draining third-spaced abdominal fluid.

4. Chest drainage: maintenance of chest tubes.

    a.   Strip chest tubes every hour or more frequently if necessary.

    b.   Do not strip chest tube too vigorously.

        1)   Too much negative pressure may cause tearing of lung or heart tissue.

    c.   Infants or small children with large chest tubes.

        1)   Large amounts of air may be sucked into chest when child is hyperventilating or screaming.

            a)   May cause pneumothorax.

            b)   Water seal drainage recommended for all ages.

        2)   Do not reverse strip; reversal may cause pneumomediastinum.

    d.   Watch for crepitus.

        1)   Caused by small leaks around chest tubes.

    e.   Replace chest drainage with colloid.

        1)   Usually cc for cc of loss.

5. Blood gases and other blood values.

    a.   Arterial blood gases as needed.

    b. Coagulation studies.
      1) Monitor at least daily, more often as needed.
      2) Immediate postoperative prolongation of coagulation usually indicates inadequate reversal post pump and can be corrected with protamine.
    c. Hematocrit, electrolytes, BUN, creatinine.
      1) Monitor serum K closely and maintain between 3.5 and 4.5, especially when patient is on digoxin.
      2) Decrease in serum Na is usually indicative of water excess rather than low Na.
    d. Sugar, calcium, and magnesium.
      1) Particularly important in infants.
    e. Replace blood samples cc for cc.
      1) Record amounts withdrawn.
      2) Withdraw smallest possible amount needed for sampling.

6. Volume status.
    a. Monitor total intake and output closely.
    b. Volume indicators:
      1) Vital signs: blood pressure, central venous pressure, pulse, respirations, left atrial pressure, pulmonary artery pressure.
      2) Pedal pulses.
      3) Warmth of extremities.
      4) Urine output.
      5) Dichrotic notch on arterial tracing.
    c. Watch volume indicators *together* as a group.
      1) In hypovolemia, vital signs may be last indicators to change.
      2) Children will shunt down peripherally to maintain pressures; only indicators may be cold extremities and loss of dichrotic notch before a sudden arrest from hypovolemia.
    d. Treatment of volume depletion with colloid.
    e. Treatment of volume overload.
      1) Colloid such as salt-poor albumin to mobilize third spaced fluid.
      2) Followed with diuretics to pull fluid from vascular space.
      3) Limit of crystalloid.
    f. Daily or twice daily weights.

7. Respiratory status (see also respiratory section).
    a. Obtain arterial blood gases and treat accordingly.
    b. Turn frequently. If chest x-ray shows atelectasis on either side, position with affected side up 75% of time (45 minutes out of every hour).
    c. Ventilatory support as needed with respirator.
    d. Daily chest x-rays.
    e. Suction as needed and at least every 1 to 2 hours to maintain tube patency.

        1) Exception: in cases of massive pulmonary edema requiring extremely high PEEP settings.

    f. Paradoxical breathing, difficulty in weaning, especially in small infants.

        1) May be due to partial paralysis of diaphragm.

        2) Often occurs with repair of transposition of great vessels but may occur with any repair.

8. Pain status.

    a. Indications of pain.

        1) Splinting or rapid respirations.

        2) Increase in monitored pressures or pulse rate.

        3) Restlessness or agitation.

    b. Control with medications as ordered.

9. Maintain tube and line placement and function

    a. Endotracheal tubes.

        1) Make sure tube is well taped.

        2) Never retape a tube by yourself.

        3) Suction as needed (at least every 2 hours).

        4) Oral tracheal tubes should be changed to nasal tracheal tubes as soon as patient is stabilized.

    b. Respirator.

        1) Increased pressure may be due to:

           a) Pulmonary edema.

           b) Increased secretions.

           c) Water in or obstruction of respirator tubing.

           d) Increased blood or stiffness in lungs.

           e) Endotracheal tube obstruction.

        2) Check exhaled volume periodically.

    c. Nasogastric tubes

        1) All patients on respirators.

        2) Check position on x-ray

        3) Usually connected to low suction.

        4) Measure and record drainage.

        5) Check patency and irrigate as needed.

        6) Tape in such a way as to minimize chance of eroding nostrils.

    d. Intravascular lines

        1) CVP, LAP, PAP, arterial lines.

           a) May be affected by positioning; be sure transducer level is the same for each reading.

           b) Check periodically for patency and function.

           c) Calibrate at least every 8 hours or as needed.

           d) Do not allow air to enter any of these lines.

           e) Arterial lines should be maintained by continuous infusion of small amounts (3 cc or less/hr) of heparinized saline.

           f) It is preferable to maintain these lines with a constant infusion pump.

10. Close observation for life-threatening complications.
   a. Tamponade
     1) Requires immediate attention.
     2) Indications:
       a) Decreasing blood pressure with narrowing pulse pressure
       b) Increasing CVP, LAP, PAP.
       c) Rapid, thready pulse.
       d) Unexpected loss of cardiac rub.
       e) Muffled heart tones.
       f) Increase in mediastinal widening or increased heart size.
       g) Sudden change in chest drainage.
       h) Pericardial fluid on echocardiogram.
   b. Tension pneumothorax.
     1) Requires immediate attention.
     2) Indications:
       a) Increased respirations.
       b) Decreased breath sounds on one side.
       c) Inequality of movement of sides of chest.
       d) Maximum heart sound further across chest than before.
       e) Decreased color and PO_2.
       f) Restlessness, apprehension.
       g) Moderate to severe respiratory distress.
11. Commonly used medications.
   (Dosages may vary slightly from institution to institution).
   a. Digoxin
     1) Preferred medication in pediatrics because of its rapid effect and short duration.
     2) Digitalizing: Always obtain limb lead electrocardiogram before first dose.
       Total digitalizing doses: (TDD).
       Premature and Newborn: TDD 30 to 50 mcg/kg IV.
       Under 2 years: TDD 40 to 60 mcg/kg IV
       Over 2 years: TDD 20 to 40 mcg/kg IV
       One-half TDD given stat, then one-fourth TDD every 4 to 8 hours times two.
     3) Maintenance.
       a) 0.20 mcg TDD IV per day (divide every 12 hours)
     4) Oral doses are 1/3 higher than IV dose.
     5) Before giving:
       a) Check heart rate; if 10 points lower than normal for age, check with doctor before giving.
       b) Be sure serum potassium is greater than 3.5 mEq/l.
   b. Furosemide (Lasix).
     1) 1 mg/kg/dose.
     2) Side effects: hypokalemia and volume depletion.

c. Procainamide Hydrochloride (Lidocaine) For control of arrhythmias.
   1) Bolus: 1 mg/kg each push up to 3 mg/kg every 10 to 20 min maximum.
   2) Intravenous drip: 1 gm/250 cc dextrose 5% in water (50 cc 2% Lidocaine in 200 cc dextrose 5% in water).
   3) Adverse reactions.
      a) Seizures (treat with Valium 0.1 to 0.4 mg/kg).
      b) Heart block.
d. Morphine: for sedation and pain control.
   1) Small doses IV every 1 to 2 hours.
   2) 0.1 to 0.2 mg/kg.
e. Diazepam (Valium):
   1) Is alternated with morphine sulfate to sedate and enhance pain control.
   2) Does not cause respiratory depression in children except rarely or when very large doses are used.
   3) 0.1 to 0.3 mg/kg IV every 1 to 2 hours.
f. Vasopressor drips.
   1) Dopamine drip: 1 mg/cc (1 cc Dopamine + 39 cc dextrose 5% in water).
      a) Should be run through central line.
      b) Should be maintained by continuous infusion pump.
      c) Run just to keep blood pressure at desired level.
   2) Levophed Regitine Drip: 8 mg Levophed and 20 mg Regitine + 250cc dextrose 5% in water.
      a) Administer through central venous line.
      b) Use infusion pump.
      c) Run to maintain blood pressure at 90 mm Hg systolic.
   3) Isuprel drip: 1 mg Isuprel + 250cc dextrose 5% in water.
      a) Watch for tachycardial arrhythmias.
      b) As for dopamine and L/R drip.
   4) Vasopressor drips should not be used on a hypovolemic patient except in an emergency. The patient should be rehydrated as soon as possible.
      a) Some drugs decrease kidney perfusion and may lead to permanent damage.
g. Potassium drips: 40 to 80 mEq/250 cc dextrose 5% in water. **Use with extreme caution.**
   1) Very corrosive and can damage peripheral veins; should be administered through central venous line only.
   2) Too rapid infusion can cause ventricular arrhythmias and cardiac arrest.
      a) Never give IV bolus push.
   3) Always get serum potassium level every two hours while running K^+ drip.

        4)   Rate of infusion: 0.25 to 1 cc/kg/hr of 80 mEq solution (varies with institution).

        5) K^+ drip should be run until serum K^+ is between 4.5 and 5.0 mEq/l serum level.

    h.   Drugs used in resuscitation (see section on cardiopulmonary resuscitation, pp. 146–148.)

12.   Continuous assessment of patient condition.

    a.   Physical assessment: touch, look, listen, smell, don't rely on monitors only.

    b.   Cardiac monitor.

    c.   Physiologic monitoring.

    d.   Vital signs and neurological status.

    e.   Intake and output from all sources.

    f.   Response to treatments.

13.   Special nursing care related to specific defect.

    a.   See specific nursing interventions for each defect.

ACQUIRED HEART DISEASE[1,2,8,11,15,18,20,21,22,24,29,30,32]

Endocardial Fibroelastosis (EFE)

1.   Incidence.

    a.   A common cause of CHF[5,21,22,24] and death in children with heart disease between ages 2 months and 1 year.

    b.   Exact etiology not known, though there are several hypotheses.

        1)   Intrauterine infection due to virus.

        2)   Increased tension in wall of heart.

        3)   Intrauterine hypoxia.

2.   Pathophysiology.

    a.   Diffuse endocardial thickening, primarily in the left ventricle and left atrium.

        1)   Frequently involves the mitral or aortic valve or both.

        2)   Involvement of right heart is rare.

    b.   Histologically similar to collagen diseases.

        1)   Hyperplasia of the elastic tissue of endocardium.

        2)   Surface layers of endocardium comprised primarily of fibrin-like fibers.

    c.   Occurs as a primary or isolated myocardial disease or more often (30 to 60% of cases) in association with other congenital heart defects, most commonly:

        1)   Hypoplastic left heart syndrome.

        2)   Coarctation of aorta.

        3)   Aortic stenosis.

        4)   Pulmonic stenosis or atresia.

    d.   Defect results in poor emptying of the left ventricle.

        1)   Elevation of diastolic pressure and impairment of systolic ejection of the left ventricle.

e. Signs and symptoms of primary endocardial fibroclastosis:
   1) Congestive heart failure–50% of patients develop symptoms in first six months, 95% within first year.
   2) Edema: peripheral, periorbital, and facial.
   3) Failure of infant to thrive.
   4) X-ray film shows left ventricular dilatation and left atrial enlargement.
   5) Electrocardiogram shows left ventricular hypertrophy.
   6) Prognosis: very poor. The younger the patient at the time of diagnosis, the worse the prognosis.
3. Therapeutic management.
   a. Control of congestive heart failure with digoxin, diuretics.
   b. Treatment of associated arrhythmias.
   c. Surgery for associated congenital heart defects is usually recommended.
   d. Long-term survivors of primary EFE may eventually need surgery for valvular involvement.
   e. Same as congestive heart failure.
   f. Postoperative nursing management.
4. Specific nursing interventions.
   a. See sections on congestive heart failure and postoperative nursing management.

Rheumatic Fever and Rheumatic Heart Disease[21,22,24]

1. Incidence and etiology.
   a. Most common cause of acquired heart disease in children.
   b. Occurs in 1 to 5 of every 1000 children between the ages of 5 and 15 years.
      1) Rarely occurs before age 2.
   c. Incidence and severity are on the decline.
   d. These patients are usually not seen in the critical care unit unless in severe CHF or for repair of valvular damage.
   e. Exact etiology unknown.
      1) Group A beta hemolytic streptococcus is implicated.
         a) Strep infection always precedes rheumatic fever, usually by 1 to 3 weeks.
         b) Exact relationship unknown; may be hypersensitivity to some product of strep.
   f. Predisposing factors:
      1) Family history of rheumatic fever.
      2) Poor socioeconomic environment.
      3) Previous attack of rheumatic fever.
2. Pathophysiology.
   a. Rheumatic changes in the heart.
      1) Verrucose endocarditis localized on the atrial surfaces of the mitral valve and the ventricular surfaces of the aortic valve.
      2) Valves are swollen, edematous, and distorted.
      3) Chordae tendineae are shortened and thickened.

    b. Most common valvular disturbance in children is mitral insufficiency, followed by aortic insufficiency.

    c. Pulmonic and tricuspid valves are rarely affected in children.

    d. Initial manifestations of rheumatic fever:

       1) Arthritis: most common presenting complaint (approximately 75%).

       2) Carditis: sole complaint in approximately 15% of cases.

       3) Chorea: sole major complaint in about 5%.

    e. Acute rheumatic carditis will occur in 40 to 50% of patients with acute rheumatic fever. They present with:

       1) Organic heart murmur, usually of mitral insufficiency and at least grade 2.

       2) Cardiac enlargement on X-ray film.

       3) Pericarditis: presence of pericardial friction rub or unequivocal effusion.

       4) Electrocardiogram shows indications of active carditis by evidence of chamber enlargement and increasing degrees of AV block.

          a) First degree block and Wenckeback phenomenon are common arrhythmias.

       5) Congestive heart failure: most common in children under 6 years of age and in recurrent attacks of rheumatic carditis.

       6) Persistent low-grade fever and elevated sedimentation rate also common.

  3. Therapeutic management and prognosis.

    a. Before antibiotics, mortality rate for rheumatic fever was 25 to 35%, with 70 to 80% of the deaths occurring in patients with gross cardiomegaly and CHF.

    b. Currently, mortality rate of first-time attacks treated with antibiotics is between 0 and 3%.

    c. Patients are still at great risk of permanent valvular damage.

    d. Treatment:

       1) Antibiotics to eradicate streptococcus.

       2) Steroids.

       3) Aspirin.

       4) Control of CHF.

       5) Bed rest.

       6) Low Na diet.

  4. Specific nursing interventions.

    a. See section on congestive heart failure.

Bacterial Endocarditis.[21,22,24]

  1. Incidence and etiology.

    a. Declining recently because of increased use of antibiotics.

    b. Primarily a disease of young adults but can occur in any age group.

       1) In children, usually found between 5 and 20 years of age.

    c. Can be caused by any organism.
      1) Alpha streptococcus enterococcus, and staphylococcus account for 95% of cases.
    d. Predisposing factors:
      1) Previous rheumatic heart disease.
      2) Congenital heart defects.
      3) Systemic/pulmonary shunts
    e. Most common congenital defects affected by alpha strep:
      1) PDA.
      2) Biscupid aortic valve.
      3) Coarctation of aorta.
      4) VSD.
      5) Aortic stenosis.
      6) Tetralogy of Fallot

2. Should be suspected in any postoperative congenital heart patient who has persistent fever after first week following surgery.

3. Pathophysiology.
    a. Usually differentiated into acute or subacute varities because of duration.
    b. Characterized by vegetative buildup of infecting organisms, which settle on the damaged valves (in patients with congenital heart defects or rheumatic heart disease) or endocardium.
      1) Mitral valve most commonly affected.
      2) In PDA: pulmonary oriface is site of vegetation.
      3) In VSD: right ventricular side of septum is usually involved.
      4) In coarctation: usually affects site of coarctations.
      5) Shunts.
    c. Vegetation may spread to chordae tendineae, and valves themselves may perforate.
    d. Infected emboli break off frequently and may be found in any organ.
    e. Acute bacterial endocarditis differs from subacute in that:
      1) Preexisting heart disease or defect is not a prerequisite.
      2) Destruction, ulceration, and perforation are much more severe with acute than subacute.
      3) General sepsis occurs in acute; cardiac involvement predominates in subacute.
      4) Acute: ends either favorably or unfavorably within two months.
    f. Signs and symptoms:
      1) Fever and malaise (40% of patients).
      2) Recent weight loss.
      3) Respiratory tract infection (20% of patients).
      4) Splenomegaly and hepatomegaly.
      5) CHF (approximately one third of patients).

      6) Lab findings: elevated sed rate (75% of patients) and decreased hemoglobin (over one half of patients).

      7) Embolic phenomena: Roth spots, splinter hemorrhages, hematuria.

  4. Therapeutic management.

    a. Early treatment before vegetations are covered by thick fibrin-platelet shield.

    b. Penicillin is often drug of choice.

These patients are usually only seen in the critical care unit when valvular damage has already occurred or when there are multiple emboli.

Pulmonary Heart Disease (Cor Pulmonale)

  1. Etiology.

    a. Most common cause of cor pulmonale in children is cystic fibrosis.

    b. Other causes, *though rare,* are:

      1) Hamman-Rich syndrome (extreme obesity).

      2) Huge tonsils and adenoids in infants (reversible).

      3) V-A shunt for hydrocephalus.

  2. Pathophysiology.

    a. Right ventricular hypertrophy associated with primary pulmonary diseases.

    b. Principle mechanism causing Cor pulmonale is hypoventilation due to:

      1) Obstructive disease.

      2) Restrictive disease.

      3) Diffusion defect.

    c. Hypoventilation causes hypoxia and acidosis, followed by pulmonary vasoconstriction, hypervolemia, and polycythemia.

    d. PO_2 in room air is usually less than 60, and PCO_2 is usually greater than 50.

    e. Symptoms are difficult to separate from those of lung disease already present.

      1) Severe dyspnea.

      2) Severe cyanosis and clubbing.

      3) Marked edema.

      4) Hepatomegaly and ascites.

      5) Distended neck veins.

      6) Ausculation of heart difficult because of rales and emphysema.

      7) Tachycardia; gallop rhythm may be present.

  3. Therapeutic management and prognosis.

    a. Prognosis very poor even with treatment.

      1) Patients with marked cardiac enlargement, edema, and high PCO_2 usually die from CHF within 1 or 2 years.

    b. Usual treatment:

1) Vigorous antibiotic treatment.
2) Careful administration of low concentrations of oxygen. Most patients are hypercapnic, and respiratory drive is initiated by anoxia alone.
3) Bronchodilators if bronchospasm is present.
4) Bed rest.
5) Low Na diet.
6) Digoxin and diuretics to support circulation.
7) Phlebotomy if Hct is greater than 65%.

4. Specific nursing interventions: most of these patients are not seen in the ICU until in CHF; see CHF section for nursing interventions. In addition:
   a. Oxygen should be administered very carefully, if at all.
   b. When giving digoxin, do not use pulse rate as a measure of digitalis effect.
      1) Anoxia causes tachycardia.
      2) Sinus slowing may not occur until digoxin toxicity is already present.

Congestive Heart Failure[1,2,3,8,18,21,22,24,30,32]

1. Incidence and etiology: CHF is a common syndrome in pediatric age groups.
   a. Usually patients with CHF are under 1 year of age and the CHF is due to congenital heart disease.
      1) 90% will occur in first year or not until adulthood.
      2) 10% will occur between 1 and 5 years.
   b. CHF occurring between 5 and 15 years is usually due to an acquired heart lesion.
   c. CHF may be caused by three major types of problems.
      1) Excessive blood pressure load. Causes include:
         a) Coarctation of the aorta.
         b) High pulmonary vascular resistance.
         c) Aortic or pulmonary stenosis.
         d) Premature closing of the foramen ovale.
         e) Cor triatriatum.
         f) Obstructed pulmonary veins.
      2) Excessive blood volume load. May be from:
         a) Large left-to-right shunts (PDA, VSD, canal).
         b) Total anomalous pulmonary venous drainage.
         c) Mitral or aortic insufficiency.
         d) Anemia.
         e) Hypervolemia.
      3) Myocardium unable to handle normal pressure or volume loads, owing to:
         a) Rheumatic heart disease.
         b) Myocarditis.
         c) Endocardial fibroelastosis.

    d) Severe tachycardia.

    e) Low calcium, magnesium, or blood sugar, or severe acidemia, especially in neonates.

  2. Pathophysiology: similar to adult CHF.

   a. CHF is the inability of heart to provide adequate circulation to provide normal tissue metabolism.

   b. Hypertrophy and dilatation of involved chambers and myocardium is caused by attempt to maintain adequate circulation to meet body tissue needs when heart is under added stress.

   c. Clinical manifestations in infants and children:

    1) Failure to thrive.

     a) Poor weight gain.

     b) Anorexia and vomiting.

     c) Lethargy or fatigue at feeding.

    2) Tachycardia and hepatomegaly.

     a) Gallop rhythm may be present, especially in infants.

    3) Tachypnea, dyspnea, and cyanosis.

     a) Frequent moist cough.

     b) May progress to frank pulmonary edema.

    4) X-ray film shows some degree of cardiomegaly and pulmonary venous congestion.

    5) Serial electrocardiogram will often show increasing right atrial enlargement.

    6) Facial edema, rather than leg edema as with adults.

    7) Hypothermia.

   d. Signs and symptoms in older children and adolescents are generally the same as in the adult.

  3. Therapeutic management.

   a. Digoxin.

   b. Diuretics, usually Lasix.

   c. Oxygen mist—30 to 40% FIO_2.

   d. Mild sedation for pulmonary edema or extreme restlessness.

    1) Morphine sulfate 0.1 to 0.2 mg/kg.

   e. Control of anemia with packed red blood cells.

    1) Especially when Hct is less than 20 mg or Hb is less than 7 gm.

   f. Antibiotics for control of bronchopneumonia.

    1) Bronchopneumonia almost always coexhists with CHF in infants and children.

  4. Specific nursing interventions.

   a. Promotion of adequate pulmonary function.

    1) Elevation of head and shoulders 30 to 45 degrees.

    2) Frequent turning, coughing, and deep breathing.

    3) Administration of humidified oxygen (FIO_2 40 to 50%).

    4) Close monitoring of arterial blood gases.

     a) Correct acidosis if present.

    5) Ventilatory support as needed for pulmonary edema.

  b. Provision for adequate rest.
   1) Bed rest (strict).
   2) Control of temperature to 37 degrees C. is desirable.
   3) Sedation with morphine sulfate for extremely restless patients.
  c. Maintenance of normal fluid volume.
   1) Daily or twice daily weights.
   2) Monitore electrolytes, hematocrit, hemoglobin.
    a) Watch potassium level closely while patient on digoxin and diuretics.
    b) Watch Hb and Hct for signs of anemia.
    c) Low Na and Cl values usually indicate excess fluid.
   3) Monitor urine output hourly.
   4) Give diuretics as ordered.
   5) Low Na diet to prevent fluid retention.
  d. Control of infection.
   1) Monitor temperature closely.
   2) Administer antibiotics and steroids as ordered.
   3) Send sputum and blood cultures when indicated.
  e. Maintenance of optimum cardiac function.
   1) Frequent assessment of patient.
    a) Listen for changes in heart sounds—gallop, muffling, pericardial rub.
   2) Continuous electrocardiogram monitoring.
   3) Give digoxin preparations as ordered.
    a) Watch for digoxin effect.
    b) Watch for signs of digoxin toxicity.
     (1) Marked slowing of heart rate.
     (2) AV dissociation, junctional rhythm, atrial or ventricular arrhythmias.
     (3) Gastrointestinal disturbances, loss of appetite, or vomiting may be early signs in the infant.
    c) Be sure serum K is above 3.5 when patient is receiving digoxin.
    d) Medications for specific arrhythmias as necessary.
    e) Maintain normal blood pressure with drugs if necessary.
    f) Correct acidosis and electrolyte imbalance.

Arrhythmias in Children[1,3,8,11,15,17,20,22,24,29,31]
 1. Heart rates: normal rates for infants and children vary according to age (See Chapter I, Normal Growth & Development.)
  a. Tachycardias.
   1) Sinus tachycardia: most common tachycardia in children.
   2) Supraventricular tachycardia: atrial more common than junctional.
    a) Usually not associated with heart disease; but often associated with fever, exercise, anemia, or shock.
    b) May come in paroxysmal attacks that begin and end abruptly.

    3) Least common types of tachycardia:
       a) Atrial flutter.
       b) Atrial fibrillation.
       c) Ventricular tachycardia.

b. Bradycardias.
  1) Relatively uncommon in infants and children.
  2) May be associated with syncope.
  3) Causes.
    a) Suctioning or vagal stimulation.
    b) Raised intercranial pressure.
    c) Myocarditis.
    d) Drugs such as digoxin, propranolol, morphine.
  4) Third degree (complete) heart block may be:
    a) Congenital: one third are associated with congenital heart defects, most often transposition.
    b) Acquired: myocarditis or postoperative cardiac procedures.

c. Infants and children may demonstrate any of the arrhythmias seen in adults, though usually less frequently. Some arrhythmias seen in children are:
  1) Paroxysmal atrial tachycardia.
  2) Adams-Stokes syndrome.
  3) Wolff-Parkinson-White syndrome.

d. Long Q-T syndromes:
  1) Characterized by:
    a) $Q\text{-}T_c$ (QT interval corrected for heart rate) of over 0.425 seconds.
    b) Episodic ventricular fibrillation.
    c) Inherited syndrome.
      (1) Romano-Ward: autosomal dominant without high frequency hearing loss; first noted in 1963.
      (2) Jervel and Lange-Neilsen: autosomal recessive with high frequency hearing loss or deaf-mutism; first described in 1957.
  2) Incidence is rare, probably from lack of recognition rather than lack of occurrence.
    a) Several hundred cases discovered since recognition by Romano and Ward.
  3) Syndrome often present in late childhood or early adolescence with syncopal episodes and seizure-like activity and, unless recognized, sudden death.
    a) Most patients seen first by neurologist for seizures before electrocardiogram reveals prolonged QT_c.
    b) Most attacks brought on by anxiety, fear, excitement, or psychic stress.
    c) Strenuous physical exercise may or may not bring on attacks.

       4) Family history almost always reveals relatives who have either died suddenly in early adolescence or who have prolonged Q-T$_c$'s.
          a) There is usually no associated organic heart disease, other than the abnormal electrocardiogram.
       5) All children with long Q-T syndromes prone to ventricular tachycardia or ventricular fibrillation.

2. Pathophysiology.
Mechanism of pathophysiology is specific to each disease noted under relative arrhythmias.

3. Therapeutic management.
    a. Aimed at prevention of ventricular tachycardia and decreasing the susceptibility of the myocardium to premature ventricular contractions.
    b. Drug treatment.
       1) Inderal: very effective in decreasing myocardial susceptibility.
       2) Dilantin: shortens Q-T interval; somewhat effective.
       3) Lidocaine and countershock: somewhat effective when child is in ventricular tachycardia or ventricular fibrillation.

4. Specific nursing interventions.
    a. Close monitoring of electrocardiogram.
    b. Provide quiet nonstimulating environment and prevent anxiety and fear-producing stimuli.
    c. Provide emotional support to patient and family.
    d. Institute immediate treatment for ventricular tachycardia or ventricular fibrillation.

CARDIOPULMONARY RESUSCITATION IN INFANTS AND CHILDREN

Etiology of Cardiopulmonary Arrest.
1. Respiratory arrest: may be caused by:
    a. Acute airway obstruction.
       1) Aspiration.
       2) Fluid, excess mucus (pulmonary edema, drowning).
       3) Marked edema or spasm of upper or lower airways.
       4) Structural defects (choanal atresia, subglottic stenosis).
    b. Central nervous system depression.
       1) Drugs.
       2) Poisons.
       3) Trauma.
       4) Electric shock.
       5) Cerebral edema.

      6) Severe hypoxia.

      7) Hypercapnia.

   c. Neuromuscular paralysis.

   d. Gross trauma to thoracic cage.

   e. Bilateral tension pneumothorax.

2. Circulatory arrest: may be caused by:

   a. Hypoxia, acidemia, or hypercapnia.

   b. Vagal stimulation.

   c. Electric current.

   d. Drugs, especially digitoxin, potassium, and anesthetics.

   e. Arrhythmias.

   f. Shock.

   g. Tamponade.

Pathophysiology of Arrest.

1. Cardiopulmonary Arrest causes:

   a. Hypoxema. ⎱ ⎰An anaerobic metabolism and lactate produc-

   b. Hypercapnia.⎰ ⎱tion cause decreased pH in blood and tissues.

   c. Increased vagal tone, which increases possibility of:

      1) Bradycardia.

      2) Asystole.

      3) Ventricular fibrillation.

2. Symptoms of impending arrest:

   a. Absent or poor chest movements.

   b. Weak or absent pulses and heart sounds.

   c. Marked bradycardia or tachycardia.

   d. Cyanosis or pallor.

   e. Loss of consciousness.

3. Arrest needs immediate treatment or death will occur.

Treatment: Basic Life Support (Cardiopulmonary Resuscitation [CPR]).

   The standardized protocols as developed by the American Heart Association serve as guidelines to the following outline of cardiopulmonary resuscitation for infants and children. Adolescents requiring basic life support can generally be treated with adult protocols.

1. Establish unresponsiveness.

   a. Gently shake shoulder.

   b. Shout near patient's ear, "Are you OK?"

      1) May use patient's name or nickname to elicit response.

2. Call for help.

3. ABC's of resuscitation.

   a. Establish **airway.**

      1) Gently tilt head in extension and lift mandible (jaw) forward.

      2) Rescuer places cheek near patient's nose and mouth, facing toward patient's chest.

      3) Look, listen, and feel for respirations.

         a) Look: for rise and fall of chest.

         b) Listen: for sounds of ventilation.

         c) Feel: for inhaled/exhaled air on cheek.

   4) If no response:
b. **Breathe** for patient.
   1) Give four (4) quick full PEEP breaths (PEEP: incremental breaths that do not allow for complete exhalation until after fourth breath, i.e., positive end expiratory pressure).
     a) Infant: cover mouth and nose with rescuer's mouth.
     b) Child: Seal rescuer's mouth over patient's mouth; pinch nostrils to prevent escape of air during ventilation.
   2) Monitor carotid pulse in child and apical pulse in infant. If they are present, continue rescue breathing.
     a) Infant: 20 ventilations per minute.
     b) Child: 15 ventilations per minute.
   3) If no pulse present:
c. Again, call for help.
d. Begin **cardiac compression.**
   1) Place infant or child in supine position with firm surface under back.
     a) Infant: Rescuer may use palm and lower arm as firm support under back.
   2) For child less than eighty (80) pounds: place heel (palmar surface) of one hand on lower half of sternum and compress 3/4 to 1 1/2 inches.
     a) Single rescuer: Administer fifteen (15) compressions to two (2) quick full breaths at a rate of 80 compressions per minute.
     b) Two person rescue: Administer five (5) compressions to one (1) quick full breath at a rate of 60 compressions per minute.
   3) For the infant: Place the index and middle fingers of one hand together (side by side) over an imaginary point of the intersecting lines drawn between the nipples, the sternal notch, and the xiphoid process.

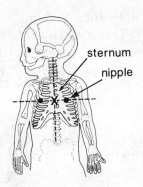

Figure 3–1. Landmarks on the infant's chest showing finger placement for cardiac compression during cardiopulmonary resuscitation.

a) One person can satisfactorily accomplish a two-person rescue procedure of cardiopulmonary resuscitation.
b) Compress the sternum at point "X", 1/2 to 3/4 inches.
c) Effect five (5) compressions to one (1) breath at a rate of 80 compressions per minute.

4. Points of caution when initiating cardiopulmonary resuscitation
   a. Check for carotid or apical pulse after one minute of Basic Life Support (CPR) and again every 4 to 5 minutes of continued CPR.
   b. Do not hyperextend the head and neck of an infant, because the trachea is very flexible and easily becomes obstructed in the hyperextended position. The most effective open airway position for an infant is described as a "sniff position" (extension of head and neck to approximately the same degree as if sniffing flowers).
   c. Avoid overinflating the lungs in order to reduce the amount of air being forced into patient's stomach and in turn reduce the complications of regurgitation with aspiration.
   d. Do not encircle an infant's chest with both hands of the rescuer and thumbs placed on "X" of sternum. Compression with this hand position has a high risk of displacement of the spine (not the sternum) and resultant spinal cord damage.

ADVANCED CARDIAC LIFE SUPPORT FOR INFANTS AND CHILDREN

As soon as basic life support is initiated and a dynamic cardiac monitor is available, prepare to have additional rescuers place electrodes on patient's chest for electrocardiographic monitoring. Have a defibrillator (DC) and completely stocked crash cart ready.

Obtain Rhythm Strip and Determine Rhythm.
Correct Base Deficit and Give Indicated Drugs.
1. Give $NaHCO_3$ (Sodium bicarbonate), 1 to 2 mEq/kg over 3 to 5 minutes. To infants under 5 Kg, give 3 to 4 ml of a 1 mEq/ml solution.
2. Repeat as needed according to arterial blood gas determinations (ABG's).
3. For neonates, dilute $NaHCO_3$ with equal amount of dextrose 5% in water because of high incidence of central nervous system bleeding if given undiluted.

SPECIFIC INTERVENTIONS FOR ARRHYTHMIAS _____

Asystole.
1. Epinephrine 1:10,000 (100 mEq/ml).
   a. Intravenous dosage:
      1) If infant is less than 4 kg., give 2 cc.
      2) Between 4 and 18 kg., give 3 cc.
      3) If child weighs more than 18 kg., give 4 cc.
2. Intracardiac injection of calcium gluconate (or gluceptate) is used as a last resort.
   a. Dose for intracardiac injection is 1 cc of a 10% solution.
   b. May damage coronary arteries.
3. Calcium gluconate (or gluceptate) 100 mg/kg IV to strengthen myocardium.
4. If no response, use temporary pacemaker.

Ventricular Fibrillation.
1. Defibrillate after acidosis is corrected.
   a. Neonate: 10 to 25 watt/sec.
   b. Infants: 25 to 50 watt/sec.
   c. Children (12 to 25 kg): 50 to 100 watt/sec.
   d. Older children (25 to 50 kg): 100 to 200 watt/sec.
2. If sinus rhythm is noted, check for effective beat. (Note pulses and correlate with heart sounds.)
   a. **Do not** take normal EKG tracing as evidence of ciculation.
   b. With sinus rhythm and weak, feeble pulse:
      1) Isoproterenol (Isuprel) 0.1 to 0.5 mcg/kg/min. by infusion pump (0.5 mg [2.5 ml] of 1:5000 solution in 100 ml of saline).
      2) Epinephrine 0.25–1 mcg/kg minute by infusion pump (under 5 kilograms, give 0.2 ml of 1:1000; for 5 kilograms and over, 0.25 ml/10 kg). This medication may be repeated two to three times at 5 to 10 minute intervals.[30]
      3) Calcium gluconate 10%: 20 mg/kg slowly, as an intravenous medication. (Under 5 kilograms, give 1.0 ml of a 10% solution. Over 5 kilograms, give 1.0 ml/10 kg.) May be repeated two to three times at 5 to 10 minute intervals.
3. If ventricular fibrillation continues, give another dose of $NaHCO_3$ and defibrillate again.
4. Multiple ectopic beats of variable form
   a. Lidocaine 1 mg/kg IV; repeat as needed.
      1) **Caution:** Excess lidocaine causes convulsions.
   b. If lidocaine is ineffective, give diphenylhydantoin (Dilantin), 2 to 5 mg/kg IV, **very slowly.**

Hypotension.
1. If not due to hypovolemia, give:
    a. Dopamine, 5 to 10 mcg/kg/min IV, diluted in solution and administered by a precision infusion pump,[30] or
    b. Levarterenol bitartrate (Levophed)/phentolamine (Regitine) drip, IV. Dosage will be individually calculated in every case because of size and variable blood pressure response.

BIBLIOGRAPHY

1. Agarwala, B., et al.: Congestive heart failure in the infant. Heart Lung, 5:63, 1976.
2. American Heart Association: A Manual for Instructors of Basic Cardiac Life Support. Dallas, American Heart Association, 1977.
3. Andreoli, K., et al,: Comprehensive Cardiac Care, 2nd ed. St. Louis, C. V. Mosby Co., 1971.
4. Argenta, Louis, et al.: A comparison of the hemodynamic effects of inotropic agents. Twelfth Annual Meeting of the Society of Thoracic Surgeons, Washington, D.C., 1976.
5. Bayer, L.: Children with Congenital Cardiac Defects. Springfield, Ill., Charles C Thomas, 1976.
6. Behrendt, D. and Austin, W.: Patient Care in Cardiac Surgery. Boston, Little, Brown & Co., 1972.
7. Benzing, G., et al.: The infant and child with cardiovascular disease: immediate post-operative care after cardiac surgery. Heart Lung, 3:415, 1974.
8. Brest, A., et al.: Congenital Heart Disease. Cardiovasc. Clin., 4, 1971.
9. Burch, G., A Primer of Cardiology, 4th ed. Philadelphia, Lea and Febiger, 1971.
10. Cooley, D., and Hallman, G.: Surgical Treatment of Congenital Heart Disease. Philadelphia, Lea and Febiger, 1966.
11. Csanady, M. and Kiss, Z.: Heritable Q-T prolongation without congenital deafness (Romano-Ward syndrome). Chest, 64:359, 1973.
12. Frater, R.: Post-operative care in the pediatric cardiology patient. Heart Lung, 3:903, 1974.
13. Guyton, A.: Function of the Human Body, 4th ed. Philadelphia, W. B. Saunders Co., 1974.
14. Hallman, G.: Surgical Treatment of Congenital Heart Disease. Philadelphia, Lea and Febiger, 1975.
15. Hanazgno, N., et al.: Heritable Q-T prolongation without deafness: the Romano-Ward syndrome. Jpn. Heart J., 14:479, 1973.
16. Hessel, E.: Surgical intervention in cardiac disease. Fourth Annual Symposium for Nurses, Washington State Heart Association, Inc., Seattle, 1971.
17. Hohn, A.: Basic Pediatric Electrocardiography. Baltimore, Williams & Wilkins, 1974.
18. James F., et al.: Congestive heart failure in infants and children. Heart Lung, 3:396, 1974.
19. Kaplan, S.: The infant and child with cardiovascular disease. Heart Lung, 3:390, 1974.
20. Karhunen, P., et al.: Syncope and Q-T prolongation without deafness: the Romano-Ward syndrome. Am. Heart J., 80:820, 1970.
21. Keith, J., et al.: Heart Disease in Infancy and Childhood, 2nd ed. New York, Macmillan, 1967.
22. Krovetz, L., et al.: Handbook of Pediatric Cardiology. New York, Harper & Row, 1969.
23. Montgomery, F.: Care of the patient with open heart surgery. In: Intensive Care Orientation Manual. Seattle,

Children's Orthopedic Hospital and Medical Center, 1978, pp. 122–135.

24. Nadas, A., and Fyler, D.: Pediatric Cardiology, 3rd ed. Philadelphia, W. B. Saunders Co., 1972.

25. Pascoe, D., et al.: Quick Reference to Pediatric Emergencies. Philadelphia, J. B. Lippincott Co., 1973.

26. Rydin, L., and Engle, M.: The infant with transposition of the great arteries. Cardiovascular Nursing, 9:27, 1973.

27. Sauvage, L., et al.: Physiologic classification of congenital heart disease. A.O.R.N. Journal, 18: 61, 1973.

28. Schwartz, D.: Cardiac catheterization in infants. Heart Lung, 3:407, 1974.

29. Schwartz, P., et al.: The long Q-T syndrome. Am. Heart J., 89:378, 1975.

30. Smith, C. (ed.): The Critically Ill Child: Diagnosis and Management, 2nd ed. Philadelphia, W. B. Saunders Co., 1977.

31. Stamm, S.: Pediatric Cardiopulmonary Handbook. Seattle, Children's Orthopedic Hospital and Medical Center, 1971.

32. Vincent, G., et al.: Q-T Interval Syndromes. Prog. Cardiovasc. Dis., 16:523, 1974.

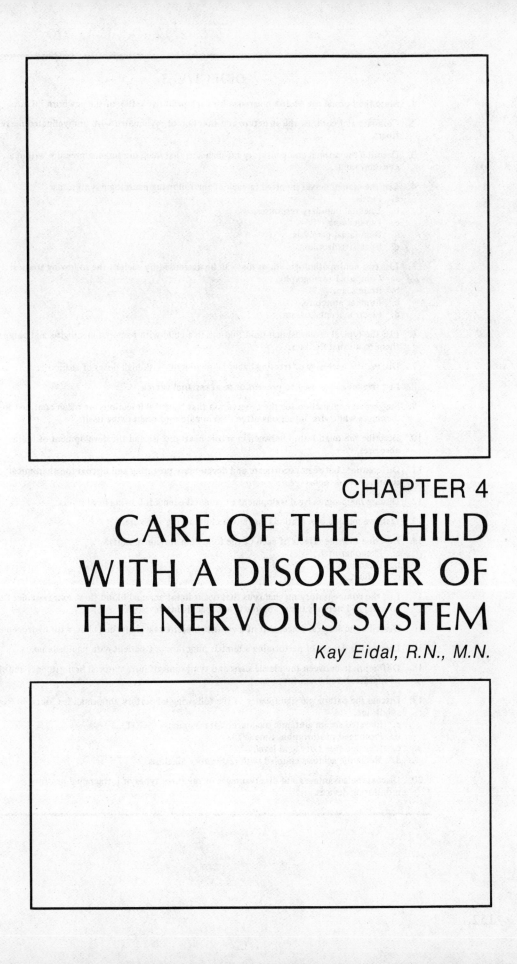

CHAPTER 4
CARE OF THE CHILD WITH A DISORDER OF THE NERVOUS SYSTEM

Kay Eidal, R.N., M.N.

OBJECTIVES

1. State the normal age of disappearance for each primitive reflex of the newborn infant.

2. Compare and contrast the structure and function of myelinated with unmyelinated nerve fibers.

3. Describe the normal compensatory mechanisms that keep intracranial pressure within a constant range.

4. List the cranial nerves involved in each of the following neurologic symptoms:
   a. Ptosis.
   b. Unequal pupillary responses.
   c. Papilledema.
   d. Hemifacial paralysis.
   e. Excessive drooling.

5. List two neuropathologic states that can be diagnosed by each of the following studies:
   a. Computed tomography.
   b. Brain scan.
   c. Lumbar puncture.
   d. Electroencephalogram.

6. List the typical cerebrospinal fluid findings in a child with bacterial meningitis and compare them to normal findings.

7. Discuss the necessity of treating bacterial meningitis with high doses of antibiotics.

8. List five measures used to prevent or treat cerebral edema.

9. Suggest an explanation for the observation that bacterial infections are often confined to the meninges while viral infections often disseminate into brain tissue itself.

10. Describe the relationship between cyanotic heart disease and the development of brain abscesses.

11. Differentiate between decorticate and decerebrate posturing and discuss the anatomical significance of each.

12. Discuss the progressive development of cerebral edema following head injury.

13. List five nursing observations made of a child having a seizure.

14. Describe the side effects of each of the following anticonvulsants:
    a. Phenobarbital.
    b. Dilantin.
    c. Valium.

15. List the compensatory mechanisms that occur in intracranial blood flow, extravascular fluid volume, and nervous tissue volume if hydrocephalus develops.

16. Describe the surgical placement of a ventriculoperitoneal shunt in a child with hydrocephalus.

17. Discuss the danger of performing a lumbar puncture in a patient with papilledema.

18. Differentiate between the classic signs and symptoms of infratentorial brain tumors and those of supratentorial brain tumors.

19. Discuss the pathologic significance of the following laboratory abnormalities found in Reye's syndrome:
    a. Elevated serum glutamic oxaloacetic transaminase (SGOT).
    b. Prolonged prothrombin time (PT).
    c. Elevated free fatty acid level.
    d. Metabolic acidosis coupled with respiratory alkalosis.

20. Discuss the advantages and disadvantages of the three types of intracranial pressure monitoring devices.

EVOLUTION OF CEREBRAL CORTICAL DOMINANCE _____

Structure and Functional State of Cerebral Cortex at Birth
1. Majority of neurons present.
2. White and gray matter of cortical hemispheres poorly differentiated.

Neurologic Functioning at Lower Levels of Central Nervous System at Birth
1. Primitive infant reflexes represent neuronal discharges from brain stem and spinal cord.
   a. Moro.
   b. Palmar and plantar grasp.
   c. Babinski.
   d. Stepping.
   e. Glabellar.
   f. Placing.
   g. Rooting.
   h. Sucking.
2. Primitive reflexes uninhibited by higher cerebral control.
3. Primitive reflexes are inhibited as higher centers begin to dominate.
   a. Disappearance occurs between 6 weeks and 2 years of age.

Development of Cerebral Cortical Dominace
1. Occurs in cephalo–caudal progression
   a. Hearing, seeing, and primitive motor skills are present at birth.
   b. Development of voluntary muscle control proceeds in the following order:
      1) Arms.
      2) Hands.
      3) Head.
      4) Legs.
      5) Bladder and bowel.
2. Ages associated with increased cortical development:
   a. 6 months: cortical development 50% complete.
   b. 2 years: cortical development 75% complete.
   c. 4 years: cortical development complete.

Central nervous system is particularly vulnerable during developmental process[1,28]

MYELINIZATION PROCESS _____

Degrees of Myelinization at Birth
1. Majority of nerve fibers are unmyelinated.

Anatomy and Physiology of Myelinization
1. Schwann cells envelop and rotate around neuronal axon, depositing myelin sheath.
   a. Myelin sheath forms multi-layered cell membrane.

2. Cell membrane contains sphingomyelin, a lipid substance.
   a. Sphingomyelin insulates cell and prevents ion flow.
3. Nodes of Ranvier: junctions between two Schwann cells.
   a. Nodes are uninsulated so ions can freely flow.
   b. Nodes are up to 500 times more permeable to ions than are unmyelinated nerve fibers.

Structure and Function in Myelinated and Unmyelinated Nerve Fibers
1. Myelinated fibers.
   a. Impulses conducted between nodes—process of saltatory conduction.
   b. Higher velocity of nerve transmission.
   c. Less metabolic energy required for ion transport.
   d. Larger in diameter.
2. Unmyelinated fibers.
   a. Impulses conducted continuously along fiber.
   b. Lower velocity of nerve transmission.
   c. Greater metabolic energy required for ion transport.
   d. Smaller in diameter.

Duration of Myelinization Process
1. Usually complete by 2 years of age.
2. Upon completion, ratio of myelinated to unmyelinated fibers is 2:1.[24]

CLOSURE OF CRANIAL SUTURES

Anatomical State of Sutures at Birth
1. Head circumference averages 34 to 35 cm.
2. Anterior fontanel measures 4 to 6 cm in each dimension.
3. Posterior fontanel measures 0.5 to 1 cm.

Progression of Suture Closure
1. Head circumference increases to 47 cm by first year and slowly to 50 cm by fifth year as cranial sutures close.
   a. Corresponds with brain growth.
2. Anterior fontanel decreases in size.
   a. Average age of complete closure is 18 months.
3. Posterior fontanel decreases in size.
   a. Average age of closure is 2 months.[10,45]

MECHANISMS FOR MAINTENANCE OF INTRACRANIAL PRESSURE

Normal Intracranial Pressure Range
1. 50 to 200 mm water.
2. 4 to 15 mm mercury.

Monro-Kellie Doctrine of Intracranial Pressure Compensation
1. Cranium is rigid and nondistensible (except in the infant).
2. Dynamic equilibrium exists between volumes of cerebral contents.
   a. Nervous tissue: volume constant.
   b. Circulating arterial and venous blood: volume variable.
   c. Cerebrospinal fluid: volume variable.
   d. Extravascular fluid in cerebral tissues: volume varible.
3. An increase or decrease in the amount of one volume must be compensated for by an equal and opposite decrease or increase in the remaining volumes.

Intracranial Autoregulation
1. Autoregulation is the automatic change in cerebral blood vessel diameter in order to maintain a constant intracranial blood flow during changes in perfusion pressure.
2. Cerebral blood perfusion pressure (CPP) equals mean arterial blood pressure minus the intracranial pressure.
   a. Normal CPP is 80 to 90 mm Hg in older children and adults, 60 to 70 mm Hg in infants and young children.
   b. Autoregulation maintains CPP at a constant level despite mean arterial pressure changes from 50 to 170 mm Hg.
3. As intracranial pressure approaches arterial blood pressure, the CPP becomes lower.
   a. Autoregulation is impaired when intracranial pressure rises to approximately 33 mm Hg (blood vessels no longer respond appropriately).
   b. Cerebral blood flow is diminished and hypoxia results.

Physiologic Factors Affecting Intracranial Pressure
1. Intra-abdominal pressure changes.
   a. Abdominal breathing.
   b. Abdominal distention.
2. Intrathoracic pressure changes.
   a. Coughing.
   b. Straining.
   c. Valsalva maneuver.
3. Chemical changes.
   a. PCO_2
      1) Elevated PCO_2 produces cerebral vasodilatation.
      2) Decreased PCO_2 produces cerebral vasoconstriction.
   b. PO_2
      1) Decreased PO_2 (hypoxemia) produces cerebral vasodilatation.
         a) Intracranial pressure can increase dramatically during intubation and airway suctioning.
4. Postural changes.
   a. Turning from side to side.
   b. Head rotation.[25,36]

HISTORY ————————————————————————————

Sources of Information
1. Child himself.
2. Parents.
3. Referral records.
4. Siblings and relatives.
5. Other child caregivers (i.e., babysitter).

Components of a Pediatric Neurologic History.
1. Chief complaint and presenting symptoms.
2. Previous medical history.
3. Family medical history.
4. Natal history.
5. Child's growth and development.
6. Child's immunization status.
7. Medication history, including allergies.
8. Evolution of present illness.

PEDIATRIC NEUROLOGIC EXAMINATION –
RECOMMENDED SEQUENCE ————————————————

General Guidelines in Performing Neurologic Examinations in Children
1. Child's age, culture, and fear may interfere with complete neurologic examination.
2. Observation alone yields valuable neurologic data about children.
3. Incorporating play into neurologic examination techniques often elicits better cooperation from child.

Observation of General Neurologic Functioning (Behavior and Mental Status)
1. Social affect.
2. Level of activity.
3. Attention span.
4. Mood.
5. Appropriateness of responses.
6. Language ability.
   a. Expressive language (talking).
   b. Receptive language (understanding).
7. Hand dominance.
   a. Usually established by 3 years of age.
8. Memory.
   a. Ability to repeat list of 4 to 5 items.
   b. Recall of recent or remote events.

9. Reading and writing ability.
   a. School-aged children.
10. Level of consciousness.
    a. General state (alert, stuporous, comatose).
    b. Orientation to person, place, and time in older children.

Physical and Growth Parameters
1. Height and weight.
2. Head and chest circumference.
3. Vital signs, including blood pressure.

Cranial Nerve Assessment
1. Olfactory nerve (I).
   a. Ability to identify familiar odors. For infants, test with whiff of alcohol swab.
   b. Presence of rhinorrhea, nasal polyps, or adenohypertrophy can influence response.
2. Optic nerve (II).
   a. Vision testing.
      1) Infants: ability to focus on small objects.
      2) Preschoolers: Snellen picture chart.
      3) School age: Snellen letter charts.
   b. Visual fields.
   c. Funduscopic examination of optic disc and vessels.
3. Oculomotor nerve (III).
   a. Pupillary size, shape, equality, and accommodation.
   b. Normal and equal elevation of eyelids.
   c. Ability of muscles to maintain eye to central position.
4. Trochlear nerve (IV).
   a. Ability to move eye downward and laterally.
5. Trigeminal nerve (V).
   a. Intactness of facial sensation except for mandibular area.
      1) Ability to sense pain and light touch.
   b. Presence of corneal reflex.
   c. Maintenance of jaw in correct alignment.
6. Abducent nerve (VI).
   a. Ability to abduct eye laterally.
7. Facial nerve (VII).
   a. Tone of facial muscles.
   b. Ability to imitate frowning, smiling, raising eyebrows, baring teeth.
   c. Facial symmetry.
   d. Presence of lacrimation and salivation.
   e. Taste identification on anterior portion of tongue.
8. Acoustic nerve (VIII).
   a. Auditory divisions (cochlear).
      1) Responses of child to a watch, rubbing or snapping fingers, crinkling paper.
      2) Older children can be asked to repeat whispered words.
      3) Bone and air conduction with tuning fork.

  b. Vestibular.
   1) Oculocephalic (doll's eye) and caloric reflexes.
    a) Used to test for intactness of vestibular function in comatose patients.
    b) Normal response depends on grossly normal rostrocaudal pathways.
    c) Abnormal responses not confined exclusively to vestibular pathology.
   2) Absence of nystagmus.
 9. Glossopharyngeal (IX) and vagus (X) nerves.
  a. Gag and swallowing reflexes.
  b. Symmetrical retraction of soft palate.
  c. Clear phonation without hoarseness or aphonia.
  d. Absence of drooling or pooling of secretions in mouth.
10. Spinal accessory nerve (XI).
  a. Ability to rotate head without weakness.
  b. Ability to elevate shoulders symmetrically.
  c. Tone of sternocleidomastoid and trapezius muscles.
11. Hypoglossal nerve (XII).
  a. Ability to protrude tongue.
  b. Absence of tongue atrophy or tremor.

Reflex Assessment

1. Stretch reflexes.
  a. Represent intactness of reflex arcs.
  b. Promote relaxation in children by distraction.
2. Primitive central nervous system reflexes as described in section on anatomy and physiology.

Signs of Meningeal Irritation

1. Nuchal rigidity.
2. Brudzinski sign.
3. Kernig sign.
4. Irritability.
5. Fever.

Sensory Functions

1. Proprioception of position of body part.
2. Identification of objects placed in hand while eyes are closed.
3. Response to pain.

Motor Performance

1. Fine motor coordination.
  a. Pincer grasp.
  b. Manipulation of toys.
  c. Ability to draw.
2. Muscle tone.
  a. Absence of atonia or rigidity.
3. Gross motor coordination.
  a. Posture.
  b. Rolling over.
  c. Crawling.

      d. Standing.

      e. Walking.

      f. Bending.

      g. Running.

      h. Absence of ataxia.

4. Observation of involuntary movements.

      a. Tremors.

      b. Chorea.

      c. Athetosis.

      d. Dystonia.

Cerebellar Functions

1. Running in place.

2. Romberg sign.

3. Heel-to-toe walk.

4. Finger to nose with eyes closed.

5. Rapidly alternating movements.

      a. Pat knees.

      b. Pronate and supinate hands.

      c. Twist hands.[8,10,13,45]

LABORATORY STUDIES

Blood

1. Chemistry.

      a. Arterial blood gases.

      b. Ammonia.

      c. Glucose.

      d. Serum glutamic oxaloacetic transaminase (SGOT).

      e. Creatine phosphokinase (CPK).

      f. Amylase.

      g. Osmolality.

      h. Blood urea nitrogen (BUN).

      i. Free fatty acids.

      j. Uric acid.

2. Hematology.

      a. Complete blood count (CBC).

      b. Clotting times.

Cerebrospinal fluid

1. Gross appearance.

2. Protein.

3. Glucose.

4. Cells.

5. Bacteria.

Urine

1. Routine urinalysis.

2. Glucose.

3. Protein.
4. Ketones.
5. Cells.
6. Uric acid.
7. Specific gravity.
8. Osmolality.

Rhinorrhea and Otorrhea
1. Glucose.

DIAGNOSTIC STUDIES

1. Computed tomography (CT).[12,23]
2. Lumbar puncture.[5,45]
3. Electroencephalography.[21,42]
4. Skull films:[45] ⎫
5. Brain scan:[34,35] ⎬ less used since the advent
6. Electromyelography:[45] ⎬ of computed tomography.
7. Echoencephalography: ⎭
8. Cerebral angiography: ⎫
9. Pneumoencephalography: ⎬ of limited use in pediatrics.[17,30,45]
10. Ventriculography: ⎭

OTHER NEURODIAGNOSTIC TESTS

1. Subdural taps.
2. Ventricular taps.
3. Transillumination.[45]

PATHOLOGIC CONDITIONS

CENTRAL NERVOUS SYSTEM INFECTIONS

MENINGITIS

Etiology and Routes of Infection
1. General.
   a. Most common mode is indirect entry following microorganism dissemination from distant site of infection.
      1) Septicemia usually present.
      2) Blood cultures yield offending organism.

   b. Direct invasion of meninges.
      1) Otitis media.
      2) Upper respiratory infection.
   c. Direct invasion following head trauma.
   d. Direct invasion via congenital sinus tracts.
      1) Myelomeningocele.
2. Pathogens responsible for meningitis.
   a. Bacterial.
      1) *Escherichia coli:* most common organism in neonatal meningitis.
      2) *Hemophilus influenzae:* ⎫ ⎧ Responsible for 95% of
      3) *Streptococcus pneumoniae:* ⎬ ⎨ cases in children over
      4) *Neisseria meningitidis:* ⎭ ⎩ 2 months of age.[19]
   b. Viral: less common pathogens.
      1) Coxsackie
      2) Polio ⎫ ⎧ Common pathogens in viral meningitis;
      3) ECHO virus ⎭ ⎩ uncommon cause of encephalitis
      4) Mumps
      5) Herpes simplex

Pathologic Progession of Untreated Meningitis

1. Infecting organism enters subarachnoid space through altered blood-brain barrier.
2. Inflammatory cells invade meninges, producing meningeal irritation.
3. Further progression leads to infection of underlying brain structures and brain cell destruction (meningoencephalitis).
4. Purulent exudate collects around base of brain.
5. Cranial nerve palsies result.
6. Cerebrospinal fluid circulation becomes obstructed.
7. Hydrocephalus develops.

Clinical Presentation

1. General signs and symptoms.
   a. Nuchal rigidity.
   b. Positive Kernig and Brudzinski signs.
   c. Petechiae or purpura, usually seen with meningococcal meningitis.
2. Signs and symptoms in infants.
   a. Fever.
   b. High-pitched cry.
   c. Irritability.
   d. Poor feeding.
   e. Vomiting.
   f. Bulging anterior fontanel.
   g. Decreased level of consciousness.
   h. Seizures.
3. Signs and symptoms in older children.
   a. Fever.
   b. Headache.

      c. Vomiting.

      d. Cranial bruits.

      e. Decreased level of consciousness.

      f. Seizures.

      g. Coma and shock.

      h. Photophobia.

4. Laboratory findings.

    a. Cerebrospinal fluid.

      1) Bacterial.

        a) Elevated cell count with a predominance of polymorphonuclear leukocytes.

        b) Elevated protein.

        c) Decreased glucose.

        d) Culture positive for infecting organism.

      2) Viral.

        a) Elevated cell count with a predominance of mononuclear cells.

        b) Elevated protein.

        c) Normal glucose.

        d) Negative bacterial culture; positive viral culture requires approximately 14 days to document.

    b. Blood.

      1) Culture positive for infecting organism in 50% of cases of bacterial meningitis.

      2) Elevated white blood cell count in bacterial disease.

      3) Decreased serum sodium may indicate inappropriate ADH secretion.

      4) Serum osmolality less than 280 mOsm/l also indicates inappropriate antidiuretic hormone (ADH) secretion.

      5) Hyperglycemia and elevated uric acid levels indicate stress response and cellular destruction, respectively.

    c. Urine.

      1) Elevated uric acid if cell destruction is pronounced.

      2) Glycosuria, ketonuria, or proteinuria reflect hormonal response to stress.

      3) Elevated urine sodium, osmolality, and specific gravity if inappropriate ADH secretion is present.

Objectives of Therapy

1. Early diagnosis.

2. Reduction of morbidity and mortality.

Therapeutic Interventions

1. Establish and maintain a patent airway and adequate ventilation.

    a. Monitor arterial blood gases frequently.

    b. Suction as needed, judiciously.

      1) Hyperventilate with 100% oxygen before and during procedure.

      2) Hypoxia from suctioning can elevate intracranial pressure.

    c.   Alter patient's position frequently.

    d.   Intubation and assisted ventilation if necessary.

        1) Control ventilation to keep arterial PCO_2 above 25 but below 30 mm Hg.

           a) Mild respiratory alkalosis is desired.

           b) Hyperventilation is an appropriate means of achieving desired PCO_2 levels.

        2) Minimal PEEP can be applied.

           a) Excessive amounts can inhibit cardiac return, increase cerebral blood flow, and promote venous congestion.

           b) Monitor child closely for development of pneumothorax.

        3) Monitor ventilator pressures closely.

           a) Pressure elevation indicates airway resistance, which will increase intracranial pressure.

        4) Administer modified chest physiotherapy.

           a) Head must remain elevated.

           b) Vibration *only* often produces less stress.

2. Administer high doses of antibiotics intravenously, based on cerebrospinal fluid culture and sensitivity test results (for bacterial organisms only).

    a.   Duration of antibiotic therapy ranges from 10 to 21 days.

    b.   Drugs of choice:

        1) Ampicillin 300 to 400 mg/kg body weight/day for sensitive organisms.

        2) Chloramphenicol 100 mg/kg body weight/day for Ampicillin-resistant organisms.

        3) Penicillin G, 200,000 to 400,000 units/kg/day for streptococcal disease.

    c.   Lumbar puncture may be repeated during treatment course to ascertain antibiotic effectiveness or if clinical improvement has been negligible.

3. Prevent, monitor, and treat cerebral edema and increased intracranial pressure.

    a.   Frequent and continuous assessment of neurologic status.

        1) Level of consciousness.

        2) Pupillary responses.

        3) Equality of movement and strength of extremities.

        4) Cranial nerve assessment.

        5) Fontanel tension in infants.

        6) Intake and output.

    b.   Restrict fluids to decrease volume of fluid in brain cells (1/2 to 2/3 of maintenance level).

    c.   Hyperventilate to control PCO_2 levels to between 25 and 30 mm Hg.

    d.   Elevate head of bed 30 degrees.

    e.   Administer osmotic diuretics if intracranial pressure remains elevated.

1) Effect is temporary, begins in minutes and lasts 6 to 12 hours
2) Dosages:
   a) Mannitol: 0.25 to 1.0 gm/kg.
   b) Urea: 0.5 to 1 gm/kg.
   c) Lasix (doses are largely variable).
3) Administer preferably through central line, as peripheral sloughing can occur.
  f. Administer steroids (usually Decadron).
   1) Effect on cerebral edema is unclear.
  g. Place intracranial monitoring device if warranted.[8]
  h. If intracranial pressure rises suddenly (as noted on monitoring device):
   1) Hyperventilate with 100% oxygen.
   2) Suction only if needed.
   3) Administer diuretics if elevation persists.
  i. Prevent patient straining.

4. Implement more drastic measures for refractory elevations in intracranial pressure.
  a. Sedate patient with barbiturates or anesthetic agents.
  b. Utilize hypothermia measures to lower body temperature to 30°C.
  c. Paralyze with a neuromuscular blocking agent (e.g., Pavulon).
  d. Drain off small amounts of cerebrospinal fluid if intraventricular monitoring device is in place.
  e. Bilaterial craniectomies may be performed as a last resort.

5. Control seizures if present.
  a. Administer anticonvulsant drugs.
  b. Protect patient from injury during seizure attack.
  c. Control hyperthermia.

6. Monitor and treat hyperpyrexia.
  a. Frequent temperature.
  b. Antipyrexic drugs.
  c. Tepid sponges if fever unresponsive to drugs.
  d. Hypothermia mattress if the first two measures fail.

7. Monitor specific gravity of urine.

8. Monitor patient closely for complications.
  a. Measure head circumference daily in children 2 years old or younger.
  b. Monitor serum electrolytes and osmolality.
  c. Monitor urine electrolytes, osmolality, and specific gravity.
  d. Accurate intake, output, and daily weights.

9. Provide emotional support to the child and his family.
  a. Allow parental contact as often as possible.
  b. Provide child with quiet environment and minimal stimulation.
  c. Maintain a realistic approach to both child and parent.

10. Plan for patient rehabilitation.
    a. Physical therapy for motor deficits.
    b. Periodic developmental and psychometric evaluation of deficits.

Complications
1. Acute.
   a. Inappropriate ADH secretion (common).
   b. Reinfection.
   c. Subdural effusion.
   d. Brain abscess.
   e. Sinusitis or mastoiditis.
   f. Hydrocephalus.
   g. Diffuse intravascular coagulation (disseminated intravascular coagulation—DIC).
   h. Coma.
   i. Death.
2. Long term sequelae.
   a. Hemiparesis.
   b. Cerebellar ataxia.
   c. Decreased IQ or other psychometric and behavioral deficits.
   d. Hearing loss.
   e. Visual deficits.
   f. Seizures.

Nursing Skills
1. Respiratory therapy.
   a. Oxygen administration.
   b. Ventilator management.
   c. Suctioning.
   d. Blood gas analysis.
   e. Chest physiotherapy.
   f. Positioning.
   g. Use of Ambu-bag.
2. Drug administration.
   a. Antibiotics.
   b. Osmotic diuretics.
   c. Steroids.
3. Intravenous fluid management.
4. Laboratory test interpretation.
5. Neurologic assessment.
   a. History and physical exam.
   b. Neurologic checks.
6. Vital sign monitoring.
   a. Intracranial pressure monitoring.
   b. Central venous pressure monitoring.
   c. Temperature monitoring and control.
   d. Cardiac rhythm interpretation.

7. Psychologic techniques.
    a. Communication.
    b. Patient and family education.
8. Emergency measures.
    a. Cardiopulmonary resuscitation.
    b. Defibrillation.[7,19,40,45]

ENCEPHALITIS

Etiology and Routes of Infection
1. General.
    a. Neural spread via peripheral nerves.
    b. Viremia.
    c. Penetration across olfactory mucosa.
2. Virology.
    a. Herpes simplex: } } Most commonly cause
    b. Arthropod-borne viruses: } } encephalitis.
    c. Mumps.
    d. Polio.
    e. Rabies.
    f. Coxsackie A and B.

Pathophysiologic Description
1. Viral or rickettsial infection involving the substance of the brain itself.
    a. These organisms demonstrate a predilection for neuronal cells themselves.
        1) Different organisms select certain types of brain tissue.
    b. Bacterial organisms are generally confined either to the subarachnoid space or to localized regions of cerebral tissue; therefore bacterial organisms are not usually involved in diffuse brain tissue infection.
2. Associated with greater morbidity and mortality than is bacterial meningitis.

Clinical Presentation
1. Signs and symptoms.
    a. Signs of meningeal irritation (see meningitis).
    b. Decreased level of consciousness.
    c. Seizures are more prevalent than in meningitis.
    d. Focal neurologic deficits.
    e. Signs of increased intracranial pressure.
        1) Cranial nerve dysfunction.
        2) Bulging fontanel in infants.
        3) Hemiparesis or hemiplegia.
        4) Abnormal posturing.
    f. Fever may or may not be present.
2. Laboratory findings.
    a. Cerebrospinal fluid.
        1) Viral study necessary for identification of organism.

      2) Normal to slightly elevated protein.

      3) Normal to moderately elevated pressure.

      4) Five to a few hundred cells with predominance of lymphocytes and polymorphonuclear leukocytes.

      5) Normal glucose.

   b. Viral cultures of blood, throat washings, and stool may yield infecting virus.

Objectives of Therapy

1. Supportive therapy.
2. Reduction of disability and death.

Therapeutic Interventions

1. Same as for meningitis.
2. Antibiotic therapy not beneficial in most instances.
3. Use vidarabine (ara-A) for herpes encephalitis.

Complications

1. Inappropriate ADH secretion.
2. Hydrocephalus.
3. Hemiparesis or hemiplegia.
4. Mental retardation.
5. Hearing loss.
6. Seizures.
7. Focal or sensory deficits.
8. Death.

Nursing Skills

1. Same as for meningitis without administration of antibiotics.
2. Intracranial pressure monitoring.[2,45]

LOCALIZED PYOGENIC INFECTIONS

Etiology and Predisposing Factors

1. Most common organisms implicated:
   a. *Staphylococcus aureus.*
   b. Non-group A or anaerobic streptococci.
   c. Mixed types of organisms or multiple bacteria.
2. Cerebral abscess.
   a. Cyanotic heart disease is common cause.
      1) Blood shunted from right to left bypasses lungs, which ordinarily serve to filter organisms.
   b. Acute and chronic otitis media and mastoiditis.
   c. Sepsis.
   d. Post-traumatic or surgical penetration.
   e. Pulmonary infections.
3. Subdural empyema.
   a. Chronic paranasal sinus infection.
   b. Postoperative infections or penetrating wounds.
   c. Bacteremia.
   d. Chronic otitis media or mastoiditis.
   e. Rupture of cerebral abscess.

    4. Epidural empyema (cerebral).
- a. Mastoiditis.
- b. Sinus infection.
- c. Osteomyelitis of the skull.
- d. Skull fracture.
- e. Postoperative infection.

Pathophysiology
1. Description.
   - a. Localized collections of pus in various locations within the cranium.
   - b. May be of sufficient size to cause increased intracranial pressure and focal deficits.
2. Classification.
   - a. Cerebral abscess.
     1) Local collection of pus within the substance of the brain itself.
     2) Fibrous capsule eventually forms around abscess.
     3) Single abscesses more common than multiple lesions.
     4) Frontal and parietal lobes are most common sites of abscess formation.
   - b. Subdural empyema.
     1) Pyogenic infection in the potential space between the dura and the arachnoid.
     2) Pus spreads rapidly over cerebral hemispheres, resulting in progressive increased intracranial pressure.
   - c. Epidural empyema (cerebral).
     1) Pyogenic infection in the space between the dura and bone of the cranium.
     2) Expansion is limited by close adherence of dura and bone.
     3) Usually presents with osteomyelitis of adjacent bone.

Clinical Presentation
1. Signs and symptoms.
   - a. Cerebral abscess (presents as a mass lesion).
     1) Headache.
     2) Nausea and vomiting.
     3) Lethargy or obtundation.
     4) Low-grade fever.
     5) Papilledema.
     6) Focal neurologic symptoms resembling those of stroke.
   - b. Subdural empyema.
     1) Swelling and erythema of overlying tissues.
     2) Headache is severe.
     3) Fever.
     4) Vomiting.
     5) Nuchal rigidity.

      6) Progressive obtundation.

      7) Local or generalized seizures and hemiparesis.

   c. Epidural abscess (cerebral).

      1) Fever.

      2) Pain and tenderness over affected area.

      3) Local neurologic signs or increased intracranial pressure are rarely manifested.

2. Laboratory findings.

   a. Cerebral abscess.

      1) CT scan shows cystic lesion with a dense rim.

      2) Increased uptake on brain scan to correspond with abscess capsule.

      3) Electroencephalogram shows slow wave focus in area of abscess.

      4) Cerebral angiography shows an avascular mass initially and a fine, ring-shaped stain later.

      5) Lumbar puncture is hazardous in the presence of papilledema, and findings are not definitive.

   b. Subdural empyema.

      1) Cerebral angiography and CT scan show mass overlying cerebral hemisphere and midline shift of cerebral structures.

      2) Cerebrospinal fluid has elevated pressure, a large population of neutrophils, normal glucose levels, and possibly infecting organisms.

   c. Epidural empyema (cerebral).

      1) Cerebrospinal fluid contains few lymphocytes and is sterile, and glucose concentration is normal.

Objectives of Therapy

1. Early recognition of disease.
2. Reduction of overall virulence.
3. Reduction of morbidity and mortality.

Therapeutic Interventions

1. Establish and maintain a patent airway and adequate ventilation (same measures as for meningitis).
2. Establish an early diagnosis.

   a. Consider intracranial pyogenic disease if history of infection is combined with neurologic signs and symptoms.

   b. Follow up on neurologic infectious diseases that fail to respond to therapy.

   c. Use appropriate diagnostic measures as described for differential diagnosis.

3. Surgically eradicate the infectious process.

   a. Surgical excision of cerebral abscess.

      1) Aspiration or surgical drainage via burr holes less effective.

   b. Surgical drainage of subdural and epidural empyemas.

   c. Instillation of antibiotics based upon organism sensitivity.

4. Administer high doses of broad-spectrum antibiotics.
   a. Chloramphenicol: ⎫ ⎧ Effective for penetration of
   b. Methicillin: ⎬ ⎨ blood-brain barrier and
   c. Penicillin: ⎭ ⎩ abscess capsules.
   d. Nafcillin: poor penetration into abscesses.
5. Monitor and treat cerebral edema and increased intracranial pressure if present.
   a. Same measures as for meningitis.

Complications

1. Cerebral abscess.
   a. Seizures.
   b. Extension of infection to surrounding brain tissue (especially if needle aspiration of abscess is employed).
   c. Continued hemiparesis
   d. Profound but usually temporary speech disturbances.
   e. Postinfection hydrocephalus.
   f. Death occurs in approximately 40% of cases.[40]
2. Subdural empyema.
   a. Diffuse pyogenic involvement of subarachnoid space and cerebral hemispheres.
   b. Cortical vein thrombosis.
   c. Infarction of cerebral tissue.
   d. Death.
3. Epidural empyema (cerebral).
   a. Epidural granuloma or abscess.
   b. Cranial nerve palsies.

Nursing Skills

1. Same as for meningitis.[4,7,40,49]

HEAD TRAUMA

General Classification and Etiology

1. Closed compression.
   a. Trauma inflicted on an immobile skull.
2. Closed acceleration.
   a. Intracranial contents move within skull in response to force.
   b. Significant brain distortion occurs.
      1) Bruising or laceration of brain.
      2) Vascular tearing from shearing force.
      3) Separation of long processes of nerve tracts from their cell bodies.
3. Open head trauma.
   a. Sharp object penetrates skull and disrupts underlying brain tissues.

Pathophysiology and Clinical Syndromes
1. Concussion.
   a. Head injury followed by temporary and reversible loss of consciousness.
      1) Hypothesis: sensory-evoked responses are interrupted.
   b. Usually follows blunt trauma.
   c. Not usually associated with pathologic changes in the brain.
      1) Severance of intracranial vessels and distortion of structures are possible.
2. Skull fracture.
   a. Denotes a break in the calvarium.
   b. Usually associated with communication between external and interior skull.
      1) Risk of infection is great.
   c. Types of skull fractures:
      1) Depressed.
      2) Linear.
      3) Stellate.
3. Contusion and laceration.
   a. Definitions:
      1) Contusion: bruising of brain tissue.
      2) Laceration: tearing of brain tissue and meninges.
   b. Bruised, torn, twisted or sheared brain tissue results in microscopic intracranial hemorrhages.
   c. Usually located directly below site of impact.
   d. Cerebral edema develops rapidly in response to:
      1) Trauma itself.
      2) Intracranial hemorrhages.
   e. Cerebral edema leads to brain compression.
4. Epidural and subdural hematomas.
   a. Result from arterial and venous vascular damage, respectively.
   b. See section on intracranial hemorrhages (p. 187).
5. Primary pathophysiologic response to trauma is cerebral edema.
   a. Cerebral edema is vasculogenic (increased cerebral capillary permeability).
      1) Hypothesis: cellular damage produces alterations in blood-brain barrier, allowing increased entry of osmotically active particles into the brain.
   b. Extent of cerebral edema dependent upon:
      1) Level of systolic blood pressure.
      2) Duration of vascular injury and increased blood-brain permeability.
      3) Extent of injured tissue.
   c. Cerebral edema acts as a mass lesion that decreases cerebral blood flow as intracranial pressure rises.
   d. Compensatory mechanisms in response to cerebral edema:
      1) Venous collapse.

        2) Cerebrospinal fluid is displaced from cranium.

        3) Cerebral arteries dilate or constrict in response to arterial blood gas partial pressures.

    e. Continued inability to compensate results in:

        1) Continuously increasing intracranial pressure.

        2) Vasomotor paralysis of cerebral vessels.

            a) Normal response to arterial blood gases (PCO_2 and PO_2) is lost.

        3) Cessation of cerebral blood flow when intracranial pressure equals systolic arterial blood pressure.

Clinical Presentation

  1. History:

    a. Nature of accident.

    b. Exact time of accident.

    c. Duration of unconsciousness is clue to severity of injury.

  2. Signs, symptoms, and diagnostic findings in concussion:

    a. Immediate but transient period of unconsciousness.

    b. Short-term impairment of higher faculties.

        1) Symptoms usually disappear in 48 hours.

    c. Transient vomiting.

    d. Post-traumatic amnesia.

    e. Complete recovery.

        1) Amnesia surrounding incident usually persists.

    f. CT scan and skull films are normal.

  3. Signs, symptoms, and diagnostic findings in contusion and laceration:

    a. Coma usually present but may vary in degree.

    b. Cushing triad (reflects increased intracranial pressure):

        1) Respiratory irregularities or arrest.

        2) Bradycardia.

        3) Hypertension.

    c. General and focal neurologic signs are related to extent and location of damage and to subsequent cerebral edema:

        1) Seizures.

        2) Cranial nerve dysfunction and palsies.

        3) Normal or abnormal pupillary response.

        4) Positive Babinski response with diffuse cortical damage.

        5) Presence or absence of oculocephalic (doll's eye) response— in comatose patients only.

            a) Positive response is normal and indicates intact vestibular function and rostrocaudal white matter tract.

        6) Hemiparesis of hemiplegia.

        7) Posturing abnormalities.

            a) Decorticate (arms and legs flexed on or toward chest; legs hyperextended.

            b) Decerebrate (all extremities hyperextended).

        8) Papilledema and retinal hemorrhages if cerebral edema is severe.

      9) Computed tomogram indicates intracranial bleeding
and cerebral edema.
    10) Skull films indicate:
      a) Bony fractures.
      b) Indriven splinters of bone and debris (glass).
    11) Cerebral angiogram indicates:
      a) Diverted or disrupted blood vessel pattern.
      b) Differentiation between extradural and intracerebral
hematomas.
    12) Electroencephalogram indicates focal brain abnormalities
and documents seizure foci.
    13) Lumbar punctures are hazardous and of little diagnostic
value.
4. Signs, symptoms, and diagnostic findings in skull fractures:
  a. Interruption in bony structures of the cranium, revealed by
examination or x-ray film (bony fracture or depression).
  b. Otorrhea or rhinorrhea.
    1) Indicative of cerebrospinal fluid leak.
  c. Fever (reflective of meningitis).
  d. Nuchal rigidity.
  e. If cerebral edema or damage to underlying brain tissue is
extensive, the signs, symptoms, and diagnostic findings of
contusion and laceration are manifested.

Objectives of Therapy
1. Reduce mortality.
2. Minimize complications of sepsis, cerebral edema, immobilization.
3. Initiate early rehabilitation focused toward a pretrauma status.

Therapeutic Interventions
1. Same as meningitis, with the following additions.
2. Intubation or tracheostomy for long-term ventilatory assistance.
3. Maintain unconscious patients in semiprone position.
4. Control intracranial bleeding prior to surgical repair.
  a. Controlled hypotension via barbiturates.
5. Keep patient NPO until fully conscious.
6. Monitor reflexes in comatose patients:
  a. Oculocephalic.
  b. Caloric.
  c. Babinski.
  d. Pupillary response.
  e. Response to pain.
  f. Corneal reflex.
7. Check otorrhea or rhinorrhea for glucose to determine whether
drainage is cerebrospinal fluid.
  a. Cerebrospinal fluid will be positive for glucose.
8. Intracranial pressure monitoring.
9. Employ corrective surgical measures.
  a. Evacuate subdural hematomas via subdural tap or burr holes.
  b. Debride compound fractures and remove foreign material.

      c. Elevate depressed skull fractures.

      d. Surgically evacuate intracerebral hematomas.

      e. Repair sources of otorrhea or rhinorrhea.

10. Clean and dress abrasions and apply antibacterial ointment.

11. Provide for adequate nutritional status of the patient if coma persists.

      a. Tube feedings.

      b. Hyperalimentation.

      c. Monitor daily weights.

12. Prevent complications of immobility.

      a. Reposition every 1 to 2 hours.

      b. Suction.

      c. Chest physiotherapy.

      d. Passive range of motion to extremities (cautiously if decerebration is present).

      e. Good skin care.

      f. "Egg carton" mattress.

13. Obtain cervical spine x-rays to rule out fractures or dislocations.

Complications

1. Cranial nerve injury.
2. Post-traumatic seizures.
3. Diabetes insipidus.
4. Defects in remote memory.
5. Cervical spine strains, sprains, dislocations, and fractures.

Nursing Skills

1. Same as those for meningitis with the following additions.
2. Intracranial pressure monitoring.
3. Tracheostomy care.
4. Range of motion exercises.[16,20,26,38,44]

SEIZURE DISORDERS

Etiology and Precipitating Factors in Children

1. Pathologic:

      a. Hypoxia.

      b. Cerebral trauma.

      c. High fever.

      d. Genetic transmission (evidence inconclusive).

      e. Perinatal injuries and birth trauma.

      f. Brain tumors.

      g. Arteriovenous malformations.

      h. Subdural hematomas.

      i. Metabolic disorders.

      j. Central nervous system infections.

      k. Lead poisoning.

      l. Idiopathic causes.

2. Nonpathologic:
   a. Sleep deprivation.
   b. Overhydration.
   c. Antihistamine drugs.
   d. Oversedation.
   e. Emotional upset.
   f. Acute alcohol intoxication.
   g. Drug abuse.

Pathophysiology
1. Descriptions:
   a. Recurrent or paroxysmal attacks of altered consciousness, usually accompanied by a series of tonic or clonic muscle spasms or other abnormal behaviors.
   b. Seizures result from abnormal electrical discharges in diseased neuronal cells of cerebral cortex and possibly of brainstem.
      1) Altered action potentials in damaged cells result in increased energy release.
      2) Normal activity of neighboring neuronal cells is altered by increased energy.
   c. Properties of epileptic cells:
      1) Variable transmembrane potentials.
      2) Chaotic electrical transmission.
   d. Variations in epileptic propensity occur in cortex, which increases or decreases the likelihood of developing seizures.
      1) Frontal and occipital regions have low epileptic propensity.
      2) Central, medial, and temporal regions of cerebral hemispheres have high epileptic propensity.
   e. Extent of seizures depends upon location and extent of abnormal neuronal discharge.
2. Seizure classification in children:
   a. Partial (beginning focally):
      1) Temporal lobe (sensory).
      2) Motor (Jacksonian).
      3) Psychomotor (complex symptomatology).
      4) Secondarily generalized (generalized seizures with focal onset).
   b. Generalized (without focal onset):
      1) Major motor:
         a) Grand mal.
         b) Tonic.
         c) Clonic.
      2) Absence (petit mal).
      3) Minor motor:
         a) Infantile spasms.
         b) Atonic/akinetic.
         c) Myoclonic.

Diagnostic Findings in Seizure Disorders
1. CT scan.
   a. Localizes some pathologic causes (tumor, A-V malformation).
   b. Documents spike waves and other abnormal impulse patterns.
2. Lumbar puncture.
   a. Not routine in seizure patients.
   b. Helpful in the diagnosis of seizures associated with lead poisoning or central nervous system infections.
3. Blood chemistry evaluation.
   a. May suggest metabolic etiology (especially Na^+, Ca^+, and glucose levels).
4. Serum drug levels.
   a. May indicate inappropriate therapeutic levels of anticonvulsants.

Objectives of Therapy
1. Complete seizure control.
2. Prevention of further cortical damage.

Therapeutic Interventions
1. Establish and maintain a patent airway and adequate ventilation.
   a. Loosen clothing around neck.
   b. Position patient on abdomen or side to prevent aspiration of pooled secretions and vomitus.
   c. Suction.
   d. Administer oxygen if cyanosis develops or seizure is prolonged.
   e. Treat pulmonary infection if aspiration does occur.
   f. Apnea or respiratory depression secondary to anticonvulsants can occur:
      1) Intubation and assisted ventilation may be necessary.
      2) Clenched teeth may make intubation difficult (child may require temporary neuromuscular paralysis).
2. Observe and record seizure characteristics.
   a. Precipitating events if evident.
   b. Presence or absence of aura.
   c. Loss of consciousness.
   d. Specific body parts involved.
      1) Jerking or deviation of eyes.
      2) Muscle groups involved and progression of seizure.
      3) Tonic or clonic movements.
   e. Respiratory changes.
   f. Incontinence.
   g. Postictal state.
   h. Duration and frequency of seizures.
3. Protect patient from injury during seizure.
   a. Avoid placing padded tongue blade or other objects between clenched teeth.
   b. Do not attempt to restrain.
   c. Pad sides and ends of crib or bed.
   d. Remove restrictive clothing.

4. Employ anticonvulsant therapy.
   a. Drugs: see Table 4–1.
   b. Ketogenic diet if patient is alert (MCT: medium chain triglycerides).
      1) Most effective in minor motor seizures.
      2) Anticonvulsant action unclear.
5. Identify cause of seizure.
   a. Appropriate diagnostic tests to rule out causes listed in pathologic conditions.
6. Monitor patient closely for drug toxicity.
   a. Anticonvulsant serum levels should remain in therapeutic range.
   b. Monitor serum anticonvulsant levels and monitor patient closely for signs of toxicity (see Table 4–1).
7. Provide emotional and psychologic support for the child and his family.
   a. Assess family's needs regarding adjustment to a potentially chronic condition.
   b. Teaching patient and parents about drug therapy and avoidance of factors precipitating seizures.

Complications
1. Drug toxicity.
2. Aspiration.
3. Cerebral hypoxia.
4. Cognitive deficits.
   a. Intelligence.
   b. Perceptual-motor.
   c. Visual-spatial.
5. Mental retardation.
6. Status epilepticus.

Nursing Skills
1. Same as for meningitis.
2. Prevention of patient injury during seizure.
3. Knowledge and administration of ketogenic diet.[3,18,22,27,35,41,42]

STATUS EPILEPTICUS

Etiology and Precipitating Factors
1. Rapid or sudden withdrawal or change of anticonvulsants: most common.
2. Intercurrent infections.
3. Meningitis or encephalitis.
4. Acute electrolyte disturbances (i.e., hyponatremia).
5. Uremia.
6. Sleep deprivation.

Table 4-1. COMMON ANTICONVULSANTS IN PEDIATRICS[18,30,39]

Drug Name Generic/Brand (Classification)	Anticonvulsant Action	Seizure Specificity	Dose/Route	Effective Serum Concentration	Side Effects
Phenobarbital/Luminal (Barbiturate)	Raises seizure threshold; Inhibits spread of discharge from epileptic focus	Grand mal Focal Psychomotor	Infant: 8 mg/kg po; Child: 3–6 mg/kg IM; Adolescent: 1–2 mg/kg IV	10–25 µg/ml	Drowsiness—dose related; Paradoxical hyperactivity; Eruptions of skin and mucous membrane
Primidone/Mysoline (Oxazolidine)	A major metabolite of the drug is Phenobarbital, therefore same as above	Grand mal Psychomotor	10–25 mg/kg po	6–12 µg/ml	Sedation; Vertigo; Dizziness; Nausea; Vomiting; Ataxia; Nystagmus
Diphenylhydantoin/Dilantin (Hydantoin)	Inhibits spread of electrical discharges from epileptic focus	Grand mal Focal Psychomotor	<20 kg: 10 mg/kg IV; 20–40 kg: 5–7 mg/kg; >40 kg: 4–6 mg/kg po	10–20 µg/ml.	Gingival hyperplasia in therapeutic doses; Cardiovascular collapse with rapid IV infusion
Ethosuximide/Zarontin (Succimide)	Raises seizure threshold	Petit mal	20–40 mg/kg po	40–100 µg/ml	Dose-related nausea; Drowsiness; Anorexia; Abdominal pain; Irritability
Carbamazepine/Tegretol (Iminostilbene)	Anticonvulsant action unclear	Psychomotor	20–60 mg/kg po Increase dosage gradually	3–10 µg/ml in adults Undocumented in children	Dizziness; Nausea and vomiting; Ataxia
Diazepam/Valium (Benzodiazepine)	Suppresses abnormal discharges; Mimics action of inhibitory neurotransmitter, glycine	Status epilepticus Refractory petit mal	Infants: .04–.2 mg/kg maximum: 5 mg; Child over 5 years: 1 mg every 5 minutes maximum: 10 mg IV; Oral dose: .12–.8 mg/kg	Not established in children	Hyperbilirubinemia; Drowsiness, Ataxia, Slurred speech; Thrombophlebitis
Clonazepam/Clonopin (Benzodiazepine)	Potentiates mechanisms that inhibit seizure discharges	Infantile spasms Myoclonic seizures Petit mal Akinetic Grand mal	.01–.2 mg/kg po	.013–.072 µg/ml	Ataxia; Drowsiness; Irritability Excess weight gain; Excess bronchial secretions
Valproic acid/Depakene	Suppresses paroxysmal activity by increasing inhibitory neurotransmitter levels	Absence seizures (only use approved by FDA for treatment)	15–30 mg/kg by mouth	50–150 µg/ml	Gastrointestinal intolerance; Sedation; Hair loss; Hepatic dysfunction

7. Structural brain lesions (tumors, hematomas).
8. Cerebral edema.
9. Genetic transmission.

Pathophysiology
1. Description (poorly understood).
   a. Recurrent generalized or lateralized seizures without regaining consciousness.
   b. Often accompanied by interference with vital functions.
   c. Nonepileptic patients in status epilepticus usually reflect acute or subacute central nervous system involvement.
2. Classifications of patients with status epilepticus and associated signs and symptoms:
   a. Nonepileptics with central nervous system involvement:
      1) Usually manifest seizures with focal or unilateral components.
      2) Tend to be more refractory to therapy.
      3) Seizures often followed by neurologic deficits.
   b. Epileptics in status epilepticus:
      1) Usually manifest generalized motor activity.
      2) Are generally more responsive to therapy.

Clinical Presentation
1. Signs and symptoms:
   a. Variable types of seizure activity.
   b. Recurrent convulsions causing prolonged loss of consciousness and cessation of adequate ventilation.
2. Diagnostic findings:
   a. Based on clinical manifestations of disease and frequency of seizures.
   b. Frequent or sustained spike and wave patterns on electroencephalogram.
   c. CT scan or other neurologic diagnostic tests may show an organic cause (tumors, A-V malformations, infectious processes).

Objectives of Therapy
1. Suppression of seizures as rapidly as possible.
2. Determination of factors predisposing to status epilepticus episode.

Therapeutic Management
1. Establish and maintain a patent airway and adequate ventilation (same measures as for meningitis).
2. Suppress convulsions rapidly.
   a. Intravenous administration of anticonvulsants in large doses.
      1) Intramuscular or small doses can prolong seizure duration and promote drug toxicity.
   b. Drugs of choice (given intravenously, 3 to 5 minutes):
      1) Valium.
      2) Phenobarbital.
      3) Dilantin.
   c. If anticonvulsants are ineffective, complete sedation, drug-induced paralysis, or general anesthesia may be required.

3. Protect patient from injury.
4. Employ general supportive measures.
   a. Intravenous hydration.
   b. Close observation of neurologic and vital signs.
   c. Antibiotics if infectious process is documented.
5. Initiate or resume daily anticonvulsant maintenance therapy.
   a. Former maintenance doses may have to be increased.
   b. Long-acting drugs intramuscularly or by mouth if feasible.
      1) Dilantin: 5 mg/kg/day.
      2) Zarontin: 250 mg two to four times a day
6. Investigate etiology of status epilepticus episode.
   a. Differential diagnosis is initiated immediately.
   b. Laboratory data:
      1) Electrolytes.
      2) Lumbar puncture.
      3) Serum levels of anticonvulsants.
      4) Serum glucose.
   c. Diagnostic studies:
      1) Computed tomography.
      2) Electroencephalogram.
      3) Lumbar puncture.
      4) Cerebral angiography.

Complications
1. Hypoxemia.
2. Drug toxicity.
3. Postepileptic paralysis.
4. Postepileptic psychosis.
5. Permanent brain damage.
6. Death.

Nursing Skills
1. Same as for seizures.[9,31,33,41]

HYDROCEPHALUS _____

Etiology and Predisposing Factors
1. Obstructive.
   a. Communicating.
      1) Ventricular dilatation in which the fluid between the ventricular system and the spinal subarachnoid space is free-flowing.
         a) Obstruction of cerebrospinal fluid flow.
            (1) Extraventricular in origin.
            (2) Commonly in subarachnoid spaces about brain stem or cerebral hemispheres.

      2) Post-traumatic obstruction of basilar cisterns from progressive fibrosis occurs with:
         a) Perinatal birth injuries.
         b) Bacterial meningitis.
         c) Toxoplasmosis.
   b. Noncommunicating
      1) Denotes obstruction of cerebropsinal fluid flow within the ventricular system.
      2) Types:
         a) Neoplasms or abscesses.
         b) Congenital malformations.
            (1) Stenosis of aqueduct of Sylvius is most common.
            (2) Absence or atresia of foramen.
         c) Arteriovenous malformations.
  2. Overproduction of cerebrospinal fluid within ventricles (rare).

Pathophysiologic Description
  1. Increased pressure gradient between intraventricular fluid and the brain.
  2. Result is abnormal enlargement of cerebral ventricles.
  3. Overproduction.
    a. Choroid plexus papilloma (rare).
  4. Defective absorption.
    a. Subarachnoid hemorrhage.
    b. Meningitis.
    c. Elevated cerebrospinal fluid protein levels.

Clinical Presentation
  1. Signs and symptoms:
    a. Infants with open sutures and fontanels:
      1) Increased head circumference.
      2) Bulging anterior fontanel.
      3) Palpably separated sutures.
      4) Increased transillumination.
      5) "Setting sun sign" in terminal phase.
         a) Eyes depressed.
         b) Increased amount of sclera is visible.
    b. All age groups:
      1) Abducent (VI) cranial nerve palsy.
      2) Vomiting.
      3) Irritability and listlessness.
      4) Visual and gait disturbances.
      5) Split sutures.
      6) Papilledema.
      7) Disturbances in muscle tone and reflex responses.
      8) Incoordination.
      9) Cranial bruits.
      10) Respiratory irregularities.

           11) Increased blood pressure.

           12) Bradycardia.

  2. Diagnostic findings:

    a. CT scan demonstrates enlargement of ventricles and can define nature of pathologic condition.

    b. Air encephalography: defines cerebrospinal fluid obstruction; most definitive study (but not often employed in children).

    c. Lumbar or ventricular puncture frequently demonstrates increased pressure and normal protein levels.

Objective of Therapy

  1. Prevention of further cerebrospinal fluid accumulation.

  2. Reduction of disability and death.

Therapeutic Management

  1. Establish and maintain a patent airway and adequate ventilation (same measures as for meningitis).

  2. Monitor neurologic status closely.

    a. Frequent neurologic and vital sign checks.

    b. Daily measurement of head circumference.

    c. Frequent assessment of fontanel tension and size.

  3. Employ surgical measures to prevent further accumulation of cerebrospinal fluid.

    a. Shunting techniques:

      1) Shunt draining cerebrospinal fluid from lateral ventricle (high-pressure space) to one of several low-pressure spaces:

        a) Right atrium.

        b) Peritoneal cavity.

        c) Pleural space.

    b. Direct, nonshunting techniques:

      1) External ventricular drainage.

      2) Choroid plexectomy (for choroid papilloma).

      3) Rickham reservoir and catheter.

  4. Evaluate postoperative function of shunt.

    a. Chest x-ray film to verify correct shunt placement.

    b. Manometric testing of ventricular pressure to verify success of surgery.

    c. Echoencephalography to ascertain ventricular size.

    d. Check shunt for adequate filling after brief compression of shunt valve.

  5. Provide for supportive care.

    a. Hydration with intravenous fluids. (Fluid restriction is usually unnecessary once ventricular drainage has been established.)

    b. Tube feedings or oral intake for nutritional needs.

      1) Patients are prone to feeding difficulties and aspiration of vomitus.

    c. Hyperalimentation if postoperative recovery is prolonged.

  6. Prophylaclic antibiotics may be administered for shunt procedures.

Complications
1. Without shunts:
   a. Neurologic deterioration if hydrocephalus is untreated.
   b. Cortical atrophy.
   c. Significant alteration in brain growth.
   d. Death.
2. With shunts:
   a. Sudden increased intracranial pressure.
   b. Shunt obstruction or malfunction.
   c. Infection.
   d. Electrolyte imbalance.
   e. Subdural hematoma following abrupt collapse of enlarged ventricles.
   f. Retardation.

Nursing Skills
1. Same as for meningitis.
2. Care of external ventricular drainage system.
3. Analysis of shunt patency.[17,45]

SPACE-OCCUPYING LESIONS

BRAIN TUMORS

Etiology
1. Basically undetermined.
2. Some brain tumors seem to be congenital.

Pathology
1. Description:
   a. Benign or malignant neoplasms developing in the brain, meninges, or skull.
   b. Clinical manifestations dependent upon type of nerve cell involved and location of tumor.
   c. Primary malignant tumors do not metastasize from the central nervous system, even though cardiac output to the brain is large and the cerebrospinal fluid flows directly into venous sinuses.
   d. Cerebral edema develops rapidly in the presence of infratentorial neoplasms.
2. Classification of brain tumor:
   a. Anatomic location of brain tumors in children:
      1) Infratentorial (66%).
      2) Supratentorial (33%).
   b. Types of tumors:
      1) Astrocytoma.
         a) Astrocytes invade brain tissue, often making complete removal impossible.

        b) May be cystic, in which case complete tumor excision is possible.

        c) Initially, tumor is benign; it may undergo malignant changes.

        d) Slow growth rate.

    2) Medulloblastoma.

        a) Develops from primitive cells within cerebellum.

        b) Highly malignant tumor; rapid tumor growth.

        c) Frequently metastasizes to subarachnoid space, cerebellum, and spinal cord.

    3) Brain stem glioma.

        a) Composed of undifferentiated, malignant glial cells.

        b) Tumor grows rapidly.

        c) Surgical excision impossible.

    4) Ependymoma.

        a) Derived from ependymal cells.

        b) Malignant.

        c) Arises from ventricular walls (usually fourth ventricle).

    5) Craniopharyngioma.

        a) Benign lesions derived from pouch in pituitary gland.

        b) Frequently calcified and contains cysts and lipid fluid.

        c) Can be mobile within cranium.

        d) Often associated with abnormal pituitary function.

Clinical Presentation

  1. General signs and symptoms (reflect cerebral edema as well as tumor mass itself):

    a. Headache.

      1) Important indication, as younger children seldom complain of headache.

      2) Usually most severe upon awakening or when recumbent.

    b. Vomiting.

      1) Often first presenting symptom.

      2) Not usually associated with nausea.

    c. Spread of cranial sutures in infants.

      1) Promotes tolerance of larger tumor burdens.

    d. Fatigue.

    e. Decreased activity level.

    f. Dispositional changes or irritability.

    g. Seizures.

      1) Seen in one third of supratentorial lesions.

      2) Rarely seen in infratentorial lesions.

    h. Strabismus or diplopia.

      1) Due to VI (Abducens) cranial nerve palsy.

    i. Papilledema.

    j. Bulging fontanel in infants.

    k. Increased head circumference in infants.

  2. Signs and symptoms more specific to infratentorial tumors:

    a. Gait disturbances, ataxia, motor incoordination.

  b. Cranial nerve dysfunction.
  c. Nystagmus.
  d. Abnormal reflex responses.
  e. Signs of generalized increased intracranial pressure may be present or absent.
3. Signs and symptoms more specific to supratentorial tumors:
  a. Paresis.
  b. Generalized signs of increased intracranial pressure.
  c. Visual disturbances and losses.
  d. Hydrocephalus.
  e. Focal neurologic deficits.
  f. Seizures (can be focal or generalized).
4. Diagnostic findings:
  a. CT scan accurately outlines abnormal intracranial structures.
    1) Posterior fossa (infratentorial) tumors more difficult to visualize.
    2) Contrast media rarely crosses into most tumor tissue.
    3) Also demonstrates extensive cerebral edema, shift of brain structures, tumor vascularity, and hydrocephalus.
  b. Cerebral angiogram defines vascular displacement and abnormal tumor vessels.
  c. Skull films identify intracranial changes from increased pressure and spread of sutures.
  d. Electroencephalogram demonstrates slowing over area of tumor and abnormalities in electrical discharge.

Objectives of Therapy
1. Total eradication of tumor if possible.
2. Palliative support if complete tumor eradication is impossible.

Therapeutic Management
1. Establish and maintain a patent airway and adequate ventilation (same measures as for meningitis).
  a. Frequent monitoring of arterial blood gases.
  b. Positioning.
  c. Suctioning.
  d. Intubation and assisted ventilation if necessary.
2. Monitor closely for signs of increased intracranial pressure.
  a. Intracranial pressure monitoring.
  b. Frequent vital sign and neurologic checks.
  c. Pre- and postoperative comparisons of neurologic status.
3. Treat cerebral edema.
  a. Corticosteroids.
    1) Decrease cerebral edema associated with brain tumors.
    2) Thought to have antineoplastic properties; activity unclear.
  b. Elevate head of bed 30 degrees.
  c. Hypertonic solutions (mannitol, urea).
    1) Most often given in acute situations while patient awaits neurosurgery or for postoperative edema.
  d. Fluid restriction (1/2 to 2/3 of maintenance).

4. Resect tumor surgically.
   a. Complete surgical excision depends upon type and extent of tumor.
   b. Surgical intervention in primary or metastatic tumors is usually only palliative.
   c. Operative drains are usually in place for 48 hours.
5. Radiate central nervous system postoperatively.
   a. Effective dose for most tumors is in upper range.
      1) 4500 to 6000 rads in daily increments of 200 rads for 5 days.
6. Chemotherapy.
   a. Common agents (drugs have difficulty penetrating blood-brain/cerebrospinal fluid barriers, making this treatment modality less effective than for other body tumors):
      1) CCNU (CeeNU) (Chloroethyl-cyclohexyl-nitrosourea)
      2) BCNU (BiCNU, carmustine) (1,3-bis-[2-chloroethyl]-1-nitrosourea), also known as NU Urea.
      3) Vincristine sulfate.
   b. Helpful for medulloblastoma, astrocytoma (grade III–IV), brainstem glioma, ependymoma.
   c. Toxicities of chemotherapeutical agents:
      1) BCNU causes nausea and vomiting, flushing of face, diuresis, pain at injection site, thrombophlebitis, myelosuppression (primarily thrombocytopenia), local necrosis with extravasation, esophagitis, dysphagia, interstitial pneumonia.
      2) CCNU causes nausea and vomiting, anorexia, myelosuppresion.
      3) Vincristine causes peripheral neuropathy, tingling or motor weakness, constipation, abdominal pain, alopecia, minimal bone marrow suppression.
7. Institute supportive measures.
   a. Anticonvulsant therapy for associated seizures or postoperative prophylaxis.
   b. Intravenous fluids for hydration.
      1) Solutions containing concentration of normal saline, to avoid danger of increasing cerebral edema.
   c. Antiemetics for severe vomiting.
8. Provide emotional support for the child and his family.
   a. Help them deal with the death process if imminent.

Complications
1. Hematoma development in the tumor bed.
2. Cerebrospinal fluid leak.
3. Wound infection and central nervous system bacterial invasion.
4. Radiation and chemotherapy side effects:
   a. Localized skin sloughing.
   b. Nausea and vomiting.

    c. Small vessel fibrosis.

    d. Cerebral atrophy.

5. Dehydration secondary to vomiting.

6. Neurologic deterioration.

7. Death.

Nursing Skills

1. Same as for head trauma.

2. Knowledge of dying and death process.[2,21,32,39,46]

INTRACRANIAL HEMORRHAGES

Etiology and Precipitating Factors

1. Rupture of congenital vascular lesions.

    a. Arteriovenous malformations.

        1) Localized vessel abnormality in which capillaries are absent and direct communication exists between involved arteries and veins.

    b. Aneurysms.

        1) Weaknesses of cerebral arterial walls, usually at points of bifurcation.

2. Blood coagulation defects.

    a. Hemophilia.

    b. Idiopathic thrombocytopenic purpura.

    c. Septic process.

3. Trauma.

4. End-stage leukemia.

5. Hemorrhage of brain tumors.

Pathophysiology and Description

1. Ruptured arteries are usual sources of intracranial bleeding, although disrupted veins may also bleed.

2. Four anatomic sites of intracranial hemorrhages and/or hematomas:

    a. Subdural space.

        1) Most often associated with meningeal tears and contusion and laceration of underlying brain tissue.

        2) Bleeding is usually venous in origin.

        3) More common type of hemorrhagic condition.

    b. Epidural space.

        1) Hemorrhage is usually due to severance of meningeal artery as a result of trauma.

    c. Subarachnoid space.

        1) Most common site for rupture of aneurysms and occasionally arteriovenous malformations.

    d. Intracerebral brain substance.

        1) Aneurysms and deep arteriovenous malformations are most often implicated in this type of hemorrhage.

3. Pathophysiology closely resembles that of adult intracranial bleeding.

Clinical Presentation

1. Epidural hemorrhage or hematoma:
   a. Child either awakens from concussion and rapidly lapses back into coma or manifests a rapid, progressive deepening of coma if consciousness has not been regained.
   b. Cranial nerve dysfunction due to rapid development of tentorial herniation.
   c. Vomiting.
   d. Irregular respiration.
   e. Increased head circumference and other signs of hydrocephalus if bleeding occurs in posterior fossa.
   f. Brain and CT scans define area of bleeding.
2. Subdural hemorrhage or hematoma:
   a. Child with severe head injury remains comatose or condition does not improve.
   b. Vomiting.
   c. Cranial nerve palsies.
   d. Papilledema.
   e. Pupillary dilatation.
   f. Hemiparesis.
   g. Convulsions.
   h. Cerebral angiogram shows avascular space between cerebral vessels and skull.
   i. Brain and CT scans define area of bleeding.
   j. Electroencephalogram shows slower amplitude on the affected side.
   k. Positive transillumination in infants.
3. Subarachnoid and intracerebral hemorrhages:
   a. Sudden severe headache.
   b. Drowsiness.
   c. Nuchal rigidity.
   d. Fever.
   e. Rapid lapse into coma.
   f. Retinal hemorrhages.
   g. Convulsions.
   h. Cranial nerve palsies.
   i. Focal neurologic signs.
   j. Intracranial bruits.
   k. Cerebrospinal fluid reveals:
      1) Persistent RBCs in sequential samples.
      2) Elevated WBCs.
      3) Initial protein elevation.
   l. CT scan and arteriogram reveal source and extent of bleeding.

Objectives of Therapy

1. Minimize neurologic deficits.
2. Minimize mortality.
3. Rehabilitate to maximum capacity.

Therapeutic Management
1. Establish and maintain a patent airway and adequate ventilation (same measures as for meningitis).
2. Monitor patient closely for deterioration in neurologic status (as previously described).
   a. Especially in children whose coma recurs or becomes progressively deeper.
3. Employ surgical intervention.
   a. Epidural hematoma:
      1) Surgical evacuation of blood from epidural space.
      2) Epidural tap and aspiration.
   b. Subdural hematoma:
      1) Surgical evacuation of blood from subdural space.
      2) Subdural tap and aspiration.
   c. Arteriovenous malformations:
      1) Surgical excision of superficial malformations.
      2) Ligation of feeding arteries (effectiveness is limited).
   d. Aneurysm:
      1) Surgical ligation or clipping of artery.
      2) Surgical webbing or prosthetic material.
4. Control bleeding if surgery is contraindicated.
   a. Controlled hypotension.
      1) Barbiturates.
      2) Arfonad.
   b. Relieve pain to prevent agitation.
      1) Avoid respiratory depressants if possible.
   c. Keep room quiet and dark.
   d. Prevent patient from becoming strained or upset.
   e. Allow parents to be with child, but monitor their effect on the patient.
   f. Avoid discussion of child's condition in his presence.
5. Monitor, control, and treat cerebral edema (as previously described).
6. Control seizures if present (as previously described).

Complications
1. Severe neurologic dysfunction.
2. Seizures.
3. Mortality rate is high in subarachnoid and intracerebral hemorrhages.

Nursing Skills
1. Same as for head injury.[2,45]

REYE'S SYNDROME _____

Theories of Etiology (Exact Cause Unknown)
1. Toxin-virus interaction.

2. Pathology of lipid metabolism.
   a. Decreased liver function results in elevated free fatty acid levels in blood.
   b. Free fatty acids inhibit metabolic processes in the brain, resulting in coma.
3. Genetic, metabolic predisposition to Reye's syndrome.
4. Viral infection of all mitochondria.
   a. Mitochondria become swollen.
   b. Most current theory of etiology.

Epidemology
1. Excessive prevalence among siblings.
2. More common in children less than one year of age.
3. Black infants are affected more than are white infants.

Pathophysiology
1. General characteristics:
   a. History of viral illness 2 to 7 days prior to onset.
     1) Influenza B and chickenpox viruses most common.
     2) Twelve viruses have been implicated.
   b. Severe encephalopathy.
   c. Fatty infiltration of the viscera, notably the liver.
2. Neurologic changes (see clinical staging):
   a. Cytotoxic cerebral edema ensues, primarily affecting the cerebral cortex.
   b. Increased intracranial pressure develops.
   c. Overactive sympathetic nervous system response.
3. Metabolic derangements:
   a. Metabolic acidosis.
   b. Respiratory alkalosis.
   c. Persistent low phosphate levels.
   d. Maximal secretion of aldosterone due to dehydration and stress.
     1) Sodium retention.
     2) Potassium loss.
4. Respiratory insufficiency:
   a. Irregular respiratory patterns.
   b. Hyperventilation.
   c. Progression to respiratory arrest can occur.
5. Cellular pathology:
   a. Diffuse cellular insult.
   b. Prominent mitochondrial abnormalities.

Clinical Staging
(Stage at admission reflects outcome to some extent.)
1. Stage I:
   a. Responds inappropriately to voice.
   b. Disoriented to place and time.
   c. Arouses to minimal stimuli.
   d. Conjugate gaze.

    e. Brisk pupillary responses.

    f. Movements are coordinated, going to ataxia and uncoordinated actions.

    g. Muscle tone normal.

    h. Lethargic.

    i. Progressive slurred speech.

2. Stage II:

    a. Delirium and agitation.

    b. Obtundation.

    c. Decorticate posturing.

    d. Deep respirations.

    e. Dilated pupils.

    f. Engorgement of optic fundi.

3. Stage III:

    a. Comatose.

    b. Increased muscle tone.

    c. Decerebrate posturing.

    d. Dilated pupils.

    e. Deep respirations; elements of Cheyne-Stokes and apneustic breathing.

    f. Seizures (variable).

    g. Positive oculocephalic response (doll's eyes).

4. Stage IV:

    a. Deep coma.

    b. Flaccid muscle tone.

    c. Absence of brain stem function.

    d. Apnea.

    e. Dilated and nonreactive pupils.

    f. Hypotension.

Clinical Presentation

1. History:

    a. Viral illness 2 to 7 days prior to onset.

    b. Protracted vomiting for 1 to 2 days.

    c. Combative or inappropriate behavior.

2. Signs and symptoms:

    a. Neurologic:

        1) Obtundation, agitation, and/or coma.

        2) Pupillary changes.

        3) Hyperreflexia.

        4) Decreased sensorium.

        5) Delirium and extreme agitation.

        6) Convulsions.

        7) Decorticate or decerebrate posturing.

        8) Diaphoresis.

    b. Cardiovascular:

        1) Slight tachycardia.

        2) Normal blood pressure until final stage.

        3) Dehydration.

    c. Respiratory:
       1) Various irregularities (see Staging).
    d. Metabolic:
       1) Hyperpyrexia.
3. Laboratory findings:
    a. Initial elevation of serum ammonia.
       1) Normal range: 40 to 80 μg/dl.
       2) Abnormal range in Reye's: 150 to 750 μg/dl.
       3) Product of initial virus-toxin interaction.
    b. Elevated SGOT.
       1) Unassociated with jaundice.
       2) Hepatomegaly inconsistently present.
    c. Prolonged prothrombin time (PT).
       1) Greater than 50% of control.
    d. Elevated serum amylase.
    e. Elevated CPK.
       1) Degree of elevation can often be correlated with severity of the disease.
    f. Hypoglycemia.
       1) More prominent in infants.
    g. Elevated free fatty acids.
    h. Elevated WBC.
       1) Usual range is 40,000 to 50,000/cu mm.
    i. Elevated BUN.
       1) Caused by abnormal protein metabolism.
    j. Variable arterial pH.
       1) Ranges from mildly acidemic to moderately alkalemic.
    k. Decreased PCO_2 initially, reflecting deep respirations.
    l. Cerebrospinal fluid essentially normal, although pressure may be elevated.
    m. Toxicology and drug ingestion screens should be negative if child has Reye's syndrome.
    n. Viral studies are negative.
4. Other diagnostic findings:
    a. CT scan usually demonstrates only cerebral edema.
    b. Electroencephalogram shows a high voltage, slow dysrhythmia.

Objective of Therapy
1. Early diagnosis.
2. Lessen morbidity.
3. Minimize sequelae.
4. Supportive care.

Therapeutic Management
1. Establish a diagnosis.
    a. Rule out other disease states such as ingestions, hepatitis, central nervous system infections.
    b. Presence of an elevated SGOT, prolonged prothrombin time (PT), increased ammonia levels, and normal bilirubin level is suggestive of diagnosis.

    c. Liver biopsy shows diffuse, fatty infiltration of parenchymal tissue; findings confirm diagnosis.

2. Monitor and treat all systems.
    a. Fluid and electrolyte balance.
       1) Restrict fluids to 50 to 75% of daily maintenance.
          a) Keep serum osmolality between 370 and 380 mOsm/l.
          b) Keep central venous pressure (CVP) between 3 and 5 cm H_2O.
       2) Supplement electrolyte losses.
       3) Monitor intake and output closely.
       4) Replace nasogastric output cc for cc with dextrose 5% in 0.45% normal saline.
       5) Administer albumin if total serum protein is below 7.5%.
       6) Administer whole blood for low hematocrit.
       7) Monitor hydration state with frequent measures of serum osmolality and BUN.
    b. Respiratory.
       1) Intubate and place on assisted ventilation (same measures required for intubation in meningitis).
    c. Cardiovascular.
       1) Place arterial line for accurate blood pressure monitoring.
       2) Monitor potassium levels closely.
          a) Losses are due to increased secretion of aldosterone.
       3) Monitor patient closely for signs of shock.
    d. Metabolic.
       1) Exchange transfusions are advocated by some to correct blood clotting abnormalities.
          a) Effective in reducing increased intracranial pressure if serum osmolality is low.
          b) Monitor patient closely for transfusion reactions.
       2) Administer $NaHCO_3$ to correct acidosis.
       3) Monitor laboratory values on a serial basis.

3. Reduce increased intracranial pressure.
    a. Assessment parameters:
       1) Level of consciousness.
       2) Pupillary responses.
       3) Deep tendon reflexes.
       4) Babinski reflex.
       5) Oculocephalic (doll's eye) response.
       6) Posturing.
    b. Place intracranial monitor:
       1) Control intracranial pressure at levels below 25 mm Hg.
       2) Intracranial pressure spikes occur with each QRS complex on electrocardiogram.
       3) Plateau waves on monitor are ominous signs.
       4) Intracranial pressure can rise rapidly to very elevated levels.
       5) Avoid injudicious flushing of monitoring system.

    c. Interventions to keep intracranial pressure at a minimum:
      1) Drug-induced paralysis (Pavulon).
        a) Eliminates activities that increase intracranial pressure:
          (1) Muscle movement.
          (2) Shivering.
      2) Central nervous system sedation (decreases metabolic demands).
        a) Pentothal.
        b) Pentobarbital.
        c) Phenobarbital.
      3) Hypothermia.
        a) Decreases metabolic demand of the brain.
      4) Craniectomy for increased intracranial pressure that fails to respond to other measures; may be used as a prophylaxis in some medical centers.
      5) Steroids have questionable effect on cytotoxic cerebral edema.

Complications
1. Hypoxia.
2. Mortality: highly variable, ranges from 15 to 75% among institutions.
3. Full recovery is more likely if diagnosis and treatment are begun in the initial stages of the disease and if patient presents in lighter stages of coma.

Nursing Skills
1. Same as for meningitis.
2. Assisting with exchange transfusions.
3. Intracranial pressure monitoring and interpretation.[14,15,47]
4. Hypothermia induction.
5. Care during recovery and rehabilitation after craniectomy.

_____ INTRACRANIAL PRESSURE MONITORING _____

Advantages
1. Provides ongoing record of intracranial pressure.
2. Allows for assessment of intracranial dynamics and early detection if pressure rises.
3. Assists in decreasing effects of disease, although it does not correct primary disease itself.
4. Allows for determination of the optimal time for surgical intervention.
5. Allows for direct measurement of treatment effectiveness.

Uses
1. If the patient's level of consciousness can be followed, intracranial pressure monitoring becomes less necessary.

2. Pathologic conditions most commonly associated with intracranial pressure monitoring:
   a. Reye's syndrome.
   b. Intracranial hemorrhages.
   c. Acute head injuries.
   d. Post-drowning encephalopathy.
   e. Encephalitis.
   f. Hydrocephalus.

Mechanics

1. Three devices are necessary for monitoring:
   a. Intracranial pressure sensor.
   b. Transducer.
      1) Picks up impulses from sensor and converts them to electrical energy.
   c. Recording device.
      1) Converts electrical energy to visible waves or numerical readings on an oscilloscope.

Types of Devices

1. Subarachnoid monitoring via screw devices (Richmond) or fiberoptic sensors.
   a. Placement:
      1) Small burr hole is made in frontal area of skull just behind hairline.
      2) Cross-shaped incision is made in dura to expose subarachnoid space (small piece of dura may be removed).
      3) Monitoring device is "screwed" into place so that proximal end is in communication with subarachnoid space.
      4) Dry sterile dressing is applied around screw or completely covering head if sensor is used.
   b. Advantages:
      1) Complicating infections (meningitis) are less severe than those associated with cannula devices.
   c. Disadvantages:
      1) Cerebrospinal fluid cannot be withdrawn.
      2) Infection produces meningitis.
      3) Marked cerebral edema can produce herniation of brain tissue into the end of the screw.
      4) A flap of dura can occlude the screw and dampen readings.
2. Ventricular monitoring via cannulas (Scott).
   a. Placement:
      1) Small burr hole is made through frontal portion of skull on nondominant side.
      2) Cannula is introduced into lateral ventricle.
      3) Dry sterile dressing is applied around area.
   b. Advantages:
      1) Cerebrospinal fluid can be withdrawn to decrease intracranial pressure.

        2) Air and contrast media can be injected to study ventricular size and patency.

        3) Intracranial compensatory mechanisms can be evaluated (see section on anatomy and physiology).

    c. Disadvantages:

        1) Infection results in ventriculitis.

        2) Cerebrospinal fluid leaks can occur.

        3) Marked cerebral edema can produce ventricular compression, which makes cannula placement more difficult.

  3. Epidural monitoring.

    a. Placement:

        1) Balloons or fiberoptic sensors with intracranial or extra-cranial transducers are inserted into epidural space following open head injury or via burr hole.

    b. Advantages:

        1) Incidence of infection is reduced as dura is not exposed.

        2) Easily inserted in emergency situations.

    c. Disadvantages:

        1) Cerebrospinal fluid cannot be removed.

        2) Heat sensitivity of intracranial transducers can produce falsely high pressure readings.

        3) Recalibration is impossible with intracranial transducers.

Physiologic Considerations

  1. Normal intracranial pressure:

    a. 4 to 15 mm Hg.

    b. 50 to 200 mm H_2O.

  2. Intracranial pressure normally rises under the following conditions:

    a. Coughing.

    b. Straining.

    c. Suctioning.

        1) Rise should be transient and of short duration.

    d. Any rise in intrathoracic or intra-abdominal pressure.

    e. Position changes, especially with head rotation.

    f. Right-sided heart failure.

  3. In children, intracranial pressures can normally fluctuate to elevated levels.

    a. Therefore one pressure reading is not very reliable

Nursing Implications

  1. Maintain patency and accuracy of monitoring system.

    a. Transducer should be along same horizontal plane as patient's head.

    b. Recalibration of monitoring system is often necessary.

        1) Watch for dampened wave forms or bizarre pressure readings when patient's condition does not appear changed.

    c. Flushing of monitoring system is highly controversial.

        1) Done primarily with screw devices.

2) No more than 0.1 cc of normal saline should be used.
   a) Even this amount can produce dramatic changes in intracranial pressure.
   b) Flushing solution usually contains an antibacterial agent (Bacitracin).
3) Use a double stopcock next to patient. If Richmond screws are being used, assemble equipment in this order: patient, screw, double stopcocks. This allows the nurse to evacuate any air that inadvertently gets into the line.

2. Change head dressing and flush solution daily under sterile conditions.
3. Assess wave forms and pressure measurements.
   a. Three types of pressure wave abnormalities:
      1) Plateau waves.
         a) Increases in intracranial pressure between 50 and 100 mm Hg for 5 to 20 minutes.
         b) Possibly denotes a combination of blood volume alterations and intermittent obstruction of cerebrospinal fluid flow.
      2) B waves.
         a) Sharp, rhythmic oscillations every 1 to 2 minutes.
         b) Intracranial pressure rises to 50 mm Hg.
      3) C waves.
         a) Intracranial pressure elevations up to 20 mm Hg occurring every 4 to 8 minutes.
         b) Associated with respiratory effects on blood pressure.
   b. Notify physician immediately of sustained rises in intracranial pressure or of prolonged elevations after procedures (i.e., suctioning).
4. Briefly hyperventilate the patient with Ambu-bag or ventilator if sudden rises in intracranial pressure occur.
   a. Call physician immediately if ineffective.

Duration of Intracranial Pressure Monitoring
1. To minimize risk of infection, devices should be left in place no longer than 48 hours.[16,25,36]

BIBLIOGRAPHY

1. Bee, H.: The Developing Child, 2nd ed. New York, Harper & Row, 1978. pp. 106-7.
2. Beeson, P., McDermott, W., and Wyngarden, J.: Textbook of Medicine, 15th ed. Philadelphia, W. B. Saunders Co., 1978.
3. Berman, P.: Management of seizure disorders with anticonvulsant drugs: current concepts. Pediatr. Clin. North Am. 21:649, 1974.
4. Black, P., et al.: Penetration of brain abscess by systemically administered antibiotics. J. Neurosurg. 38:705, 1973.
5. Blount, M., et al.: Obtaining and analyzing cerebrospinal fluid. Nurs. Clin. North Am. 9:632, 1974.

5a. Browne, T.: Drug therepy: Valproic acid. N. Engl. J. Med., *302*:661, 1980.

6. Bruce, D.: Intracranial Pressure Monitoring. Third Annual Symposium on Critical Care Medicine, Portland, Oregon, 1976.

7. Butler, I., and Johnson, R.: Central nervous system infections. Pediatr. Clin. North Am. *21*:649, 1976.

8. Carini, E., and Owens, G.: Neurological and Neurosurgical Nursing. St. Louis, C. V. Mosby Co., 1974.

9. Carter, S., and Gold, A.: Status epilepticus. *In* Smith, C. (ed.): The Critically Ill Child: Diagnosis and Management, 2nd ed. Philadelphia, W. B. Saunders Co., 1977.

10. Chinn, P., and Leitch, C.: Child Health Maintenance. St. Louis, C. V. Mosby Co., 1974.

11. Clipper, M.: Nursing care of patients in a neurologic intensive care unit. Nurs. Clin. North Am., *4*:211, 1969.

12. Computed tomography. Med. Lett. Drugs Ther., *18*:79, 1976.

12a. Conn, H. (ed.): Current Therapy 1980. Philadelphia, W. B. Saunders, 1980, pp. 713–720, 767–770.

13. DeJong, R., et al.: Essentials of the Neurological Examination. Philadelphia, Smith Kline, 1974.

14. Deliberti, J.: Reye's syndrome. Third Annual Symposium on Critical Care Medicine. Portland, Oregon, 1976.

15. DeVivo, D., and Keating, J.: Acute encephalopathy with fatty infiltration of the viscera. Pediatr. Clin. North Am., *23*:527, 1976.

16. DeVivo, D., and Dodge, P.: The critically ill child: diagnosis and management of head injury. Pediatrics, *48*:1129, 1971.

17. Donohoe, K., et al.: Cerebrospinal circulation and cerebral angiography. Nurs. Clin. North Am., *9*:623, 1974.

18. Drugs for Epilepsy. Med. Lett. Drugs Ther., 18:25, 1976.

19. Feigin, R., and Dodge, P.: Bacterial meningitis: newer concepts of pathophysiology and neurologic sequelae. Pediatr. Clin. North Am., *23*:541, 1976.

20. Feuer, H.: Early management of pediatric head injury. Pediatr. Clin. North Am. *22*:425, 1975.

21. Fewer, D, et al.: The chemotherapy of brain tumors. J.A.M.A., *222*:549, 1972.

22. Fish, I.: The electroencephalogram in clinical pediatrics. Pediatr. Clin. North Am., *18*:191, 1971.

23. Gomez, M., and Reese, D.: Computed tomography of the head in infants and children. Pediatr. Clin. North Am., *23*:473, 1976.

24. Guyton, A.: Textbook of Medical Physiology, 5th ed. Philadelphia, W. B. Saunders Co., 1976.

25. Hanlon, K.: Description and uses of intracranial pressure monitoring. Heart Lung, *5*:277, 1976.

26. Hendrick, B., et al.: Trauma of the central nervous system in children. Pediatr. Clin. North Am., *22*:415, 1975.

27. Hooshmand, H.: Toxic effects of anticonvulsants: general principles. Pediatrics, *53*:551, 1974.

28. Horowitz, S.: Neurologic Problems. *In* Klaus, M., and Fanaroff, A.: Care of the High-Risk Neonate. Philadelphia, W. B. Saunders Co., 1973.

29. Hudak, C., et al.: Critical Care Nursing. Philadelphia, J. B. Lippincott Co., 1973.

30. Kinney, A., et al.: Cerebrospinal fluid circulation and encephalography. Nurs. Clin. North Am., *9*:611, 1974.

31. Kutt, H.: The use of blood levels of antiepileptic drugs in clinical practice. Pediatrics, *53*:557, 1974.

32. Lampkin, B., et al.: Response of medulloblastoma to vincristine sulphate; a case report. Pediatrics, *39*:761, 1967.

33. Lombroso, C.: The treatment of status epilepticus. Pediatrics, *53*:536, 1974.

34. Mandrillo, M.: Brain Scanning. Nurs. Clin. North Am., *9*:633, 1974.

35. Menkes, J.: Diagnosis and treatment of minor motor seizures. Pediatr. Clin. North Am., *23*:435, 1976.

36. Mauss, N., and Mitchell, P.: Increased intracranial pressure: an update. Heart Lung, 5:919, 1976.

37. Nellhaus, G.: Neurologic and neuromuscular disorders. *In*: Current Pediatric Diagnosis and Treatment. Los Altos, Lange Medical Publications, 1976.

38. Parsons, L.: Respiratory changes in head injury. Am. J. Nurs., 71:2187, 1971.

39. Rosenblum, M., et al.: Chloroethylcyclohexyl-nitrosourea (CCNU) in the treatment of malignant brain tumors. J. Neurosurg., 39:306, 1973.

40. Samson, D., and Clark, K.: A current review of brain abscess. Am. J. Med., 54:201, 1973.

41. Schmidt, R., and Wilder, B.: Epilepsy. Philadelphia, F. A. Davis Co., 1968.

42. Sibley, W.: Diagnosis and treatment of epilepsy: overview and general principles. Pediatrics, 53:531, 1974.

43. Smith, D., et al.: Bacterial meningitis: a symposium. Pediatrics, 52:586, 1973.

44. Swift, N.: Head injury: essentials of excellent care. Nursing '74, 4:26, 1974.

45. Vaughn, V., McKay, R., and Behrman, R. (eds.): Nelson Textbook of Pediatrics, 11th ed. Philadelphia, W. B. Saunders Co., 1979.

46. Walker, M.: Diagnosis and treatment of brain tumors. Pediatr. Clin. North Am. 23:131, 1976.

47. Weeks, H.: What every intensive care nurse should know about Reye's syndrome. Am. J. Matern. Child Nurs., 1:(4):231-38, 1976.

48. Wehrle, P., et al.: The critically ill child: management of acute bacterial meningitis. Pediatrics, 44:991, 1969.

49. Wright, L., and Ballantine, T.: Management of brain abscess in children and adolescents. Am. J. Dis. Child., 114:113, 1967.

50. Young, J.: Recognition, significance, and recording of the signs of increased intracranial pressure. Nurs. Clin. North Am., 4:223, 1969.

CHAPTER 5
CARE OF THE CHILD WITH A DISORDER OF THE RENAL SYSTEM

Anita Stoeppel, R.N., M.S.N.
Annalee Oakes, R.N., M.A.

OBJECTIVES

1. State five areas to include when taking the history.

2. State four causes of acute renal failure.

3. Discuss the pathophysiology of hemolytic uremic syndrome, acute tubular necrosis, renal trauma, and acute uric acid nephropathy.

4. State the definitions of renal contusion and renal hematoma.

5. List five causes of chronic renal failure.

6. State four laboratory findings in chronic renal failure.

7. Discuss the complications of renal failure, dialysis, and transplantation.

The following review includes special pediatric considerations in normal renal anatomy and physiology.

Structure
1. Infant.
   a. Kidneys located low in lumbar region.
   b. May be readily palpated.
   c. Kidneys are lobulated.
2. Children.
   a. Kidneys assume their higher adult position.
   b. Perirenal fat is extremely scanty until the age of 10 years.
      1) Child is more vulnerable to trauma.

Function
1. Infant.
   a. Glomerular filtration rates are low due to:
      1) Relatively impermeable basement membrane.
      2) High intrarenal vascular resistance.
      3) Low net driving force for filtration.
   b. Tubular transport capacity is proportionally even lower.
      1) Results in urinary losses of glucose, amino acids, phosphate, and calcium.
   c. Act of urination is a lower arc reflex.
2. Child.
   a. Kidneys reach functional maturity during second year of life.
   b. Urination becomes a conscious function by 30 months.
      1) Cerebral control.
      2) Inhibitory influence during sleep.
3. Average urinary output
   a. See Growth and Development, Chapter 1.

CLINICAL ASSESSMENT

History
1. Abnormal patterns of micturition.
   a. Polyuria.
   b. Nocturia.
   c. Urgency.
   d. Incontinence.
   e. Dysuria.
   f. Hesitancy.
2. Gastrointestinal disturbances are frequently associated by way of the solar plexus.
3. Trauma.
4. Failure to thrive.
5. Fever of undetermined origin.
6. Flank pain.

7. Ingestions of poisonous chemicals.
8. Prenatal and postnatal periods.
9. Family history.
   a. Polycystic disease.
   b. Genital malformations.
   c. Rubella infection.
   d. Oligohydramnios or polyhydramnios.
   e. Single umbilical artery.
10. Other congenital anomalies.
    a. Absence of abdominal muscles.
    b. Aganglionic megacolon.
    c. Aniridia.
    d. Imperforate anus.

Physical Examination

1. Inspection.
   a. Dehydration.
      1) Dry, inelastic skin.
      2) Sunken eyes.
      3) Depressed anterior fontanel.
      4) Dry mucous membranes.
   b. Edema.
      1) Generalized.
      2) Periorbital.
2. Palpation.
   a. With any generalized enlargement or hardening, the normal lobulated form is more pronounced and palpable.
   b. Abdominal mass.
3. Percussion.
   a. Bladder of infant felt and percussed to level of the umbilicus.
4. Vital signs.
   a. Temperature.
   b. Blood pressure.

Laboratory Studies Specific to Children

1. Children over 2 years of age have results similar to adults.
2. Tests involving concentrations (specific gravity, osmolality) give the same results regardless of patient's size.
3. Tests involving quantities per minute (glomerular filtration rate) correlate roughly with renal mass, which is related to body size. The most suitable criterion of body size for this purpose is surface area.
4. Blood studies.
   a. Plasma urea: 10 to 20 mg% in first year.
   b. pH: mean 7.34 in first 2 weeks.
   c. PCO_2: mean 37 mm Hg in first 2 weeks.
   d. Total CO_2: mean 22 mmol/l in first 2 weeks.

    e. Albumin.
       1) 3 to 4 g/dl: premature.
       2) 3 to 8 g/dl: term.
       3) 4.2 to 5.6 g/dl: to 1 year.
       4) 4.6 to 4.9 g/dl: 1 to 4 years.
       5) 4.2 to 5.8 g/dl: 5 to 12 years.
       6) 4 to 7 g/dl: 12 to 15 years.
    f. Total serum protein.
       1) 4 to 5 g/dl: premature.
       2) 5.1 to 5.7 g/dl: term.
       3) 5.8 to 6.4 g/dl: to 1 year.
       4) 6.4 to 7.5 g/dl: 1 to 4 years.
       5) 6.7 to 7.9 g/dl: 5 to 12 years.
       6) 7.2 g/dl: 12 years.
    g. Inorganic phosphorus.
       1) 5 to 6.7 mg/dl: newborn.
       2) 4 to 5 mg/dl: to 2 years.
       3) 3 to 4 mg/dl: 2 to 15 years.
    h. Electrolytes.
    i. Blood urea nitrogen (BUN).
  5. Urine studies.
    a. Glomerular filtration rate.
       1) 5 to 7 ml/min: full term infant (25 to 50% of the adult
          figure).
       2) Normal by 6 months.
    b. Specific gravity in early infancy (first few months).
       1) 1.001 to 1.006: spontaneous levels.
       2) 1.016: maximum concentration.
    c. Creatinine.
       1) 15 to 20 mg/kg/24 hours: 0 to 6 years.
       2) 20 to 30 mg/kg/24 hours: 6 to 12 years.
    d. Culture and sensitivity.
    e. Urinalysis.

		newborn	infant	child
1)	Protein	tr.	0	0
2)	RBC/HPF	0.1	0	0
3)	WBC/HPF	0-5	2-4	2-4

    f. Osmolality.

Other Tests
  1. Renal biopsy.
  2. Ultrasound.
  3. X-ray film.
  4. Intravenous pyelogram.
  5. Renal angiography.

PATHOLOGIC CONDITIONS

ACUTE RENAL FAILURE

Definition: Abrupt loss of renal excretory function due to impaired blood supply to the kidney or intrarenal blood flow and characterized by changes in creatinine clearance. Causative factors may be shock, toxic agents, allergic phenomena, and/or obstructive uropathy because of stones or tumor. The conditions here described precipitate acute renal failure.

HEMOLYTIC UREMIC SYNDROME

Incidence
Predominantly seen in young infants. In the United States the mean age is 4 1/2 years.
Pathophysiology
1. Sudden onset of intravascular hemolysis and acute renal failure.
2. Diffuse intravascular clotting followed by fibrin deposits.
3. Injury to red blood cells and platelets attempting passage through damaged vessels.
Cinical Presentation
1. Signs and symptoms.
    a. Clinical signs of hematuria and decreased urine output develop after several days of acute gastroenteritis.
    b. Mild to severe neurologic signs, i.e., irritability, ataxia, seizures, coma.
    c. Complications of thrombocytopenia: petechiae and ecchymoses.
2. Laboratory findings.
    a. Fibrin found in glomerular capillaries and arterioles when studied by electron microscopy.
    b. Thrombocytopenia.
    c. Anemia, increased reticulocyte count.
    d. Negative Coombs' test result.
    e. Hyperglycemia may be present.
    f. Triangular or "helmet-shaped" red cells present during the crisis phase.
    g. Electrolyte disturbance − decreased sodium or increased potassium.
Objectives of Therapy
1. Early diagnosis of cause.
2. Reverse acute renal ischemia.
3. Supportive therapy during neurologic coagulation crisis.
4. Extrarenal removal of metabolic wastes.
Therapeutic Management
1. Blood and platelet transfusions and possible exchange transfusions.
2. Heparin therapy controversial.

3. Dialysis.
4. Control of seizures.
5. Fluid regulation.

Complications
1. Multiple intrarenal infarcts leading to chronic renal failure.
2. Hemorrhage.

Nursing Skills
1. Careful monitoring of vital and neurologic signs.
2. Knowledge of dialysis complications.
   a. Hemodialysis: infection, cannula separation and bleeding, AV shunt occlusion, arrhythmias.
   b. Peritoneal: infections, dialysate retention, respiratory changes.

ACUTE TUBULAR NECROSIS

Incidence
Rare under 10 years of age.[8]

Pathophysiology
1. Patchy necrosis, commonly affecting the terminal portions of the proximal convoluted tubules through the distal convoluted tubules.
2. General disruption at the basement membrane; impaired and incomplete regeneration.

Clinical Presentation
1. General signs and symptoms:
   a. Oliguria to anuria.
   b. Interstitial renal edema which causes kidney swelling.
2. Laboratory findings:
   a. Specific gravity: 1.008 to 1.014.
   b. Proteinuria, protein casts.
   c. Low serum sodium.
   d. Urine sodium and chloride: 50 to 90 mEq/l.
   e. Urine urea nitrogen: 300 to 400 mg/dl.
   f. Urine osmolality: 300 to 350 mOsm/l.

Objective of Therapy
1. Extrarenal removal of excess body water and metabolic wastes.
2. Minimize residual damage.

Therapeutic Management
1. Frequent and early dialysis, as indicated by:
   a. Progessive hyperkalemia.
   b. Decreased carbon dioxide combining power to 12 mEq/l.
   c. BUN of 125 to 150 mg/dl.
   d. Excessive fluid retention.
   e. Clinical signs of progessive uremia.
2. Specific treatment for contributing cause, such as shock, septicemia, or transfusion reaction.
3. Control of fluid balance and thirst.

    4. Control of hyperkalemia.

    5. Control of seizures.

Complications

    1. Infection.

    2. Coma.

    3. Death.

Nursing Skills

    1. Same as for hemolytic uremic syndrome.

RENAL TRAUMA

Incidence

    1. Majority of injuries are due to blunt trauma to the abdomen.

    2. Less common are injuries from fractured reticulocytes because of immediate post blood pump machine use and cardiopulmonary bypass procedures.

Types of Injuries

    1. Contusion: inflammation of the parenchymal tissue.

       a. Parenchymal blood flow is decreased as a result of inflammation, resulting in decreased urine output.

       b. Hematuria may persist for days or weeks.

       c. Self-resolution is the rule.

    2. Renal hematoma: damage to the capsule of the kidney, resulting in a break in the renal capsule.

       a. Bleeding into the surrounding area occurs.

       b. Hematuria is present, flank mass may be present.

       c. Self-resolving.

    3. Acute disruption of the collecting system.

       a. Leakage of urine into the surrounding area.

       b. Stagnant urine and blood produce excellent culture media, making abscess formation probable.

    4. Vascular injuries.

       a. Renal vessel laceration.

          1) Blood supply to the kidney is decreased; ischemia and necrosis are likely to occur.

          2) Necessitates immediate diagnosis and treatment if the kidney is to be saved.

       b. Clot formation.

          1) Occurs secondary to the trauma of the tunica intima.

          2) Surgery is the only treatment.

Clinical Presentation

    1. General signs and symptoms:

       a. Shock (most striking symptom).

       b. Pain and tenderness.

       c. Flank mass.

       d. Inspiratory pain.

       e. Pallor.

    f. Nausea and vomiting.

    g. Abdominal rigidity, guarding.

    h. Oliguria or anuria.

2. Laboratory findings:
   a. Decreased hemoglobin.
   b. Hematuria, microscopic or gross; quantity is not indicative of the severity of the injury.
3. Other diagnostic findings:
   a. IVP is the diagnostic procedure of choice.
   b. Radiologic evidence includes:
      1) Extravasation of dye.
      2) Any distortion of the contour of the kidney or the calyceal system.
      3) Obliteration of the shadow of the psoas muscle.

Objectives of Therapy

1. Control of hemorrhage and shock.
2. Relief of obstruction.
3. Repair of intraperitoneal trauma.
4. Drainage of infection.

Therapeutic Management

1. School or employment is allowed as long as bilateral kidney function is demonstrated and the patient's vital signs are stable, even though signs of renal damage are present.
2. Antibiotics and bedrest.
3. Surgical management: vessel or ureter repair or partial or complete nephrectomy.

Complications

1. Sepsis, infection.
2. Shock.
3. Residual scarring and impaired urine excretion.

Nursing Skills

1. Same as for hemolytic uremic syndrome.
2. Wound care and dressing.

ACUTE URIC ACID NEPHROPATHY

Incidence

A serious iatrogenic complication of leukemia and lymphoma treatment.

Pathophysiology

1. Cause: intrarenal crystallization of uric acid.

Clinical Presentation

1. History of disease, ie., leukemia, lymphoma.
2. Chemotherapy and medications history.
3. General signs and symptoms are similiar to those of acute tubular necrosis.
4. Laboratory findings.
   a. Urine contains microscopic uric acid crystals and casts.

5. Other diagnostic findings.
   a. X-ray film may show opacities.
   b. Delayed renal tubule filling and excretion studies.

Objectives of Therapy

1. Focus: prevention of renal complications of leukemia and lymphoma therapy.

Therapeutic Management

1. Prior to and during treatment of leukemia and lymphoma:
   a. Hydrate and alkalinize the urine.
   b. Administer allopurinol.
2. Diuresis with mannitol or high doses of diuretics is recommended by some.
3. Peritoneal dialysis.

Complications

1. Continual deterioration of tubules and eventually of parenchymal tissue of kidneys.
2. Retention of metabolic wastes with related fluid electrolyte and protein derangement.

CHRONIC RENAL FAILURE

Etiology

1. Recurrent urinary tract infections, pyelonephritis.
   a. In children under 2, the symptoms are more likely to be systemic: shaking chill, abrupt onset of fever, restlessness, apathy, or prostration.
   b. Chronic urinary infection may be asymptomatic.
2. Hypersensitivity diseases (glomerulonephritis, acute lupus nephritis).
3. Hypertensive cardiovascular diseases.
4. Congenital disorders (cystic disease, congenital nephritis).
5. Miscellaneous.
   a. Urinary calculi.
   b. Neuromuscular disorders (neurogenic bladder).

Pathophysiology

1. Chronic long-term destruction of the kidney filtration and collection mechanisms, with related deterioration of parenchymal tissue.
2. Amount and severity of damage is dependent on the kind and duration of pathology.

Clinical Presentation

1. General signs and symptoms:
   a. Edema.
   b. Decreased muscle mass.
   c. Hypertension.
   d. Nausea and vomiting.
   e. Growth failure.

    f. Polyuria, nocturia.

    g. Bleeding.

    h. Intolerance to cold.

    i. Increased skin pigmentation.

2. Laboratory findings:

    a. Azotemia.

    b. Anemia.

    c. Acidosis.

    d. Increased serum inorganic phosphorus.

    e. The kidneys in children with renal failure are generally able to maintain sodium and water balance under ordinary circumstances, but they lack the flexibility to handle additional stresses imposed by disease or injudicious therapy.

Objectives of Therapy

1. Minimize progression of deterioration.

2. Reduce incidence and severity of complications.

Therapeutic Management

1. Diet to minimize renal solute load and control mild hypertension (generous water intake, high carbohydrate, high fat, minimal protein, low sodium).

2. Transfusion of packed red cells.

3. Minimize osteodystrophy with aluminum hydroxide, Basaljel calcium, and vitamin D.

4. Antihypertensives: reserpine, Aldomet, Apresoline, diazoxide (see complications); diuretics: Diuril, Lasix, Aldactone.

5. Sodium citrate to control severe acidosis.

6. Dialysis to control severe acidosis, hyperkalemia, and hyperhydration.

7. Insertion of shunts and formation of fistulas for hemodialysis. Pediatric shunts should be used so that more distal vessels can be used and less blood is shunted, in order to prevent high-output cardiac failure.

8. Transplantation.

Complications of Chronic Renal Failure, Dialysis, and Transplantation

1. Profound anemia: child is left with no reserve to survive an unexpected major hemorrhage.

2. Hypertensive crisis.

    a. Often related to fluid overload.

    b. Renin-mediated.

    c. Treated with rapid (over 30 seconds or less) intravenous diazoxide, 2 to 5 mg/kg. Transient tachycardia lasting 10 to 15 minutes may occur after diazoxide injection.

    d. If response is unsatisfactory after 30 minutes, establish an IV drip for administration of Apresoline or Aldomet.

    e. Maintain fluid infusion at the most minimal volume and lowest sodium chloride content.

    f. Diuretics or dialysis may be required to remove a volume of fluids equal to infusate.

g. Central venous pressure (CVP) monitoring may be used to gauge rate of infusion.

3. Infections.
    a. Septicemia (major cause of death).
    b. Hepatitis.
    c. Pericarditis, with or without effusion.
    d. Cytomegalovirus syndrome (has occured within two months following transplantation).
        1) Presenting symptoms include:
            a) Fever persisting up to three weeks and associated with leukopenia.
            b) Lymphocytosis.
            c) Hemolytic anemia.
            d) Thrombocytopenia.
        2) Treated with cytosine arabinoside.
        3) Complication: hepatic dysfunction.
    e. Other infections caused by *Clostridium perfringens, Pneumocystitis carinii, Nocardia asteroides, Aspergillus,* and Candida.
4. Clotting of AV shunts is the most common complication of hemodialysis in the pediatric age group.
5. Hypotension shock: administer vasoconstrictor such as Levophed, 1 ml in 250 ml dextrose 5% in water at an individually adjusted rate. More frequently, dopamine, 10 mcg/kg/min, is being used to increase cardiac output and normalize blood pressure.
6. Acid-base imbalance.
7. Air embolus.
8. Arrhythmia.
9. Hemolysis.
10. Transfusion reaction.
11. Seizures.
12. In patients with dialysis encephalopathy syndrome: mixed dysarthria, apraxia of speech, myoclonus, dementia, focal seizures, and abnormal electroencephalogram.
13. Hepatic dysfunction due to cytomegalovirus or Imuran toxicity.

――――――――――――― **HEMODIALYSIS** ―――――――――――――

Advantages
1. More efficient, especially in severely catabolic patients.
Disadvantages
1. Requires access to circulation; in small children this may be very difficult.
2. Technically more difficult than peritoneal dialysis.
3. Sepsis.
4. Air embolism.

Indications
1. Prophylactic use in critically ill and multi-injured patients who may have oliguria resulting from the severe stress placed on kidney function.
2. Central nervous system symptoms: lethargy, coma, irritability, seizures.[16]
3. Congestive heart failure.
4. Severe hypertension.
5. Gastrointestinal or skin bleeding.
6. Uncontrollable hyperkalemia, hyponatremia, or acidosis.
7. In the absence of symptoms, a BUN greater than 80 to 100 mg/dl.
8. Severe oliguria for 24 to 48 hours in any patient, regardless of symptoms or BUN level.[16]

Physiologic Considerations for Pediatric Hemodialysis
1. Weight changes.
   a. Weigh initially and monitor constantly during dialysis.
   b. Infants and small children must have blood lines taped to insure correct weight measurements.
2. Vital signs are labile with rapid fluid and electrolyte changes in the patient undergoing dialysis.
3. Saline infusion if blood pressure suddenly falls. May need to remove the ultrafiltration and place head of bed in tilted-down position. Turn down blood pump.
4. Albumin infusion if patient is edematous and has a low serum albumin.
5. Extracorporeal blood volume should be approximately 8% or 80 ml/kg of ideal body weight.
6. Type of dialyzer membrane system depends on size of child; the single pass dialysis is usually considered for poisonings.
7. Temperature of dialysis bath is kept at 37°C, except for very young children for whom the bath is put at 38°C to decrease the heat loss. Infants lose body heat rapidly; dialysate bath should be kept at 39°C.
8. Heparinization.
   a. Obtain hematology consultation when:
      1) The platelet count is less than 50,000.
      2) The prothrombin time (PT) and partial thromboplastin time (PTT) are abnormal prior to starting dialysis.
      3) Any bleeding problem is present.
   b. Regional heparinization is usually done for very small children, if patient is bleeding, is going to surgery, or has been to surgery in the past five days.
   c. May need greater heparin dosage if blood flow is less than 100 ml/min and the dialysis time is less than 4 hours.
9. Length of time on the dialysis:
   a. No more than 2 to 3 hours for a stable patient with chronic renal failure who is undergoing dialysis for the first time.

      b.   Usually dialysis lasts less than six hours, especially when the patient is in acute distress.

10.   If the following laboratory values do not gradually return to normal range, notify the physician immediately:
      a.   Elevated phosphorus.
      b.   Low calcium.
      c.   Low hemoglobin.
      d.   Elevated potassium (over 6 mEq/l).
      e.   Elevated BUN.
      f.   Great weight gain.

11.   If air is accidently infused into the patient, **immediately** tip patient's head down and position on left side. Stop dialysis and notify physician.

12.   Patient and family may indicate or demonstrate emotional changes during dialysis; these should be reported to the psychiatric nurse consultant or social worker.

13.   Monitor electrocardiogram continuously during and immediately after dialysis.

14.   One unit of washed packed red cells should be on hand for transfusion.

Special Nursing Care of Infants and Children During Hemodialysis

Careful, accurate interpretation of vital signs is of the utmost importance. However, with infants and small children, changes may be symptomatic before vital signs vary. It is therefore recommended that the nurse scrutinize and document all changes. The most important signs are facial expressions, color, and level-of-consciousness responses. If the central color (face, lips, buccal mucosa) becomes pale, dusky, or mottled, any one of the following may be causative: blood is being stolen by the dialyzer; the infant or small child is in shock owing to the rapid ultrafiltration; there is a change in cardiac status; the body temperature has dropped; or there is increasing respiratory distress. In each of these events, the nurse should obtain the patient's weight and blood pressure, check the cardiac monitor for any rhythm or rate changes, and note variances of the trans-membrane pressure.

If the patient gives a sudden sharp cry or has a startled expression, this may mean he is experiencing abdominal cramping. Likewise, a sudden drop in blood pressure usually causes the patient to vomit or stool. Pulse and respiratory changes are associated with these changes. Abrupt agitation in the infant should be a signal to the nurse that the patient is most likely hypertensive from fluid overloading. This occurs from arterial spasm and the resulting action of blood being dumped from the dialyzer into the infant. Aspiration of feedings is common because the patient is weak and may not cough or gag. Throughout the dialysis procedure, a critically ill patient must be continuously observed for cardiac arrest, as this event is all too common.

PERITONEAL DIALYSIS

Advantages
1. Can be instituted quickly.
2. Requires a minimum of equipment.
3. Is relatively simple and safe to perform.

Disadvantages
1. Dialysis time is generally longer than with hemodialysis.
2. Risk of peritonitis and general sepsis.
3. Risk of shock.
4. Hypernatremia and hyperglycemia.
5. Protein loss.
   a. Hypoproteinemia.
   b. Hypogammaglobulinemia with ascites.
   c. Poor wound healing.
   d. Susceptibility to infection.
6. Hypoventilation.
   a. Atelectasis.
   b. Pneumonia.

Indications
1. See indications for hemodialysis.
2. May be used when hemodialysis is contraindicated, AV shunt sites are closed, or circulation is not accessible.

Physiological Considerations for Pediatric Peritoneal Dialysis
1. Record of exact time of beginning and ending of dialysis is necessary to determine amount infused, amount recovered, and balance.
2. Solutions should be warmed to approximately body temperature.
   a. Increases solute clearance.
   b. Increases patient comfort.
   c. Controls heat loss.
3. Gravity flow of dialysate into patient takes 5 to 10 minutes. If flow takes longer, patient may need to be repositioned.
4. Solution usually remains in patient 25 to 30 minutes.
5. Draining for larger children is accomplished within 10 minutes and collected in a run-off bag; for smaller children, use a urimeter (for less than 300 cc).
6. Unpredictable flow of dialysate may run in more than ordered or run off more than desired. Large losses could cause shock in the patient.
7. Leaking of solution can occur around the peritoneal catheter and soak the dressing. If leakage is excessive, this loss must be accounted for in determining fluid balance.

8. Blockage of the peritoneal catheter is a common problem; it slows or prevents flow of dialysate into the peritoneal cavity or interferes with complete drainage out of the cavity.
9. Preoperative and postoperative weight is necessary to determine body fluid loss.
10. Respiratory distress or abdominal pain may indicate fluid shifts in and out that are excessive for that patients.

-------------------------- **TRANSPLANTATION** --------------------------

Objectives of Therapy: Preoperative
1. Control of hypertension.
2. Correction of anemia.
3. Adequate hydration.
4. Reduction of risk of infection.

Objectives of Therapy: Postoperative (in Addition to Routine Postsurgical Care)
1. Reverse isolation for four to seven days to decrease risk of infection: single room, sterile linens, gown, mask, strict handwashing used with patient contact. Some units do not require personnel to wear gown and mask, but all persons must be free of infection and adhere to correct handwashing. Visitors are generally limited to immediate family members (parents) for one week.
2. Immunosuppressive therapy: antilymphocytic globulin, antimetabolites, corticosteroids.
3. Central venous line to monitor effect of fluid loss on circulating blood volume and to determine replacement therapy. Readings are done every hour. A peripheral route is used for fluid replacement.
4. Foley catheter for bladder decompression and urine output measurement.
   a. Closed drainage system.
   b. Observe for kinks or anything that may obstruct flow.
   c. Bladder catheter, if clogged, is irrigated by physician under strict aseptic technique.
   d. Bladder catheter is removed at the discretion of physician or urologist.
   e. Urine output is measured and tested for specific gravity and protein.
5. Fluid replacement.
   a. Done hourly; determined by output of the previous hour.
   b. Potassium is not added to IV solutions until serum volume is in normal range and there is adequate urine output.

    c. Serum and urine electrolytes are used to monitor patient's chemical balance.

    d. Observe for signs of hyponatremia, hypokalemia, and hypotension. This is especially important in children, in whom serious fluid shifts can occur rapidly.

    e. Daily weight.

    f. Replace nasogastric suction loss of the day before with 1/2 N/S + KC1 20 mEq/1.

6. Observe for signs of transplant rejection.

    a. Fever.

    b. Hypertension.

    c. Swollen, tender kidney; tenderness in operative area.

    d. Oliguria and weight gain.

    e. Increased BUN or creatinine; decreased creatinine clearance.

7. Antibiotics.

8. Pain medication.

Nursing Skills

1. Care of AV fistula.

    a. Elevate the extremity for 48 hours postoperatively to decrease edema.

    b. Observe capillary refill in the affected extremity.

    c. Check for bruit.

    d. Aid distention of the veins by:

        1) Use of warm compresses.

        2) Hand exercises. (Blood pressure cuff is placed snugly around upper arm for 15 minutes, four times a day. The patient squeezes a rubber ball with the cuff in place. The cuff should be snug enough to cause distention of the veins.) Exercising should not be done the first 4 or 5 days after the fistula is created.

    e. Do not draw blood or take blood pressure in arm with fistula.

2. Care of AV shunt: Check for patency hourly, using one or more of the following methods:

    a. Listen for bruit at the end of the arterial shunt tubing.

    b. Feel shunt for warmth.

    c. Gently squeeze the shunt tubing. Pulse should be felt as pressure is released.

    d. Squeeze the arterial end of the tubing and with the other hand milk the blood about 2 cm toward the venous end. Release the tubing, and blood should quickly flow through the tube toward the venous end.

3. Infection control.

    a. Meticulous housekeeping of transplantation patient's environment.

    b. Culture and sensitivity tests of all invasive materials, once removed from patient.

    c. Aseptic technique for all patient procedures.

BIBLIOGRAPHY

1. Alfrey, A., et al.: The dialysis encephalopathy syndrome. N. Eng. J. Med. *294*: 184, 1976.

2. Barnett, H., (ed.): Pediatrics, 15 ed. New York, Appleton-Century-Crofts, 1972.

3. Bois, M. et al.: Nursing care of patients having kidney transplants. Am. J. Nurs. *6*:1238, 1968.

4. Dolan, P., and Greene, H., Jr.: Renal failure and peritoneal dialysis. Nursing 75, *5*:40, 1975.

5. Fine, R., et. al.: Hemodialysis in infants under one year of age for acute poisoning. Am. J. Dis. Child. *116*:657, 1968.

6. Hansen, G. (ed.): Caring for Patients with Chronic Renal Disease, A Reference Guide for Nurses. Philadelphia, J. B. Lippincott Co. 1974.

7. Harrison, J., et al. (eds.): Campbell's Urology, 4th ed. Philadelphia, W. B. Saunders Co., 1970, Volume 2.

8. Holmes, J.: Acute tubular necrosis and its management. Surg. Clin. North Am., *43*:2, 1963.

9. Knepshield, J.: Dialysis of poisons and drugs: annual review. Am. Soc. Artif. Intern. Org. *19*:590, 1973.

10. Linder, A., and Curtis, K.: Morbidity and mortality associated with long-term hemodialysis. Hosp. Pract. *9*:143, 1974.

11. Loggie, J.: Hypertension in children and adolescents. I. Causes and diagnostic studies. J. Pediatr., *74*:331, 1969.

12. Loggie, J.: Systemic hypertension in children and adolescents: causes and treatment. Pediatr. Clin. North Am. *18*:1273, 1971.

13. Loggie, J., and Van Maanen, E.: The autonomic nervous system and some aspects of the use of autonomic drugs in children. I. J. Pediatr. *81*:2 1972.

14. Loggie, J., and Van Maanen, E.: The autonomic nervous system and some aspects of the use of autonomic drugs in children. II. J. Pediatr., *81*:432, 1972.

15. O'Neill, M.: Symposium on care of the patient with renal disease. Nurs. Clin. North Am., *10*:411, 1975.

16. Smith, C., (ed.): The Critically Ill Child, 2nd ed. Philadelphia, W. B. Saunders Co., 1977.

17. Snydman, D., et al.: Prevention of nosocomial viral hepatitis, type B (hepatitis B). Ann. Intern. Med., *83*:838, 1975.

18. Steinberg, S., et al.: Hemodialysis for acute anuric uric acid nephropathy. Am. J. Dis. Child. *129*:956, 1975.

19. Symposium on pediatric hemodialysis and renal transplantation. Clin. Proc. Child. Hosp. Nat. Med. Cent. *30*:8, 1974.

20. Symposium on Pediatric Hemodialysis and Renal Transplantation. Clin. Proc. Child. Hosp. Nat. Med. Cent. *30*:9, 1974.

21. West, C.: Electrolyte Imbalance and Parenteral Fluid Therapy. Cincinnati, Cincinnati Children's Hospital, 1971.

22. Willey, M.: Care of the patient with a kidney transplant. Nurs. Clin. North Am., *8*:127, 1973.

23. Williams, D., (ed.): Pediatric Urology. New York, Appleton-Century-Crofts, 1968.

24. Winbert, C., and Roehm, M.: Sawyer's Nursing Care of Patients with Urologic Diseases, 2nd ed. St. Louis, C. V. Mosby Co., 1968.

25. Wolf, Z.: What patients awaiting kidney transplant want to know. Am. J. Nurs., *76*:92, 1976.

26. Ziai, M., (ed.): Pediatrics, 2nd ed. Boston, Little, Brown & Co., 1975.

Additional Reading

Altshuler, A., et al.: Even children can learn clean self-catheterization. Am. J. Nurs., *77*:97, 1977.

Cross, P.: Ureteral reimplantation: Nursing care of the child. Am. J. Nurs., *76*:1800, 1976.

Gittes, R.: Retrograde renal and ureteral brush biopsy. Am. J. Nurs., *78*:410, 1978.

Juliani, L.: Assessing renal function. Nursing 78, *8*:34, 1978.

Juliani, L., and Reamer, B.: Kidney transplant: your role in aftercare. Nursing 77, 7:46, 1977.

Kobrzycki, P.: Renal transplant complications. Am. J. Nurs. 77:641, 1977.

Living with End-Stage Renal Disease. Department of Health, Education, and Welfare, U.S. Government Printing Office, 1976, #017-026-00043-7.

Nelson, B. A nursing approach to patients with long-term renal transplants: a practical application of nursing theory. Nurs. Clin. North Am., *13*:155, 1978.

Wheeler, D.: Teaching home-dialysis for an eight-year-old boy. Am. J. Nurs. *77*:273, 1977.

Wood, R.: Catheterizing the patient with an ileal conduit stoma. Am. J. Nurs. *76*:1592, 1976.

CHAPTER 6
CARE OF THE CHILD WITH DIABETES MELLITUS

Anita Stoeppel, R.N., M.S.N.

OBJECTIVES

1. Describe essential components of the normal anatomy of the pancreas.

2. Relate the pancreas structure to the normal function of this endocrine system.

3. State the abnormal chemistry findings in ketoacidosis.

4. State the different physical signs present when there is 5% or 15% weight loss.

5. Describe priority nursing and medical management of ketoacidosis, including the low-dose insulin infusion treatment.

6. State the major hazards of insulin therapy.

7. Describe the progression of pathophysiology known as Somogyi syndrome.

8. State four areas of infection to which children with diabetes are prone.

NORMAL ANATOMY AND PHYSIOLOGY OF THE PANCREAS

Structure
1. A 12.5 cm long, 5 cm wide lobular structure located beneath and behind the stomach.
2. Types of tissue:
   a. Acini tissue.
   b. Islets of Langerhans: collections of cells scattered through the pancreas; cells are of three types: alpha, beta, and delta.

Function
1. Exocrine: acini tissue secretes alkaline pancreatic fluid through the pancreatic duct into the duodenum. This fluid contains trypsin, amylase, lipase, and chymotrypsin, which hydrolyze protein, starch, and fat during digestion.
2. Endocrine:
   a. Alpha cells secrete glucagon, which is a catabolic agent that increases the release of glucose, fatty acids, and amino acids into the blood stream. Hyperglucagonemia is present in most patients with diabetes mellitus.
   b. Beta cells secrete insulin, which is an anabolic agent that increases the storage of glucose, fatty acids and amino acids. Insulin also causes potassium to enter cells, resulting in a decrease of extracellular potassium concentration.
   c. Delta cells secrete somatostatin, which inhibits the secretion of insulin and glucagon.

INCIDENCE AND ETIOLOGY OF DIABETES MELLITUS

Precipitating Factors in Juvenile Diabetics
1. Heightened activity of the beta cells with resultant exhaustion: may be due to increased stimulation from growth hormone, adrenocortical hormones, disorders of insulin binding, and an abnormal and less effective insulin.
2. Destruction of beta cells by immune mechanism.
3. Impaired adenylcyclase activity of the beta cells.
4. An altered responsiveness of both alpha and beta cells.

Frequency of Diabetic Ketoacidosis in Children and Adolescents
1. Severe attacks are prevalent during the first 5 years of known diabetes, regardless of age at diagnosis.
2. Severe ketoacidosis is prevalent in the teen years regardless of duration.
3. Onset may be rapid.
4. Can follow severe psychologic stress in the absence of other causative factors.
5. Some juvenile diabetics experience wide and often rapid swings in blood sugar levels.

PATHOPHYSIOLOGY OF INSULIN INSUFFICIENCY AND GLUCOSE EXCESS

With little to no insulin secretion, carbohydrate utilization in peripheral tissue is impaired, especially in muscle and adipose tissue. The liver decreases synthesis of glycogen and increases glucose output from the alternate source of amino acids. The result of these two mechanisms is an elevated blood glucose level (hyperglycemia), which causes osmotic diuresis. Body water and electrolytes are lost through the kidneys, causing total body water depletion and circulatory insufficiency.

To further complicate this derangement, protein catabolism and lipolysis produce urea and organic acids, especially ketones. Only a partial amount of ketones may be utilized by muscle and other organs; the excess combines with plasma to cause metabolic acidosis. This phenomenon is termed ketoacidosis of diabetes.

CLINICAL ASSESSMENT

History
1. Evolution of present symptoms.
2. Past medical history, including allergies.
3. Family medical history.
4. Growth and developmental stage.
5. Medication history.

Physical Examination
1. Increase in depth and rate of respirations when serum carbon dioxide is less than 15 mM/l.
2. Kussmaul acidotic breathing when serum carbon dioxide is less than 10 mM/l.
3. Weight loss of 5% or more is manifested by:
   a. decreased skin turgor.
   b. softened eyeballs.
   c. dry mucous membranes.
4. Weight loss of 15% or more is manifested by:
   a. circulatory insufficiency.
      1) Hypotension.
      2) Tachycardia.
   b. Circulatory collapse and death.
5. Vomiting, absence of fluid and caloric intake.
6. Candida infection of perineal area, particularly in girls.
7. Signs of infection in:
   a. Sites of insulin injection.
   b. Finger and toe nails.
   c. Oral cavity.
      1) Carious teeth.
      2) Red or swollen gums.

Laboratory Examination
1. Serum ketones present (by Acetest)
2. pH less than 7.30.
3. Serum K+.
4. Blood glucose levels (above 150 mg%).
5. Urine ketones and glucose present.

PSYCHOSOCIAL ASSESSMENT OF DIABETIC CHILDREN AND ADOLESCENTS

Attitude—May Go Through Four Phases:
1. Initial acceptance.
2. Experimentation.
3. Denial during the age of peer culture.
4. Resignation.

Potential Problems
Some studies suggest three characteristics that may exist in sufficient degree to disturb the patient and may interfere at times with good management and desired physiologic course of the disorder.[2,8,9,16]
1. Excessive drive for self-assertion.
   a. Rebellion against authority, hostility directed first toward parents and later toward teachers and employers.
   b. Diabetes may aggravate usual teen-age drive toward recognition, because disease can result in rejection of the patient by parents or others, or the disease induces anger or frustration in the patient.
2. Severe hidden anxiety.
   a. Difficulty in accepting the fact of the diagnosis.
   b. Denial and persistent refusal to carry out diabetic tasks or to discuss the diabetes with others.
   c. Failure to seek medical advice when diabetes is out of control until ketosis has advanced and requires frequent hospitalization, which induces discouragement.
   d. Denial of disease because of unrealized anxiety related to the pressure of having a formidable condition.
3. Overt anxiety.
   a. Expressions of insecurity concerning the future.
   b. Worry by boys regarding role as men, by girls regarding role as wives and mothers.
   c. Fear of complications that may occur in the future.

Body Image Changes and Concerns Related to Skin and Other Tissue Disorders such as:
1. Necrobiosis lipoidica diabeticorium.
2. Lipoatrophy.
3. Lipohypertrophy
4. Xanthomata.

5. Vaginal moniliasis.
6. Toughness and discoloration of the skin at the site of insulin injections.

Parental Attitudes
1. Tolerant, relaxed, not outwardly aggressive or punitive. Parents may boast of how well they manage; some may feel excessively sorry for child. Regulation is usually satisfactory and adjustment good.
2. Overcontrolled perfectionism: all tasks become expressions of the mother's absolute power to do the right thing. Aggressive and subduing in dealing with the child. Tends to crush the child's personality, although diabetes may be satisfactorily regulated; child acts out by stealing, poor schoolwork, or sudden rebellion.
3. Erratic or persistently poor cooperation with medical regimen; mother's attitude may be self-pity, self-blame for the child's illness, or open hostility and rejection. Satisfactory regulation in this group is difficult; most children are poorly controlled or demonstrate marked fluctuation in the degree of regulation.

OBJECTIVES OF THERAPY

1. Early diagnosis.
2. Management that produces healthy control of glucose metabolism.
3. Reduction of systemic complications.
4. Establishment of good mental health regarding chronicity of disease.

THERAPEUTIC MANAGEMENT

Immediately upon Admission to Emergency Room
1. Dextrostix for blood glucose, Clinitest for urine sugar, and Acetest for urine ketones.
2. Electrolytes, blood urea nitrogen (BUN), glucose, Ca, P, creatinine, serum ketones, and capillary blood gases.
3. Electrocardiogram lead II rhythm strip.
4. Begin IV fluids:
   a. Normal saline, 200 cc over one hour for a 10 kg child, to provide fluids for maintenance and for extracellular losses.
   b. If pH is between 7.1 and 7.2, give 40 mEq/m^2 of sodium bicarbonate over two hours; if pH is less than 7.1, give 80 mEq/m^2 of sodium bicarbonate over two hours. Then reevaluate the patient's arterial pH.

    c. Obtain repeat blood gases until management has stabilized pH
to near normal.

5. Give regular insulin, 0.1 unit/kg by IV push.

6. Obtain additional studies as needed:

    a. Cultures.

    b. Chest.

    c. X-ray film.

7. Transfer to critical care unit.

Upon Admission to Critical Care Unit

1. Regular insulin may be administered subcutaneously according to
the patient's response.

2. The trend in several hospitals is toward intravenous low-dose
insulin infusion, as described here.

    a. Give priming dose of 0.1 unit/kg regular insulin intravenously.
(This dose may have been given in the Emergency Room;
please observe carefully.)

    b. Beginning with the second hour, give 0.1 unit/kg/hr regular
insulin by continuous intravenous infusion.

    c. To make insulin infusion for a 10 kg child, add 10 units of
regular insulin to 100 cc normal saline. Flush 50 cc through
the tubing to saturate the insulin binding sites. Infuse at
10 cc/hr.

    d. When the blood glucose level approaches 300 mg/dl, discon-
tinue the regular insulin infusion. Change the intravenous
fluid to dextrose 5% in 1/2 normal saline and begin a "sliding
scale" regular insulin therapy.

    e. If blood glucose level drops below 250 mg/dl, change IV fluids
to dextrose 2.5% in one-half normal saline as noted above, with
potassium chloride 10 mEq/m^2 for three hours.

    f. Discontinue insulin infusion when serum is negative for ketones
by Acetest and blood glucose is less than 250 mg/dl.

    g. Immediately upon stopping insulin infusion, give regular
insulin, 0.2 to 0.5 U/kg. Use a lower dose in new diabetics and
in children under 5 years; use a higher dose in adolescents and
children on a high dose of insulin (greater than 1.0 unit/kg/day).

    h. Obtain urine sugar and acetone every four hours and give
regular insulin according to previous response.

    i. Remember that the major hazards of insulin therapy are
hypoglycemia and relative hypokalemia.

    j. After correction of acidosis, beware of the Somogyi syndrome,
in which excessive hypoglycemia, glycosuria, and ketonuria may
result from excessive insulin dosage.

Prevention and Alleviation of Emotional Problems

1. Set up an individualized program of diet, urine testing, and
insulin to control the patient's diabetes.

2. Maintain an interested, flexible, but reasonably firm relationship with the child.
3. Teach the child and the parents about diabetes and techniques involved in best living with it.
4. Investigate the parental attitudes in the family and the child's reactions to them.
5. Make suggestions aimed at redressing any imbalance of mutual respect in the family relationships.
6. Refer the family for psychiatric help if the family relationships are so disturbed or the child's reactions so uncooperative that a reasonable diabetic regimen cannot be maintained.

COMPLICATIONS

1. Volume depletion and osmotic changes between compartments.
2. Acid-base disequilibrium progressing to acidosis and buffer depletion.
3. Nutritional deficiency.
4. Sepsis.

NURSING SKILLS

1. Support parents, who may feel guilty if child is newly diagnosed because of the inherited nature of the disease.
2. A patient who is a known diabetic may have a feeling of failure in carrying out the prescribed regimen.
3. Establish trusting relationship with child or adolescent.
   a. Learn whether episodes of acidosis are an expression of need for attention or a means of self-assertion.
4. Begin patient-family education if child is a new diabetic.
5. Reinforce knowledge about ketoacidosis in a known diabetic.
6. Plan for followup care in the diabetic clinic.
7. Home visit for diabetic teaching by nurse.
8. Referral to public health nurse, if indicated.

BIBLIOGRAPHY

1. Barnett, H. (ed.): Pediatrics. New York. Appleton-Century-Crofts, 1972.

2. Benoliel, J.: Social consequences of diabetes mellitus in adolescence. American Nurses' Association, Seventh Nursing Research Conference, Atlanta, Ga., 1971.

3. Bruck, E., and MacGillivray, M.: Post-hypoglycemic hyperglycemia in diabetic children, J. Pediatr., 84:672, 1974.

4. Brunner, L., and Suddarth, D. (eds.): Lippincott Manual of Nursing Practice, 2nd ed. Philadelphia, J. B. Lippincott Co., 1978.

5. Cerasi, E. and Luft, R. (eds). Pathogenesis of Diabetes Mellitus. Nobel Symposium 13. New York, John Wiley & Sons, 1970.

6. Drop, S.L., et al.. Low-dose intravenous infusion versus subcutaneous insulin injection: A controlled comparative study of diabetic ketoacidosis. Pediatrics, *59*:733, May, 1977.

7. Gamble, D., et al.: Viral antibodies in diabetes mellitus. Br. Med. J. *3*:627, 1969.

8. Knowles, H., et al.: The course of juvenile diabetes treated with unmeasured diet. Diabetes, *14*:239, 1965.

9. Missildine, W. (ed.): Emotional Problems of Diabetic Children: Feelings and Their Medical Significance. Ross Laboratories, Columbus, Ohio, Volume 5, 1963.

10. Muller, W., et al.: Abnormal alpha-cell function in diabetes. N. Engl. J. Med. *283*:109, 1970.

11. Nerup, J., et al.: Anti-pancreatic cellular hypersensitivity in diabetes mellitus. Diabetes, *20*:424, 1971.

12. Owen, J.: The Insulin Revolution. Hospital Formulary, July 1976, p. 343.

13. Singal, D.: Histocompatibility (HLA) antigens, lymphocytic antibodies, and tissue antibodies in patients with diabetes mellitus. Diabetes, *22*:429, 1973.

14. Smith, C. (ed.): The Critically Ill Child, 2nd ed. Philadelphia, W. B. Saunders Co., 1977.

15. The once and future diabetic. Emerg. Med., *8*:26, Sept., 1976.

16. White, P.: Fourth Allied Post-graduate course in Diabetes, American Diabetic Association in cooperation with Vanderbilt University, Nashville, Tennessee, April 1972.

Additional Reading

Ganong, W.: Review of Medical Physiology, 8th ed. Los Altos, Lange Medical Publications, 1977.

Keyes, M.: The Somogyi phenomenon in insulin-dependent diabetics. Nurs. Clin. North Am., *12*:439, 1977.

McCarthy, J.: Somogyi effect: Managing blood glucose rebound. Nursing 79, *9*:38, 1979.

Petrokas, J.: Commonsense guidelines for controlling diabetes during illness. Nursing 77, 7:36, 1977.

Wolfe, L.: Insulin: paving the way to a new life. Nursing 77, 7:38, 1977.

CHAPTER 7
CARE OF THE CHILD WITH A DISORDER OF THE ALIMENTARY TRACT

Cara Q. Brown, R.N., M.S. and
Annalee Oakes, R.N., M.A., CCRN

OBJECTIVES

1. Name the major structures of the alimentary system.

2. List two functions for each accessory organ to the alimentary system.

3. Compare stomach capacity and 24 hour caloric needs of a normal infant at each of the following body weights:
   a. 7 pounds.
   b. 10 pounds.
   c. 13 pounds.

4. Describe "planned intake" for a small, dehydrated child by a care plan example.

5. Outline one method of weighing a patient with gastrointestinal pathology.

6. Describe the reasons why neonates have a high risk of jaundice.

7. Explain the mechanisms of bilirubin light therapy.

8. Note three reasons why it is advantageous to assign the same nurse to a patient having long-term hyperalimentation.

STRUCTURE

Alimentary Tube
1. Extends from lips to anus; each section has a specific name and special anatomic characteristics.
2. Sections, in descending order:
    a. Oral cavity.
    b. Pharynx.
    c. Esophagus.
    d. Stomach: cardiac sphincter at proximal opening, pyloric sphincter at distal opening.
    e. Small intestine: extends from pylorus to ileocecal orifice, arranged in coils, divided into three parts.
        1) Duodenum.
        2) Jejunum.
        3) Ileum.
    f. Large intestine: extends from pylorus to ileocecal valve to anus.
        1) Cecum.
        2) Vermiform appendix.
        3) Colon.
            a) Ascending: cecum to undersurface of liver to hepatic flexure.
            b) Transverse: crosses upper part of abdominal cavity to splenic flexure.
            c) Descending: splenic flexure to brim of pelvis and sigmoid.
            d) Sigmoid: extends from descending colon to rectum.
        4) Rectum: extends to anus.
3. Microscopic anatomy: walls are composed of four main layers:
    a. Mucous membrane (innermost): has three components:
        1) Epithelial lining: varies in structure according to function of part of tube it lines — protective in esophagus, secretory in stomach, absorptive in small intestine.
        2) Lamina propria: supports the epithelium and connects it with underlying submucosa.
        3) Muscularis mucosa.
    b. Submucosa: connects mucous membrane with outer muscular layer.
    c. External muscular layer: thoroughly mixes the contents of the lumen with the digestive juices; moves them by peristaltic waves.
    d. Serosa (adventitia): mostly fibrous in nature.

FUNCTION

Ingestion
1. Mastication.
2. Salivation.
   a. Cleansing.
   b. Excretory.

Digestion and Secretion
1. Deglutition.
2. Chemical restructuring.
3. Mechanical changes.
4. Concentration or dilution of food to attain compatibility with normal body fluid, pH, components, and consistency.

Absorption
1. Into capillaries.
   a. Amino acids.
   b. Minerals.
   c. Sugars.
   d. Glycerol.
   e. Some fatty acids and vitamins.
2. Into lacteals.
   a. Glycerides and some fatty acids.
   b. Fat-soluble vitamins.
3. Into large intestine.
   a. Water.
   b. Salts.

Elimination
1. Storage of feces.
2. Defecation.

Synthesis of Vitamins, e.g., B and K.

MOVEMENTS

Oral Cavity
1. Mastication.
2. Rolling of food into bolus.

Pharynx
1. Projection of food.
2. Neurostimulation
   a. Lifts palate, thereby preventing passage of food into nose.
   b. Closes glottis, preventing passage of food into larynx.

Esophagus
1. Peristalsis: muscle coats are stimulated by (intrinsic) Auerbach's plexus.
2. Food bolus in esophagus stimulates nerve endings in wall, thus causing the vagus nerve to relax the cardiac sphincter.

Stomach

1. Filling causes bulging and lengthening (receptive relaxation).
2. Tonus exerts constant slight pressure on food, squeezing the food toward pylorus.
3. Peristalsis: vigorous contractions that mix the food.
4. Emptying occurs by neurogenic and humoral stimulation.

Small Intestine

1. Segmentation: rhythmic alternating contractions and relaxations; myogenic type of movement.
    a. Mixing: "shuttling."
2. Peristalsis: constriction behind bolus with relaxation of muscle in front; neurogenic type of movement.
    a. Propelling.
3. Emptying through ileocecal valve is initiated by autonomic neurogenic control.

Large Intestine

1. "Tone waves": a myogenic movement that sweeps contents backward and forward.
2. Mass peristalsis: strong waves at infrequent intervals that start at upper end of ascending colon and sweep feces through descending colon.
3. Defecation (emptying) occurs when feces distend the rectum wall, causing stimulation of the sympathetic and parasympathetic nerves of the abdominal muscles and colon. For children aged 24 to 30 months, these sensations rise to the level of consciousness, and defecating is a voluntary decision.

Accessory Organs

1. Tongue: helps in mastication and swallowing.
2. Teeth: dentition begins about 6 months (1 tooth each month up to 20 teeth); deciduous teeth are lost between 6 and 13 years. Permanent teeth begin at approximately age 6 and continue erupting to approximately age 17 or until child has 32 regular teeth. "Wisdom teeth" may erupt at any adolescent or adult age and are not counted in the 32.
3. Salivary glands.
    a. Parotid: serous secretions.
    b. Submandibular: serous secretions.
    c. Sublingual: mucous secretions.
4. Liver lies mostly in right hypochondriac and epigastric regions.
    a. Production of bile — both secretion and excretion.
    b. Conversion of glucose to glycogen and storage of latter.
    c. Deamination.
    d. Desaturation.
    e. Phagocytosis.
    f. Production of heparin.
    g. Production of plasma proteins.
5. Pancreas: has both endocrine and exocrine functions; pancreatic juices are emptied into duodenum.

APPLICATION TO CHILD

Stomach and Intestinal Tract
1. Underdeveloped at birth, but normal full-term infant has functional capacity to propel, digest, and absorb each of the main food types in liquid form (amino acids, fats, carbohydrates) except complex sugar.
2. Greater diameter of the anterior surface; the intestinal mass is transverse in the newborn and vertical in the adult.
3. Weight of tract: 1/10 of the adult weight.
   Length in adult: twice that in the newborn.
4. Surface area of intestinal tract increases four times birth size between birth and adulthood.
5. Thin wall at birth is due to comparatively weak development of its musculature.
6. Well-developed secretory and absorbing surfaces.

Ascending, Transverse, Descending and Sigmoid Colons
1. Have certain features in common at birth that differ from those in adults.
2. Teniae coli not well developed at birth.
3. Walls are thin owing to poor muscular development, and their external surfaces are smooth.
4. Rectum is relatively longer in the newborn than in the adult.
5. Anal canal is relatively longer in the newborn than in the adult.
6. Anus in the newborn is located a little posterior to its position in the adult.
7. Muscular part of the wall in the rectum is relatively very thin at birth.

Liver
1. Weight increases 12 to 13 times between birth and adulthood.
2. Relative weight to total body weight:
   a. At birth, constitutes 4.0%.
   b. In childhood, constitutes 3.0 to 4.0%.
   c. In adulthood, constitutes 2.5 to 3.5%.
3. Is the largest gland of the body.
   a. Composed of sinusoids and vessels filled with blood.
   b. Consists of flexible and compressible parenchyma.
   c. Shape is directly influenced by adjacent structures.
4. Appears to be structurally mature at birth but functionally immature (transient physiologic jaundice, variable vitamin K production and usage.)
5. Low level of hematopoietic activity at birth.

Pancreas
1. Weight of pancreas in adult is over 30 times that of newborn.
2. Subdivisions are clear in adult; no sharp demarcations at birth.
3. Exocrine function of gland is not achieved at birth.
   a. Pancreatic islets in newborn – 120,000; in adult – 800,000.

NOURISHMENT AND CALORIC NEEDS

Concerns for Alimentary Tract Capacity
1. Concept of "feeding on demand" (depending on infant to communicate hunger) is not always applicable with sick or premature infants. The nurse needs to monitor improvement in sick infant so as to allow demand feeding when baby is ready. Table 7–1 is a recommended guideline for infant feeding.

Table 7–1. TYPICAL AMOUNTS OF FORMULA TO OFFER IN A SELF–DEMAND REGIMEN

Infants Age and Average Weight	Typical Daily Quantity	Typical Number and Amounts of Feedings
Up to 1 month (up to 9 pounds)	20 to 24 fl oz	6 to 8 bottles (of 3 to 4 fl oz)
1 to 2 months (9 to 10 pounds)	24 to 28 fl oz	5 or 6 bottles (of 4 to 5 fl oz)
2 to 3 months (10 to 13 pounds)	26 to 32 fl oz	5 bottles (of 5 to 6 fl oz)
3 to 4 months and over (13 pounds and up)	32 fl oz (1 quart)	4 or 5 bottles (of 6 to 8 fl oz)

Alimentary Tract Capacity and Developmental Level
1. The younger the child, the shorter the attention span during large feedings or big meals; therefore, give small amounts and frequent feedings.
2. The younger the child, the sooner stomach capacity is reached; over-filling causes regurgitation. Sphincters at proximal and distal ends of stomach gradually develop sensitivity and tone over the first year of life.
3. Review information about stomach capacity as presented in Chapter 1, Growth and Development.

Food Selection and Quantity
1. Child tends to choose nourishing foods when presented with foods from the basic seven requirements.
2. Children select amounts to satisfy hunger demands if they are not forced to clear plate of all food served.

Factors Influencing Alimentary System Function
1. Child's total nutritional status; present nutritional state may be affected by an acute or chronic nutritional condition.
2. Growth rate has hereditary and environmental influences and is affected by periodic spurts and lax phases.
3. Activity and level of motor development (i.e., large muscle strength).
4. Level of tolerance for particular food that is offered.

5. Child's age and capacity to understand food choices.
6. Child's involvement in planning, feeding self, making charts with eating patterns, and other interesting activities.
7. Child's development and interest in good smells and appealing visual displays as a motive to ingest food.

Caloric Requirements

1. Review information about caloric requirements as presented in Chapter 1, Growth and Development.
2. A general broad guide may be employed by starting with a base of 1000 calories and adding 100 calories for each year of age. Begin at age 24 hours and continue to add until child is 10 or 11 years old.
3. Table 7–2 provides a comparison of caloric needs for maintenance and selected types of stress.

Table 7-2. GUIDELINES FOR CALORIC REQUIREMENTS IN INFANTS AND CHILDREN

Body Weight (kg)	Calorie Requirement	Type of Stress*	Cal/kg	Protein (g/kg)
1	120	A	120	2.0
2	240	A	120	2.0
	350	B	175	3.0
5	500	A	100	1.5
	800	B	160	2.5
10	800	A	80	1.0
	1400	B	140	2.0
20	1200	A	60	0.6
	2400	B	110	1.2
30	1350	A	45	0.5
	2250	B	75	1.0

*A: maintenance for children, adjusted for age
 B: trauma plus growth, adjusted for age

Water Requirements

1. Refer to Chapter 1, Growth and Development, for specific amounts for each age level. Use as a guide, not as an absolute standard, since each child requires individual consideration.
2. For infants, a general guideline is 130 cc of water/kg/24 hours.
3. If using actual weights, a general guideline is:
   a. 100 cc/kg if weight is 10 kg.
   b. 50 cc/kg for weights between 10 and 20 kg, using 100 cc/kg for first 10 kg. E.g., for a 15 kg child:

   $$\begin{array}{ll} 1000 \text{ cc for } 10 \text{ kg} \\ \underline{250 \text{ cc for } 5 \text{ kg}} \\ 1250 \text{ cc} 15 \text{ kg} \end{array}$$

    c. 20 cc/kg for weights between 20 and 70 kg, using 100 cc/kg for first 10 kg. E.g., for a 35 kg child:

$$
\begin{array}{ll}
1000 \text{ cc} & \text{for 10 kg} \\
\underline{500 \text{ cc}} & \text{for 25 kg} \\
1500 \text{ cc} & \quad\;\; 35 \text{ kg}
\end{array}
$$

CLINICAL ASSESSMENT

HISTORY

Growth and Development Before Current Illness or Trauma

1. Age, weight, height.
2. Pattern of gaining or losing weight.
3. Allergies to food or ingested materials (medications).
4. Differentiate signs and symtoms of normal gastrointentinal tract function that has been interrupted as compared with the sick child's gastrointestinal tract function that has been interrupted.
5. Feeding habits and preferences.
6. Hereditary influences.

Presenting Illness

1. Note any report of dysphagia, abdominal pain, bleeding, or melena.
2. Frequency, quality, and quantity of feedings and meals.
   a. Note time of last retained feeding.
   b. Obtain description of last 24 hours of eating and drinking, and determine who has fed patient each meal.
   c. Ask whether patient has an appetite.
3. Differentiate between regurgitation and "spitting vomiting," and have parent or caretaker describe reaction of patient to ingested items.

Elimination and Excretion

1. Note changes in voiding.
   a. Number of wet diapers in 24 hours.
   b. Frequency in older children.
   c. Describe odor, appearance, any differences from normal for that child (as observed by parent or caretaker).
   d. Ask to have wet diaper available for inspection at the time of history taking.
2. Note changes in defecation.
   a. Number, amount, quality of stools.
   b. Color, odor.
   c. Presence or absence of mucus, blood, fat globules.

PHYSICAL EXAMINATION

Inspection
1. Size, symmetry of abdomen, contours, bulges.
2. "Rippling" of peristalsis as noted on external abdominal wall.
3. Position of comfort or discomfort that child assumes for examination.
4. Skin turgor, condition of mucous membranes, rashes, color of buccal membranes.
5. Protrusions, retractions; note uniform contours of orifices.
6. Odors.
7. Color of feces.

Palpation
1. Tender points, rigidity.
2. Abnormal placement of abdominal organs: extra, displaced, or extended protrusions, bulges.
3. Changes in body temperature: heat or cold associated with any location along the alimentary tract, specifically in oral cavity or rectum.
4. Movement of intestinal contents.
5. Movement or fixation of organs and structures when manual rectal examination is performed.

Percussion
1. Tympany.
2. Changes in peristaltic waves (sound changes) that result from stroking.
3. Dull sounds over organs that are within normal boundaries; note changes of size and shape if misplaced or enlarged or if there are any suspicious findings.

Auscultation
1. Changes in sound and location of peristalsis.
2. Note pulsations of abdominal aorta.

Vital Signs, Height, Weight, Temperature
Rectal temperatures for infants, oral temperatures for children who can cooperate; if only glass thermometers are available, defer their use until child fully understands safe use.

LABORATORY AND OTHER DIAGNOSTIC PROCEDURES

Stool
1. pH: obtained by sample smeared on pH paper and compared with color chart. Normal range: 5.5 to 7.5.
2. Occult blood.
3. Microscopic smears for ova, parasites, motile bacteria.
4. Culture for ova and parasites, yeast.
5. Chemical analysis for suspected losses of fat (steatorrhea), excess glucose, vitamins, hormones, pigments, or blood.

X-ray Film
1. Dye contrast studies for portions of intestine and gall bladder.
2. Horizontal and upright views to visualize trapped air beneath diaphragm or changes in specific abdominal organ placement.
3. Scans and isotope studies of liver.

Hematology and Blood Chemistries
1. Complete blood count, including differential.
2. Electrolytes: Na^+, K^+, Cl^-, Ca^{++}, P^+, Mg^{++}.
3. CO_2 content.

Arterial Blood Gases
1. If acid-base imbalance suspected.

Urinalysis: microscopic, specific gravity, pH, color, and quantity of individual voiding

PATHOLOGIC CONDITIONS _____

ACUTE DEHYDRATION DUE TO DIARRHEA

Etiology and Incidence
1. Infections: bacterial, viral, parasitic.
2. Psychological: stresses of fear, anger, hostility.
3. Mechanical, e.g., hyperperistalsis.
4. Chemical imbalances due to ingestion of toxic products.

Pathophysiology
1. Definition: excessive losses of water, salts, vitamins, and trace elements from the gastrointestinal tract.
2. Critical condition: fluid volume equal to approximately 10% of total body weight is lost in a period of 24 to 48 hours.
3. Vomiting and anorexia usually accompany the diarrhea and complicate the fluid and electrolyte disturbances.
4. Dehydration should be considered in two categories:
   a. Disturbances of Na balance: extracellular fluid (saline) excess or extracellular fluid (saline) depletion.
   b. Disturbances of water balance. Low osmolality (indicated by low serum Na^+ or water excess): both intracellular and extracellular water are elevated in relation to solute. High osmolality (indicated by high serum Na^+ or water depletion): both intracellular and extracellular compartments are under-hydrated.

Clinical Presentation
1. Signs and symptoms.
   a. Diarrhea and/or vomiting of gastrointestinal contents, occurring at frequent intervals; may be induced by suggestion or actual ingestion of fluid or food.
   b. Anorexia.
   c. Dry, cracked mucous membranes, poor skin turgor.

    d. Sticky, thick saliva.

    e. Dark discoloration around eyes; eyes often appear sunken in the ocular cavities.

    f. Depressed fontanels in infants.

    g. Oliguria or anuria.

    h. Increased specific gravity of urine to 1.040.

    i. Tachycardia.

    j. Progressive hypovolemia with symptoms of shock, i.e., disturbances in consciousness.

    k. Hypertonicity of muscles; increased reflexes in hypernatremia.

    l. Marked thirst.

    m. Hyperpnea when acidemic.

    n. Abdominal distention, muscular weakness, and diminished reflexes when intracellular ion deficits are present.

    o. Extremities show cyanosis, mottling, and diminished temperature.

    p. Marked loss in body weight.

2. Laboratory findings

    a. Serum sodium concentrations (for patients hospitalized in North America):

        1) Isonatremic dehydration: approximately 65% of patients.

        2) Hypernatremic dehydration: approximately 20 to 25% of patients.

        3) Hyponatremic dehydration: approximately 10% of patients.

        4) Values vary with different regions, changing seasons, kinds of feeding practices.

    b. Countries promoting the use of dry whole milk for low-cost infant feeding have a higher incidence of hypernatremic dehydration.[17]

    c. Values: Serum sodium level greater than 150 mEq/1 is considered hypernatremic dehydration; serum sodium level less than 132 mEq/1 implies hyponatremic dehydration when compared with the relative clinical status. When a low serum sodium level accompanies the obvious signs of body fluid losses, there is a greater degree of total volume loss. This includes fluids from the extracellular and intracellular compartments.

    d. Blood urea nitrogen elevated above 20 mg/dl.

    e. Serum K^+ is not a good indicator of intracellular K^+ levels in infants and small children because of poor glomerular filtration during oliguric phase. Potassium loss may be appreciated only when hydration begins.

    f. Increased H^+ concentration of blood, elevated owing to HCO_3 losses through stools, starvation metabolism causing increased production of keto-acids, increased lactic acid production from tissue with diminished perfusion, and impaired renal excretion of nonvolatile acids. If vomiting losses equal diarrhea losses, H^+ ions may still be slightly elevated but serum Cl^- values will show a moderate drop.

    g. Calcium levels may fluctuate widely during dehydration, especially with hypernatremia.

Objectives of Therapy

1. Rehydration.
2. Correction of cause.
3. Teaching parents to reduce recurrence of cause.

Therapeutic Management

1. Initial hydration.
   a. Volume infusion to expand the intravascular compartment.
   b. Suggested solutions, in order of common acceptance by practitioners:
      1) Hypertonic glucose (10%) with sodium 75 mEq/l, bicarbonate 20 mEq/l, and chloride 55 mEq/l.
      2) Albumin: useful for patients in shock complicated by hypernatremia.
      3) Balanced electrolyte solutions, i.e., Ringer's lactate.
      4) Whole blood and single donor plasma.[16]
2. Replacement therapy.
   a. Rate adjusted water volume with appropriate electrolytes for individual patients.
   b. Add potassium when urine formation has been established.
   c. Administer on a planned outline; expect only one-half correction in first 24 hours.
   d. If patient has hypernatremic dehydration, rate of fluid administration must be slower than usual and monitored to avoid rapid expansion of the intravascular space.
3. Maintenance phase (early).
   a. Frequent weighings are necessary to determine success of therapy.
   b. For severely dehydrated patients, replacement solutions are continued over 24 hours. Additional losses are quantified into a replacement-plus-maintenance plan.
   c. Recovery from critical dehydration usually allows oral intake. Balanced electrolyte and glucose solutions should be continued, with addition of protein as soon as patient is ready.
   d. Hyperalimentation may be indicated depending on the state of nutrition, etiology of diarrhea and/or vomiting, duration of disorder, general state of health prior to dehydration (i.e., presence of chronic diseases), and other factors.[16]

4. Therapy plan and basic allowances.
   a. Average basic allowances in adults have been modified as a guide to water and electrolyte therapy for children:
   b. Average basic losses in adult:

Loss of	Water (ml/day)	Electrolytes (mEq/day)		
		Na^+	Cl^-	K^+
urine	1500	50	90	40
sensible/ insensible	100	0	0	0
gastric	previous volume	90	100	10

If urine pH is less than 4, replace Na^+ to one-half of total Cl^- losses.

   c. Modification of allowances for children:

Weight in kg	% of adult allowances
15	50
25	75
45	100

   d. Basic losses of urine water and electrolytes in infants and children:

	Water (ml/kg/24 h)	Electrolytes (mEq/kg/24 h)
Minimum	15	Na^+ 3
Average	45	K^+ 2
Maximum	120	Cl^- determined by acid-base status

   e. Basic losses of obligatory sensible and insensible fluids:

	Fluids (ml/kg/24 h)	Electrolytes (mEq/kg/24 h)
Premature and newborn in mist	15	0
not in mist	25	0
Infants over 2 months inert	25	0
ill		
afebrile	50	0
febrile	75	1–2

   f. Gastrointestinal losses:

	Fluids (ml/kg/24 h)	Electrolytes (mEq/kg/24 h)		
		Na^+	Cl^-	K^+
Gastric	25–200	50–100	100	10–20
Diarrhea	50–400	60	45	30

5. Hyperalimentation – Total parenteral nutrition (TPN) – takes place beyond the ordinary route of ingested nourishment, i.e., bypassing the alimentary canal. Intravenous infusions are high caloric, glucose-protein hydrolysate solutions with numerous electrolyte and vitamin additives. More recently, fat suspension solutions have also been used for hyperalimentation. The goal of the practitioner is to provide a normal intake of nutrients.
    a. Indications for use.
        1) When gastrointestinal tract, because of disease or immaturity, is rendered incompetent or conventional modes are inconvenient or hazardous, provision of nutrient intake for normal growth and development is accomplished by the parenteral route, central or peripheral.
            a) Peripheral used when central alimentation is contraindicated or cannot be maintained.
            b) May be used routinely in older children but is very difficult to continue in infants.
            c) Alimentation for less than two weeks.
            d) When patient is making a transition from central alimentation to oral intake.
        2) Moral and ethical considerations.
            a) When intravenous nutrition becomes a life support system, decisions to continue or discontinue may be required; i.e., cost must be balanced against preservation and quality of life.
            b) Benefits of hyperalimentation (TPN) are greater than risks when patients are carefully selected for therapy. Thus, not every candidate with vomiting or diarrhea may meet the criteria for hyperalimentation.
    b. Management of hyperalimentation program.
        1) Will vary slightly from center to center.
        2) Caloric requirements of the sick infant or young child:
            a) Infants (general rule): 120 calories and 130 cc of water per kg/24 hours.
            b) Older child or adolescent (general rule): 40 to 45 calories per kg and 20 cc of water per kg/24 hours. This rule applies to children between 20 and 70 kg.
        3) Extra electrolytes (potassium and sodium chloride) are necessary for most patients.
            a) Standard infusates of 20%, 8%, or 5% glucose; 10 to 25% TPN solutions "A" and "B" have established levels of electrolytes. Note Table 7–3.
        b) Adding 30 mEq of NaCl and 20 mEq of KCl per liter to the standard infusate will adequately begin replacement and will not overburden the normal kidney or cardio-vascular system.[17]

Table 7–3.   ELECTROLYTES (amount per liter in the
Standard Solution of Freamine II)

TPN SOLUTION "B" (For patients under 10 kg)			TPN SOLUTION "A" (For patients over 10 kg)		
Each 1000 ml TPN contains:			Each 1000 ml TPN contains:		
Dextrose	10–25%		Dextrose	10–25%	
Freamine II	2.125%		Freamine II	4.25%	
NaCl	25	mEq	NaCl	25	mEq
Na acetate	2.5	mEq	Na acetate	5	mEq
KCl	5	mEq	KCl	5	mEq
K phosphate	15	mEq	K phosphate	10	mEq
$MgSO_4$	4	mEq	$MgSO_4$	4	mEq
Ca gluconate	8	mEq	Ca gluconate	8	mEq
Vitamin K	0.5	mg	Vitamin K	0.5	mg
Folic acid	0.5	mg	Folic acid	0.5	mg
Vi-syneral	1.5	ml	Vi-syneral	0.5	ml
Berocca C	0.5	ml	Berocca C	0.5	ml

    c) Children with reduced renal function or other metabolic disorders are cautiously given electrolyte additions (sodium and, particularly, potassium).

4) Vitamins and trace elements.

    a) Vi-syneral and Berocca vitamins are added to the standard solutions of Table 7–3 and meet all vitamin requirements except those for folate, B_{12}, and vitamin K.

    b) Other standard glucose-protein hydrolysate solutions are laboratory prepared and contain all essential vitamins and trace minerals.[17]

    c) Essential fatty acid requirements may be satisfied by a once-a-week infusion of Intralipid (10% fat solution, isotonic, administered in peripheral vein) or daily application of sunflower seed oil to the child's back and chest.[11]

    d) Iron requirements can be met by intramuscular injections of iron dextran weekly or by whole blood transfusions.

c. Specific considerations when administering TPN.

1) Hypertonic infusates must be administered through a central venous catheter to avoid peripheral inflammation and thrombosis.

2) Constant and correct flow rate of infusion is maintained for the amount of solution calculated as emergency or replacement volume.

3) An infusion pump is routinely used to maintain correct TPN infusion rate.

4) TPN lines should contain no stopcocks and should be free of kinks.

5) Flow rates require frequent evaluations to allow for minor adjustments. *Do not try to "catch up"* if infusion is discontinued or slowed for a time.

6) Each new bottle of solution requires complete new tubing for administration; tubing and bottle should be changed every 24 hours.

7) Strict intake and output recording is necessary; daily weights are made at the same time each day on the same scale with the same amount of patient clothing; notations are kept regarding unusual incidents that may influence weight fluctuations.

8) Fractional urine checks are done every 4 to 6 hours and any urine sugar and/or acetone is reported.

9) Vital signs are monitored every 2 to 4 hours and changes of blood pressure and temperature are reported.

10) Guidelines for other medications and solutions infused through the TPN central catheter:

   a) Antibiotics and other medications may *not* be administered.

   b) Blood and blood products may *not* be administered.

   c) Intravenous solutions and plasma may be administered.

   d) Any questions regarding compatibility of solutions or acceptability of sharing the site for other infusions should be discussed with pharmacist and medical team.

11) Strict sterile technique is imperative when caring for a patient's central venous catheter and TPN solutions.

   a) No TPN solution should be infused or be exposed for more than 24 hours.

   b) All dressing and equipment changes require that the nurse gown, mask, glove, and keep a sterile field.

   c) When TPN tubing is disconnected from catheter, patient should be in Trendelenburg position or, if this is not tolerated, with head of bed flat and horizontal. Disconnection and reconnection of tubing with central venous catheter *must* be accomplished during expiratory phase of ventilation to insure that no air is "sucked" into venous circulation.

   d) TPN system is never used to measure central venous pressure (CVP) or to obtain blood samples.

   e) Antibiotics are not administered prophylactically when patient is placed on TPN. They may be given if indicated by child's primary illness.

12) Management of potential infection is required when patient becomes febrile or deteriorates without other specific cause.

       a) Culture the nutritional solution, TPN catheter, catheter sites.

       b) Obtain blood cultures from peripheral vein.

       c) Change bottle and tubing; observe patient for 6 to 12 hours.

13) Nursing responsibilities.

       a) Maintain aseptic techniques and protective isolation.

       b) Standardize optimal care by staffing TPN patients with the same nurse (same relief nurse), who is on call for special problems.

          (1) Same nurse provides continuity and oversees the TPN program.

          (2) Families develop trust more quickly with nurse who knows individual patient problems and is expert in TPN therapy.

          (3) Hardware (tubing, machinery, pumps, and infusates) is specialized; therefore, more economical use is made of nurse time when one or two people are uniquely educated to evaluate and "trouble-shoot."

          (4) One nurse establishes and maintains a daily routine for critically ill patients, who need an opportunity for balanced sleep and stimulation.

          (5) The TPN nurse should not be required to assist with painful and intrusive procedures that may cause distrust in the patient. Since the TPN nurse must maintain a long-term relationship of trust with patient and family, the health care team should protect this relationship.

       c) Peripheral venous feedings require some special nursing considerations.

          (1) Large volumes of hypertonic solutions easily cause fluid overload and must be monitored frequently.

          (2) Heparin therapy may be indicated to reduce risk of thrombophlebitis.

          (3) A micropore filter is placed in line just below the bottle of hypertonic (amino acid–glucose) solution, and the entire set plus bottle is changed every 24 hours.

          (4) Careful observations must be made to detect infiltration and phlebitis, which will necessitate immediate change of infusion site. (Length of effective use of intravenous site is usually 24 to 48 hours.[17])

    (5) Intralipid solution and glucose solutions cannot be mixed and require separate bottles and tubing. A single intravenous site is permissible if the Intralipid solution enters the circuit carrying the glucose solution close to the venous entry site.

    (6) All solutions for infants and children should be administered with an infusion pump.

    (7) Bacterial filters are not used when administering Intralipid because they snag the fat emulsion and clog the screening material.

    (8) Intralipid therapy is begun with 15 ml/kg/day and increased by 5 ml/kg/each day, if no lipemia is demonstrated in the patient's serum, until individual maintenance levels are achieved.

    (9) Exogenous insulin is usually unnessary in the nondiabetic child, but blood sugar levels are obtained as a guide to therapy.

    (10) Frequent urine sugar determinations are required. Consistent results of 3+ may signal osmotic diuresis due to septicemia, especially in the child who has undergone therapy without glycosuria for several days.

14) Complications:
  a) Glucose intolerance and hyperglycemia.
  b) Osmotic diuresis.
  c) Postinfusion hypoglycemia.
  d) Essential fatty acid deficiency.
  e) Selected avitaminosis due to nonassimilation.
  f) Hyperammonemia in infants less than 6 months old.[17]
  g) Metabolic acidosis.
  h) Copper deficiency (hypocupremia).
  i) Occasionally, seizures due to hypomagnesemia.
  j) Amino acid toxicity.
  k) Fluctuating calcium and phosphorus levels, which swing out of normal range on both high and low ends.
  l) Transient liver enlargement, liver dysfunction, and questionable results of liver function studies.
  m) Patients receiving Intralipid have a strong tendency to develop eosinophilia.
  n) Candida albicans (yeast) and bacterial infections are the greatest threat to TPN patients.

Complications of Acute Diarrhea
1. Convulsions, seizure activity.
2. Profound shock, death.

Nursing Skills
1. Calculation of body fluid balance.
2. Basic nutrition.
3. Infection control.

NEONATAL JAUNDICE

Etiology
1. Physiologic jaundice of newborn.
2. Primary liver disease.

Pathophysiology
1. Neonatal jaundice (sometimes termed "physiologic jaundice of newborn"): increased unconjugated hyperbilirubinemia due to decreased bilirubin uptake and excretion; disturbance of enteric circulation.
2. Primary liver disease: elevation of conjugated serum bilirubin due to a variety of causes.
   a. Anatomic:
      1) Biliary atresia, intrahepatic or extrahepatic.
      2) Tumor.
      3) Pyloric stenosis.
   b. Metabolic:
      1) Parenteral hyperalimentation.
      2) Carbohydrate (sugar) and lipid metabolism.
      3) Medications (sulfas, aspirin, some antibiotics, tranquilizers).
   c. Functional:
      1) Familial syndromes (nonhemolytic unconjugated hyperbilirubinemia).
      2) Parasitic diseases.
      3) Viral hepatitis.
      4) Bowel obstruction.
      5) Bacterial sepsis.
3. Hemolytic disease of newborn (erythroblastosis, Rh or ABO incompatibility).

Clinical Presentation
1. Signs and symptoms:
   a. Normal or "sick" looking infant with petechiae and ecchymoses over any area of body.
   b. Deep reddish-yellow appearance of skin; jaundice (yellow skin) is particularly noticeable when skin of child's nose or over sternum is depressed and released quickly.
   c. *Acholic* or *clay-colored* stools with jaundice due to impairment of bile flow (either intrahepatic obstruction or extrahepatic biliary obstruction), or *very darkly colored* feces due to impaired excretion of urobilinogen by liver.

     d. Drowsiness.

     e. Irregularities of respiration.

     f. Muscular "twitchings," hypertonia.

     g. Cry may be shrill and high-pitched.

     h. Hepatomegaly, occasional splenomegaly.

     i. Seizures, opisthotonos.

     j. Appearance of jaundice in first 24 hours of life.

     k. Jaundice lasting longer than first seven days in a full-term newborn.

     l. Edema, pleural and pericardial effusion, ascites.

     m. In intrahepatic atresia patients, pruritus, steatorrhea, and bleeding tendencies.

     n. Sometimes, xanthoma of hands, feet, ears, eyes, nose.

     o. Generalized atherosclerosis.

     p. Osteoporosis.

2. Laboratory findings:

     a. Serum bilirubin levels greater than 12 mg/dl in full-term infants.

     b. Serum bilirubin levels increasing more than 5 mg/dl per day (taken in serial progression).

     c. Direct bilirubin greater than 1.5 mg/dl.

     d. Urine urobilinogen is greater than 4 mg/24 hr.

     e. May show anemia with a variety of abnormal red cell formation, i.e., elliptocytosis, pyknocytosis, spherocytosis.

     f. May show decreased serum albumin and reduced globulin binding capacity.

     g. May have polycythemia owing to transfusion therapy.

Therapeutic Management

1. Surgical repair for obstructions, extrahepatic atresia, tumors.

2. Phototherapy: use of intense fluorescent light (blue more effective than white) to decompose bilirubin by photo-oxidation.

     a. Blue light obscures the appearance of cyanosis. Infants or small children being treated with blue light phototherapy must be observed in bright room light or daylight to assess true skin color. Place a white sheet or paper next to child as reference for skin color determination.

     b. No information available on optimal or maximal safe dose of photolight or duration of therapy. (Energy output in blue range of phototherapy is 425 to 475 nm.)

     c. Photolamps produce radiant heat, so patient must have temperature monitored every four to six hours.

     d. Greater amounts of insensible water losses occur owing to increased metabolism, increased per cent of stool water, and elevation of body temperature. Replacement fluids are necessary to maintain correct body water balance.

     e. Protect eyes from photolight with shields.

     f. Plexiglas shield should be placed between photolight and patient to protect the skin from ultraviolet radiation.

    g. There is no documentation that phototherapy causes adverse effects on growth and development, bone age, intelligence level, vision, or blood amino acids.

    h. Measure serum bilirubin levels every 12 hours, or more frequently if indicated.

    i. Obtain daily hematocrit level, especially if jaundice is due to hemolytic disease.

    j. Discoloration of skin, serum, and urine may occur after phototherapy, particularly in black infants, and has not been proven harmful.

    k. Loose stools may be frequent; greenish-brown color is probably due to photodegradation products.

3. Nonsurgical treatment of intrahepatic atresia.

    a. Phenobarbital, 5 to 10 mg/kg/24 hours, which lowers serum bilirubin concentration by enhancing bile flow and increasing biliary excretion of bile salts.

    b. Cholestyramine therapy, which prevents intestinal reabsorption of bile salts.

4. Exchange transfusion.

    a. To correct anemia occurring because of hemolytic disease.

    b. To avert or treat hyperbilirubinemia.

    c. General criteria indicating need for exchange transfusion:

      1) Serum bilirubin level of 10 mg/dl by 24 hours or 15 mg/dl by 48 hours (after birth) or 20 mg/dl at any age.

      2) Decreasing hemoglobin and hematocrit (less than 35%).

    d. Requires careful monitoring during transfusion.

      1) Cardiorespiratory status.

      2) Vigorous treatment of asphyxia, acidosis, hypoglycemia, and hypothermia.

      3) Circulatory overload.

    e. Post-transfusion complications:

      1) Thrombocytopenia.

      2) Possible coagulation disorders.

      3) Bleeding from any puncture sites.

      4) Hypervolemia (vascular compartment); circulatory overload due to colloid osmotic pressure changes incurred with whole blood transfusion.

    f. Watch for early rebound of bilirubin due to compartmental shifting of bilirubin with partial equilibration, and continued heme breakdown from the patient's sensitized red cells and from hemolysis of transfused blood.

    g. Albumin (1 g/kg of 25% salt-poor albumin, or substitution of 12.5 g [50 ml] of albumin for 50 ml of plasma in the donor blood) is usually administered with the exchange transfusion. Restricted to repeat transfusions. *Do not use* for patients with severe anemia or congestive heart failure.

Complications
1. Kernicterus.
2. Hepatic coma.
3. Necrotizing enterocolitis after exchange transfusion.
4. Subtle changes in neurologic, psychologic, or intellectual development.

Nursing Skills
1. Calculation of body water and electrolyte balance; replacement.
2. Seizure precautions and protection of patient during seizure.
3. Management of patient and materials during transfusion.
4. Use of photolight equipment.
5. Postsurgical care for patient at high risk of bleeding.

BIBLIOGRAPHY

1. Allen F.: Bilirubin in the Newborn. Proceedings: symposium on the placenta, its form and functions. National Foundation Birth Defects Original Article Series, Vol. 1, No. 1, 1965.

2. Ament, M.: Pediatric gastroenterology. Pediatr. Ann., Volume 11, 1976.

3. Brobeck, J.: Best and Taylor's Physiological Basis of Medical Practice, 9th ed. Baltimore, Williams & Wilkins, 1973.

4. Crelin, E.: Functional Anatomy of the Newborn. New Haven, Yale University Press, 1973.

5. Dodge, P., et al.: Nutrition and the Developing Nervous System. St. Louis, C. V. Mosby Co., 1975.

6. Fishman, A. (Ed.): Symposium on Salt and Water Metabolism New York, American Heart Association, 1960.

7. Francis, D., and Dixon, D.: Diets for Sick Children. Blackwell Scientific Publications. Philadelphia, J. B. Lippincott Co., 1974.

8. Goldberger, E.: A Primer of Water, Electrolyte and Acid-Base Syndromes, 5th ed. Philadelphia, Lea & Febiger, 1975.

9. Creisheimer, F.: Physiology and Anatomy. Philadelphia, J. B. Lippincott Co., 1963.

10. Heird, W., and Winters, R.: Total parenteral nutrition. J. Pediatr., 86:2, 1975.

11. Press, M., et al.: Correction of essential fatty acid deficiency in man by cutaneous application of sunflower seed oil. Lancet, 1:579, 1974.

12. Schiff, L. (Ed.): Diseases of the Liver, 4th ed. Philadelphia, J. B. Lippincott Co., 1975.

13. Schubert, W.: Liver disease in infancy and childhood. In Schiff, L.: Diseases of the Liver, 2nd ed. Philadelphia, J. B. Lippincott Co., 1975, pp. 1173-1245.

14. Scribner, B. (Ed.): Teaching Syllabus for the Course on Fluid and Electrolyte Balance, 7th ed. Seattle, University of Washington, 1969.

15. Silverman, A., et al.: Pediatric Clinical Gastroenterology. St. Louis, C. V. Mosby Co., 1975.

16. Sleisenger, M., and Fordtran, J.: Gastrointestinal Disease, 2nd ed. Philadelphia, W. B. Saunders Co., 1973.

17. Smith, C.: The Critically Ill Child, 2nd ed. Philadelphia, W. B. Saunders Co., 1977.

18. Taitz, L. S., and Byers, H. D., High caloric/osmolar feeding and hypertonic dehydration. Arch. Dis. Child., 47:257, 1972.

19. Total Parenteral Alimentation Protocol. Seattle, Children's Orthopedic Hospital, 1977.

20. White, P., and Selvey, N.: Let's Talk About Food. Littleton, Massachusetts, Publishing Sciences Group, Inc., 1974.

21. Winters, R. (Ed.): The Body Fluids in Pediatrics. Boston, Little, Brown & Co., 1973.

CHAPTER 8

CARE OF THE CHILD WITH A HEMATOPOIETIC DISORDER

Anita Stoeppel, R.N., M.S.N.

OBJECTIVES

1. Discuss three components of blood (erythrocytes, leukocytes, and platelets) and their origin, cell development, and function.

2. Discuss the vascular factors involved in clotting.

3. Discuss the classic and "cascade" theories of the blood clotting mechanism.

4. Discuss four laboratory tests of coagulation.

5. Discuss five disorders (acute lymphocytic leukemia, disseminated intravascular coagulation [DIC], aplastic anemia, hemophilia, and sickle cell disease) and their pathophysiology, clinical presentation, and medical and nursing management.

BLOOD COMPONENTS

Erythrocytes
1. Origin: formed in the red bone marrow after birth.
2. Structure: homogeneous, biconcave, circular discs without nuclei.
3. Cellular development:
   a. Hemocytoblast in the red marrow → basophilic erythroblast → polychromatophilic erythroblast (more hemoglobin formed) → normoblast (nucleus disappears) → reticulocyte (few enter the blood stream) → erythrocyte.
   b. Amino acids, folic acid, iron, copper, zinc, vitamin B_{12}, and enzymes are needed.
4. Hemoglobin.
   a. Structure.
      1) Two pairs of identical polypeptide chains.
      2) Heme group is situated between the loops of the chain.
   b. Synthesis occurs in the cytoplasm of maturing red cells.
5. Functions.
   a. Carry oxygen to cells.
   b. Carry carbon dioxide from cells.
   c. Aid normal acid-base balance.
   d. Determine viscosity and specific gravity of the blood.

Leukocytes
1. Neutrophils.
   a. Origin: formed in the red bone marrow.
   b. Cellular development:
      1) Hemocytoblast → myeloblast → promyelocyte → neutrophilic myelocyte → metamyelocyte → band cell → segmented cell → neutrophil.
2. Eosinophils.
   a. Origin: formed in the red bone marrow.
   b. Cellular development:
      1) Hemocytoblast → myeloblast → promyelocyte → eosinophilic myelocyte → eosinophil.
   c. Give evidence of adrenal function.
3. Basophils.
   a. Origin: red bone marrow.
   b. Cellular development:
      1) Hemocytoblast → myeloblast → promyelocyte → basophilic myelocyte → basophil.
   c. Contain large amounts of histamine.
4. Lymphocytes.
   a. Origin: primary lymphoid tissue of the lymph nodes and spleen, bone marrow.

  b. Cellular development.
   1) Primary lymphoid tissue → lymphoblast →
    prolymphocyte → lymphocyte.
  c. Functions to wall off chronic infections and produce antibodies.
 5. Monocytes.
  a. Origin: chiefly the lymph glands and spleen.
  b. Cellular development:
   1) Primary lymphoid tissue → monoblast → promonocyte →
    monocyte.
 6. Functions of leukocytes.
  a. Protect the body from pathogenic organisms.
  b. Promote tissue repair.

Platelets (Thrombocytes)

  a. Fragments of cells formed in the bone marrow.
  b. Cellular development:
   1) Hemocytoblast → megakaryoblast → promegakaryocyte →
    megakaryocyte → thrombocyte.
  c. Function: plays a role in control of bleeding.

BLOOD COAGULATION

Factors

 1. Factor I: fibrinogen.
 2. Factor II: prothrombin.
 3. Factor III: thromboplastin.
 4. Factor IV: calcium.
 5. Factor V: proaccelerin.
 6. Factor VII: proconvertin.
 7. Factor VIII: antihemophilic factor (AHF).
 8. Factor IX: plasma thromboplastic component (PTC).
 9. Factor X: Stuart-Prower factor.
10. Factor XI: plasma thromboplastin antecedent (PTA).
11. Factor XII: Hageman factor.
12. Factor XIII: Fibrin stabilizing factor.

Mechanism of Clotting

 1. Vascular aspects.
  a. After injury to vessel there is an immediate reflex contraction.
  b. This is reinforced by an aggregation of platelets and the release
   of serotonin, a vasoconstrictor.
 2. Blood coagulation mechanism.
  a. Classic theory.
   1) Thrombin is formed by two systems.
    a) Intrinsic system:
     (1) Plasma thromboplastin (intrinsic) is formed by the
      interaction of platelets with factors V, VIII, IX, X,
      XI, and XII.

       (2) Plasma thromboplastin, in the presence of ionized calcium, converts prothrombin to thrombin.

   b) Extrinsic system:

       (1) Tissue thromboplastin (extrinsic) is formed by the interaction of tissue extract (incomplete thromboplastin) with factors V, VII, and X and ionized calcium.

       (2) Tissue thromboplastin, in the presence of ionized calcium, converts prothrombin to thrombin.

  2) Extrinsic thromboplastin is formed in seconds, intrinsic thromboplastin in minutes.

  3) Extrinsic system is important following tissue damage, intrinsic when there is no tissue damage.

  4) Both must be intact for normal hemostasis.

  5) Thrombin then converts fibrinogen to fibrin.

  6) Fibrin in the presence of factor XIII forms an insoluble fibrin clot.

  b. "Cascade" theory: a stepwise sequence in which precursors of enzymes are activated, which in turn activate subsequent enzyme precursors. Eventually this "cascade" brings about the conversion of prothrombin to thrombin, which converts the fibrinogen to fibrin.

    1) Intrinsic system:

       a) Factor XII is activated by contact with glass, collagen, or some fatty acids to form a complex with factor XI.

       b) This complex (factors XII–XI) activates factor IX.

       c) Activated factor IX forms a complex with plasma to activate factor X.

       d) Activated factor X forms a complex with factor V and platelet factor 3 to split prothrombin and form thrombin.

    2) Extrinsic system:

       a) Tissue factor protein activates factor VII.

       b) Tissue factor and active factor VII form a complex that activates factor X.

       c) Activated factor X plus tissue factor phospholipid plus factor V form a complex that converts prothrombin to thrombin.

PEDIATRIC HEMATOPOIETIC ASSESSMENT _____

History
1. Anorexia and irritability.
2. Previous medications.
3. Ingestion of poisonous chemicals, such as lead.

4. Infections.
5. Bleeding.
6. Family history of hematologic problems.

Physical Examination
1. Inspection.
   a. Pallor.
   b. Ecchymosis.
   c. Petechiae.
   d. Icterus.
2. Palpation for hepatosplenomegaly.

Laboratory
1. Complete blood count.
2. Reticulocyte count: normal count is 0.5–1.4%; elevation indicates an increased production of red blood cells (RBCs).
3. Bone marrow aspiration and biopsy.
4. Serum bilirubin: indicates breakdown of hemoglobin.
   a. Normal values (consult local laboratory):
      1) Direct: 0.0–0.5 mg/dl.
      2) Total: 0.2–1.0 mg/dl.
5. Coombs' test.
   a. Direct: used to check RBCs for presence of antibodies that coat the cells.
   b. Indirect: used to test for the presence of antibodies to the RBC antigens.
6. Sickle cell preparations: exposure of RBCs to reducing substances that cause RBCs with hemoglobin S to sickle.
7. Hemoglobin electrophoresis.
8. Serum iron: normal range is 56 to 180 μg/dl.
9. Tests of coagulation.
   a. Extrinsic system:
      1) Prothrombin time.
   b. Intrinsic system:
      1) Prothrombin consumption.
      2) Partial thromboplastin time.
   c. Bleeding time: time required for a small pinpoint to cease bleeding; normal time is 3 to 6 minutes.
   d. Coagulation time: normal time is 10 to 12 minutes.
10. Chest x-ray film to detect cardiomegaly.

PATHOLOGIC CONDITIONS

ACUTE LYMPHOBLASTIC LEUKEMIA

Etiology and Precipitating Factors (Theories)
1. Chronic ionizing irradiation.

2. Exposure to nuclear bomb.
3. Genetic factors.
4. Viruses.

Pathophysiology
1. Malignant disruption of blood cell precursors.
2. Deficient production of all blood cells.
3. Accumulation of abnormal blasts in the bone marrow and other reticuloendothelial tissue.
4. Replacement of normal bone marrow cells by leukemic cells.

Clinical Presentation
1. General signs and symptoms:
   a. Insidious onset, usually lasting six weeks.
   b. Effects of anemia: weakness, excessive fatigue, malaise, decreased exercise tolerance, progressive pallor.
   c. Bleeding: epistaxis, hematuria, blood in stools, petechiae, bleeding mucous membrane.
   d. Infection: otitis media, pharyngitis, pneumonia.
   e. Pain in bone or abdomen.
   f. Enlarged lymph nodes.
   g. Fever (50% of patients).
   h. Hepatosplenomegaly.
2. Laboratory findings:
   a. Hemoglobin under 12 g/dl.
   b. Platelet count under 100,000/cu mm.
   c. Variable white count.
   d. Neutropenia.
   e. Presence of blast cells in peripheral smear.
3. Diagnosis:
   a. History and physical findings.
   b. Peripheral blood smear.
   c. Bone marrow aspiration and biopsy.
   d. Lumbar puncture.

Objectives of Therapy
1. Reduction of morbidity and mortality.
2. Palliative therapy if disease is progressive.

Therapeutic Management
1. Chemotherapy (see also complications):
   a. Induction.
   b. Maintenance.
   c. Central nervous system prophylaxis.
      1) Radiation to cranium: 2000 to 2400 rads.
      2) Intrathecal methotrexate (5 doses).
2. Supportive treatment:
   a. Administration of packed red cells.
   b. Administration of platelets.
   c. Treatment of pneumonia, fungal and viral infections.
3. Bone marrow transplantation:
   a. Pre- and post-transplant immunosuppression.

1) Two days of high-dose cyclophosphamide followed by 1000 rads of total body irradiation (for leukemic patients).
2) Four days of high-dose cyclophosphamide only (for aplastic anemia patients).
3) Low-dose methotrexate four times during the first 11 days after grafting and once weekly for 3 months after.

b. Protective isolation (type varies in differenct centers).
c. Control of nausea and vomiting due to the irradiation.
d. Control of fluid overload, if necessary.
e. Control of allergic reaction, if necessary.
f. Support until graft is established (10 days to 3 weeks).
1) Platelets.
2) IV antibiotics.
3) White cell transfusions.
g. Control of diarrhea.
h. Treatment of septic shock.
i. Control of graft-versus-host disease (GVHD).

Complications

1. Anemia.
2. Hemorrhage.
3. Infection.
4. Central nervous system complications: headache, vomiting, diplopia, seizure, and personality change.
5. Bone involvement: pain, osteoporosis, infarction.
6. Gastrointestinal bleeding.
7. Hyperuricemia (see renal disorders).
8. Chemotherapy complications.
   a. Hematologic:
   1) Neutropenia.
   2) Hyperuricemia (prednisone).
   b. Neurologic (vincristine).
   c. Gastrointestinal.
   d. Cardiovascular.
   1) Hypertension (prednisone).
   2) Cardiac toxicity (Adriamycin).
   e. Anaphylaxis (bleomycin, L-asparaginase): have adrenalin, Benadryl, and Solu-Cortef at hand; check BP every 10 minutes for one hour, then every half hour for six hours.
   f. Urologic.
   1) Hemorrhagic cystitis (Cytoxan).
      a) Encourage intake of fluids by mouth.
      b) Have patient void frequently.
      c) Give Cytoxan in morning.
   2) Renal tubular damage (high-dose methotrexate).
   g. Hepatic (6-mercaptopurine, methotrexate).
9. Graft-versus-host disease (GVHD).
   a. Occurs when lymphocytes of the bone marrow graft recognize the host as foreign and "reject" the host.

    b. Skin involvement occurs with an erythematous rash. This
        may lead to severe sloughing.
    c. Liver involvement may occur.
    d. Gastrointestinal involvement occurs, ranging from mild
        diarrhea to severe sloughing of intestinal mucous membranes.
    e. Treatment: IM injections of antithymocyte globulin.

Nursing Skills
1. Vital sign monitoring.
    a. Temperature.
      1) Elevation may indicate infection associated with sudden
          drop in blood pressure, may indicate gram-negative shock.
      2) Hypothermia mattress, if necessary.
      3) To avoid trauma to rectal mucosa, do not take rectal
          temperatures.
    b. Pulse.
      1) May be elevated with increased temperature, low
          hemoglobin, hemorrhage, or congestive heart failure.
    c. Respiratory.
      1) Distress may be due to:
        a) Congestive heart failure.
        b) Hepatosplenomegaly.
        c) Enlarged lymph nodes around trachea.
2. Observe for transfusion reactions.
3. Positioning and skin care.
    a. Handle child gently.
4. Good oral hygiene.
5. No IM injections.
6. Test urine, emesis, and stool for blood.
7. Strict aseptic technique.
8. No vaccines to be given.

DISSEMINATED INTRAVASCULAR COAGULATION

Etiology and Precipitating Factors
1. Toxic substances such as those occurring in hemolytic uremic
    syndrome, infection by gram-negative microorganisms, leukemia,
    and severe burns.
2. Activated by pathological mechanisms and substances that
    accompany some diseases.

Pathophysiology
1. Clotting throughout the vascular network.
    a. Most common in arterioles, capillaries, and venules.
2. Gradual depletion of platelets and major clotting factors,
    leading to thrombocytopenia and hemorrhage.
3. Hemorrhage with widespread deposition of fibrin in small blood
    vessels, resulting in local tissue necrosis.
4. Massive intravascular clotting.

5. Clot lysis and multiple small areas of hemorrhage.
6. Sporadic and variable reestablishment of patent small vessels.

Clinical Presentation
1. General signs and symptoms:
   a. Severe bleeding at multiple sites.
2. Laboratory findings:
   a. Depletion of plasma clotting factors V and VIII.
   b. Deficiency of fibrinogen and prothrombin.
   c. Decreased platelets.
   d. Elevation of fibrin split products.

Objectives of Therapy
1. Early recognition of predisposing problems.
2. Supportive care.
3. Aggressive therapy for underlying cause.

Therapeutic Management
1. Observation of urine, stools, and mucous membranes for bleeding.
2. Anticoagulants: heparin, coumarin.
   a. Antidotes:
      1) Protamine sulfate for heparin.
      2) Vitamin K for coumarin.
   b. Increased anticoagulant requirements:
      1) With diarrhea.
      2) With administration of multivitamin supplements that contain vitamin K.
3. Daily or frequent laboratory monitoring.
   a. Coagulation screens, including:
      1) Platelet count.
      2) Prothrombin time, partial thromboplastin time.
      3) Fibrinogen level.
      4) Fibrin split products level.
4. Treat shock as necessary.

APLASTIC ANEMIA

Etiology of Types
1. Congenital (Fanconi's anemia):
   a. Autosomal recessive trait.
   b. Often associated with other conditions, such as:
      1) Bronze pigmentation of skin.
      2) Dwarfism.
      3) Mental retardation.
      4) Skeletal, renal, and cardiac malformations.
2. Acquired:
   a. Idiopathic.
   b. Toxins such as chloramphenicol, DDT, methotrexate, 6-mercaptopurine (most common cause: compounds containing benzene ring).

c. Radiation.

d. Malignancies.

Pathophysiology

1. Pancytopenia resulting from aplasia of the bone marrow.
2. Failure in later stage division of hematopoiesis and inability to release cell into circulation (maturation arrest).

Clinical Presentation

1. General signs and symptoms:
   a. Bruises.
   b. Epistaxis.
   c. Petechiae.
   d. Fever.
   e. May have rash.
   f. Sore throat and mouth.
   g. Malaise, fatigue, muscle weakness.
2. Laboratory findings:
   a. Peripheral pancytopenia.
   b. Normocytic, normochromic anemia.
   c. Leukopenia.
   d. Thrombocytopenia.
   e. Hypocellular bone marrow.

Objectives of Therapy

1. Removal or reduction of cause.
2. Supportive therapy with hope of improved bone marrow function.

Therapeutic Management

1. Prevent infection.
2. Medications.
   a. Steroids.
   b. Testosterone.
   c. Other marrow stimulants.
3. Supportive therapy.
   a. Blood transfusions.
   b. Administration of platelets during hemorrhage.
   c. Antibiotics for infection.

Complications

1. Infection.
2. Nutritional deficiencies resulting from malabsorption of dietary components.

Nursing Skills

1. Reverse isolation technique.
2. Early recognition of toxicities.
   a. Known high-risk medications.
   b. Common benzene ring compounds.
3. Monitoring for complications of steroid therapy.
4. Identification and warning of patient's medication reactions.
   a. Personal identification card or tag.
   b. Medical and personal records clearly marked in red ink with name of toxic substance.

5. Avoidance of offending medication or closely related ones.
6. Patient and family instruction regarding nutritional deficiencies, hemorrhage, and the avoidance of infections.

HEMOPHILIA

Etiology
1. Hereditary.
   a. Factor VIII deficiency is an X-linked recessive trait (i.e., males are affected almost exclusively).
2. Acquired.
   a. Trauma, e.g., shock, burns.
   b. Disease, e.g., malignancy.

Pathophysiology
1. Uncontrolled bleeding due to intrinsic pathway deficiencies of factor VIII.
2. Nonproduction of factor IX.

Clinical Presentation
1. General signs and symptoms:
   a. Bruisability.
   b. Oozing from wounds.
   c. Excessive bleeding from circumcision.
   d. Excessive bleeding from tooth eruption.
   e. Hemarthrosis.
   f. Spontaneous bleeding: hematuria, epistaxis.
2. Laboratory findings:
   a. Prolonged clotting times.
   b. Prolonged partial thromboplastin time.

Objectives of Therapy
1. Supportive therapy through periods of hemorrhage.
2. Periodic restoration of missing coagulation factors.
3. Assist patient with self-administration of factor.
4. Observation for allergic response.
5. Patient and family teaching of safety measures in activities of daily living.

SICKLE CELL DISEASE

Etiology
1. An autosomal recessive trait.

Incidence
1. In American blacks, 7 to 9% are carriers, while 0.3 to 1.5% are affected by the disease. May also occur in people of Mediterranean origin.

Pathophysiology

1. Abnormal hemoglobin (hemoglobin S) is synthesized.
2. Isoelectric point of the hemoglobin molecule is shifted and the following occurs:
   a. Low pO_2 and/or low pH causes RBCs to sickle.
   b. The sickled cells cause vascular occlusion at the capillary level.
   c. The blood is also viscous owing to the presence of crystallized hemoglobin S.
   d. Stasis results, leading to increased deoxygenation and increased sickling.
3. Decreased life span of the RBCs (10 to 25 days).

Clinical Presentation

1. General signs and symptoms:
   a. Joint pain, swelling, redness.
   b. Multiple thromboses and infarcts of organs.
   c. Variety of acute abdominal emergencies.
2. Laboratory findings:
   a. Blood smear shows RBC sickling.
   b. Positive sickle cell preparation.
   c. 50% or more hemoglobin S, as demonstrated by hemoglobin electrophoresis.
   d. Hemoglobin: 5 to 9 mg/dl.
   e. Reticulocytosis.
   f. Leukocytosis.
   g. Platelets are slightly increased.
   h. Direct bilirubin is increased.
3. Types of crises:
   a. Aplastic: cessation of erythropoietic activity.
   b. Sequestration: pooling of blood in spleen leading to hypovolemic shock.
   c. Vaso-occlusive or thrombotic: occlusion of vessels by sickled cells.

Objectives of Therapy

1. Reduction of morbidity.
2. Support during crisis.

Therapeutic Management

1. Hydration, intravenously and by mouth.
2. Analgesics, rest.
3. Treatment of complications.
4. Hypertransfusion in special circumstances, to lower production of RBCs with sickled hemoglobin.
5. Prophylactic antibiotics.

Complications

1. Congestive heart failure as a result of prolonged anemia.
2. Infarction of any organ (spleen, brain, kidneys, heart, lungs, skin, bones).

3. Chronic leg ulcers.
4. Aseptic necrosis of femoral head.
5. Septic arthritis.
6. Fat emboli.
7. Gallstones.
8. Retinopathy.
9. Narcotic addiction.

Nursing Skills

1. Test specific gravity of urine for adequate hydration; should be 1.001 to 1.003.
2. Prevent chilling.
3. Observe for complications.
4. Patient teaching and genetic counseling.

BIBLIOGRAPHY

1. Abildgaard, C, et al.: Prothrombin complex concentrate (Konyne) in the treatment of hemophilic patients with factor VIII inhibitors. J. Pediatr., 88:200, 1976.
2. Baehner, R.: Disorders of leukocytes leading to recurrent infection. Pediatr. Clin. North Am., 19:935, 1972.
3. Barnett, H. (ed.): Pediatrics, 15th ed. New York, Appleton-Century-Crofts, 1972.
4. Beland, I.: Clinical Nursing: Pathophysiological and Psychosocial Approaches, 2nd ed., New York, Macmillan, 1970.
5. Bettner, E.: Your Child and Hemophilia: A Manual for Parents. New York, Medical and Scientific Advisory Council, The National Hemophilia Foundation, 1975.
6. Binger, C., et al.: Childhood leukemia: emotional impact on patient and family. N. Engl. J. Med., 280:414, 1969.
7. Bloom, G.: Disorders of bone marrow production. Pediatr. Clin. North Am., 19:983, 1972.
8. Burgert, E.: Emotional impact of childhood acute leukemia. Mayo Clin. Proc., 47:273, 1972.
9. Buschman, P.: The child with leukemia: group support for parents. Am. J. Nurs., 76:1121, 1976.
10. Corrigan, J.: Oral bleeding in hemophilia: treatment with epsilon aminocaproic acid and replacement therapy. J. Pediatr., 80:124, 1972.
11. Crosby, M.: Control systems and children with lymphobastic leukemia. Nurs. Clin. North Am., 6:407, 1971.
12. Eisenhauer, L.: Drug-induced blood dyscrasias. Nurs. Clin. North Am., 7:777, 1972.
13. Fleming, J.: The child with sickle cell disease. Am. J. Nurs., 65:88, 1965.
14. Fochtman, D.: Leukemia in children. Pediatr. Nurs., May-June, 1976, 2:8–13.
15. Foley, G., and McCarthy, A.: The child with leukemia: the disease and its treatment. Am. J. Nurs., 76:1108, 1976.
16. Foley, G., and McCarthy, A.: In a special hematology clinic. Am. J. Nurs., 76:1115, 1976.
17. French, R.: Nurse's Guide to Diagnostic Procedures, 4th ed. New York, McGraw-Hill, 1975.
18. Gaston, M.: Screening for sickle cell disease. South. Med. J., 67:257, 1974.
19. Gilchrist, G.: Platelet disorders. Pediatr. Clin. North Am., 19:1047, 1972.
20. Githens, J., and Hathaway, W.: Hematologic disorders. In Kempe, C., et al. (eds.): Current Pediatric Diagnosis

and Treatment. Los Altos, Lange Medical Publications, 1974.

21. Greene, P.: Acute leukemia in children. Am. J. Nurs., 75:1709, 1975.

22. Greene, T.: Symposium on cancer in children. Nurs. Clin. North Am., 11:1, 1976.

23. Guyton, A.: Textbook of Medical Physiology, 5th ed. Philadelphia, W. B. Saunders Co., 1971.

24. Hann, H., and London, W.: Studies of parents of children with acute leukemia. J. Nat. Cancer Inst., 54:1299, 1975.

25. Hathaway, W., and Hays, T.: Hypercoagulability in childhood cancer. J. Pediatr. Surg., 10:893, 1974.

26. Holland, J.: Chemotherapeutic goals in acute leukemia. N. Engl. J. Med., 280:216, 1969.

27. Holton, C.: Clinical study of daunomycin and prednisone for induction of remission in children with advanced leukemia. N. Engl. J. Med., 280:171, 1969.

28. Hubbard, S., and Devita, V.: Chemotherapy research nurse. Am. J. Nurs., 76:560, 1976.

29. Judak, C., et al.: Critical Care Nursing. Philadelphia, J. B. Lippincott Co., 1973.

30. Hughes, W.: Fatal infections in childhood leukemia. Am. J. Dis. Child., 122:283, 1971.

31. Hughes, W., and Feldman, S.: Infections in children with leukemia. Hosp. Med., 8:68, December 1972.

32. Isler, C.: Care of the pediatric patient with leukemia. R.N., 72:30, 1972.

33. Isler, C.: Children are surviving leukemia and lymphoma. R.N., 35:20, 1975.

34. Jackson, B., and Armenaki, D.: A tumor classification system. Am. J. Nurs., 76:1320, 1976.

35. Keaveney, M., and Wiley, L.: Hodgkin's disease...the curable cancer. Part I: diagnosis and treatment. Nursing 75, 5:48, 1975.

36. Kevitt, M.: Combination sequential chemotherapy in advanced reticulum cell sarcoma. Cancer, 29:630, 1972.

37. Krakoff, I.: L-asparaginase. Am. J. Nurs., 70:9, 1970.

38. Lampkin, B., et al.: Treatment of acute leukemia. Pediatr. Clin. North Am., 19:1123, 1972.

39. Marino, E., and LeBlance, D.: Cancer chemotherapy. Nursing 75, 5:22, 1975.

40. Martinson, I.: The child with leukemia: parents help each other. Am. J. Nurs., 76:1120, 1976.

41. Mattsson, A.: Long term illness in childhood: a challenge to psychosocial adaptation. Pediatrics, 50:801, 1972.

42. Mattsson, A., and Agle, D.: Group therapy with parents of hemophiliacs — therapeutic process and observation of parental adaptation to chronic illness in children. J. Am. Acad. Child Psychiatry, 11:558, 1972.

43. Mauer, A.: Pediatric Hematology. New York, McGraw-Hill, 1969.

44. McCurdy, P., and Mahmood, L.: Intravenous urea treatment of the painful crisis of sickle-cell disease. N. Engl. J. Med., 285:992, 1971.

45. McFarlane, J.: The child with sickle cell anemia. Nursing 75, May, 1975, 29–36.

46. Moore, T., et al.: Spontaneous perforation and closure of the small intestine in association with childhood leukemia. J. Pediatr. Surg., 10:955, 1975.

47. Nagao, T., et al.: Maintenance therapy in acute childhood leukemia. J. Pediatr., 76:134, 1970.

48. Nirenberg, A.: High-dose methotrexate. Am. J. Nurs., 76:1776, 1976.

49. Oski, F.: Fetal hemogloblin, the neonatal red cell, and 2,3-diphosphoglycerate. Pediatr. Clin. North Am., 19:907, 1972.

50. Patterson, P., and Schumann, D. (eds.): Symposium on patients with blood disorders. Nurs. Clin. North Am., 7:709, 1972.

51. Peterson, K.: Current Practice in Oncology Nursing, Vol. 1. St. Louis, C. V. Mosby, 1976.

52. Phillips, J., and Gerald, B.: Incidence of cholelithiasis in sickle cell disease. Am. J. Roentgen. Radium Ther. Nucl. Med., *113*:27, 1971.

53. Pinkel, D.: Treatment of acute leukemia. Pediatr. Clin. North Am., *23*:117, 1976.

54. Piomelli, S.: Diagnostic approaches to anemia. Pediatr. Clin. North Am., *18*:3, 1971.

55. Pochedly, C.: Sickle cell anemia: recognition and management. Am. J. Nurs., *71*:1948, 1971.

56. Rapaport, S.: Introduction to Hematology. New York, Harper & Row, 1971.

57. Rodman, M.: Anticancer chemotherapy. Parts I, II, III. R.N., *35*:45, 61, 49, 1972.

58. Rogers, J.: Hodgkin's disease: hope is the key to nursing care. Part 2, nursing needs. Nursing 75, *5*:55, 1975.

59. Schwartz, E.: Hemoglobinopathies of clinical importance. Pediatr. Clin. North Am., *19*:889, 1972.

60. Scipien, G., et al.: Comprehensive Pediatric Nursing. New York, McGraw-Hill, 1975.

61. Smith, C.: Blood Disease of Infancy and Childhood. St. Louis, C. V. Mosby Co., 1972.

62. Smith, C.: The Critically Ill Child, 2nd ed. Philadelphia, W. B. Saunders Co., 1972.

63. Spinetta, J., et al.: Anxiety in the dying child. Pediatrics, *52*:841, 1973.

64. Strauss, H.: Diagnosis and treatment of inherited bleeding disorders. Pediatr. Clin. North Am., *7*:711, 1972.

65. Vaughan, V., et al. (eds.): Nelson Textbook of Pediatrics, 11th ed. Philadelphia, W. B. Saunders Co., 1979.

66. Widmann, F.: Clinical Interpretation of Laboratory Tests. Philadelphia, F. A. Davis Co., 1973.

67. Wiley, L. (ed): DIC. Nursing 74, *4*:66, 1974.

68. Ziai, M., et al. (eds.): Pediatrics. Boston, Little, Brown & Co., 1969.

Additional Reading

Bochow, A.: Cancer immunotherapy: what promise does it hold? Nursing 76, *6*:50, 1976.

Burns, N.: Cancer chemotherapy: a systemic approach. Nursing 78, *8*:56, 1978.

Desotell, S.: A brighter future for leukemia patients. Nursing 77, *77*:18, 1977.

Donley, D.: Nursing the immunosuppressed patient. Am. J. Nurs., *76:* 1619, 1976.

Doswell, W.: Sickle cell anemia: you can do something to help. Nursing 78, *8*:65, 1978.

Greene, P.: Teaching aid for children with sickle cell disease. Am. J. Nurs., *77*:1953, 1977.

McElligott, D.: My nursing experience with Bobby was brief . . .but intense. Nursing 77, *7*:52, 1977.

McFarlane, J.: Sickle cell disorders. Am. J. Nurs., *77*:1948, 1977.

Nysather, J., et al.: The immune system: its development and functions. Am. J. Nurs., *76*:1614, 1976.

Rossman, M., et al.: Phoresis therapy: patient care. Am. J. Nurs., *77*:1135, 1977.

Scarlato, M.: Blood transfusions today: what you should know and do. Nursing 78, *8*:68, 1978.

Varricchio, C.: Nursing care during total body irradiation. Am. J. Nurs., *77*:1314, 1977.

Walker, P.: Bone marrow transplant: a second chance for life. Nursing 77, *7*:24, 1977.

Zimmerman, S., et al.: Bone marrow transplantation. Am. J. Nurs., *77*:1311, 1977.

CHAPTER 9
CARE OF THE MULTI-INJURED CHILD

Donalda Parkes, R.N., B.Sc.N. and
Carmelle Sylvestre-Simon, R.N., B.Sc.N.

OBJECTIVES

1. List 10 characteristics of the pediatric patient that should be considered in the care of a multi-injured child.

2. Outline the "6B" approach in patient care management and state the signs and symptoms of at least three possible diagnoses for each system.

3. Outline the nursing actions for each of the above diagnoses selected.

4. Describe at least three possible "special" complications of the multi-injured child and the nursing actions suited to each.

Definition of Multiple Trauma
1. Multiple trauma generally refers to injuries involving more than one body region.
2. However, any child who has only one injury but one which has the potential of being life-threatening should also be considered as, and handled similarly to, the child with multiple injuries.[26]

General Features
1. Typically involves the 6- to 8-year old who has been hit by a car.
2. Obvious injuries are characteristically distributed along one side of the body, and major intrathoracic or intra-abdominal lesions are usually on the same side as the extremity injuries.[26]
3. The triad of head injury, blunt trauma to the trunk, and a limb fracture, usually the femur, is common.[26]

Incidence
1. Major trauma is the leading childhood killer in the United States and Canada, particularly of children over the age of 2 years.[22]
2. Over two million in the United States and a half million in Canada yearly are injured, many with permanent disabilities.[22]
3. More males than females are injured, particularly in the 6- to 16-year age group.[26]
4. Extensive trauma to two major systems results in a mortality rate of over 30%; damage to the brain, chest, and liver has a mortality rate often higher than 50%.[26]

Etiology and Precipitating Factors
1. Child is commonly struck by a motor vehicle, may be a passenger in a motor vehicle accident and thrown against something or out of the vehicle.
2. Falling from a considerable height, e.g., high-rise apartments in urban centers.
3. Crushing injuries when caught inside, between, or under objects.

Clinical Assessment
1. Breathing.
2. Bleeding.
3. Brain.
4. Bowel.
5. Bladder.
6. Bone.
7. Other special complications.

Patient Care Management
1. An organized approach with well-established priorities is essential. The "6B priorities," breathing, bleeding, brain, bowel, bladder, and bone, can be a very useful outline.[26]
2. Special Nursing Skills Required
   a. Ability to work quickly under stress in an organized way.
   b. Ability to work with many medical disciplines and with complex equipment and procedures.
   c. Ability to make astute observations, in-depth assessments, and quick decisions.

    d. Ability to support the child and parents through crises despite the great amount of physical care required; this demands patience, insight, considerable explanation, and a gentle approach.

3. Characteristics of the Pediatric Patient that Influence Patient Care Management.[26,32]

    a. Fear and pain make it hard for the child to cooperate. An inability to explain pain and localize symptoms can make diagnosis and treatment difficult.

    b. The margin for error in diagnosis and treatment of the infant and young child is narrow. They can change quickly and with little warning.

    c. Although children generally do not have preexisting illnesses as do adults, they may have congenital abnormalities.

    d. Children rarely sustain penetrating injuries, but much harm can come from the "hidden injuries" of blunt trauma that are common to children.

    e. Children's tissues are highly elastic, thus there is a lower incidence of serious injury. Children generally tolerate surgery well, have good healing qualities, and can recuperate rapidly with fewer of the adult complications.

    f. Breathing

       1) The child's thorax is very flexible, making him or her less susceptible to rib and sternal fractures and rupture of the diaphragm, but the chest organs are then more vulnerable to contusions.

       2) Smaller lung volumes and smaller respiratory passages make the child less tolerant of any interference with gas exchange.

       3) Clinical signs are subtle; thus the child needs more frequent chest x-ray and blood gas studies.

    g. Bleeding

       1) Direct cardiovascular injuries and thoracic aneurysms are rare. Organs can rupture from stress injuries, but children are more prone to vascular spasm because their soft, muscular vessels are heavily innervated by the sympathetic nervous system.

       2) The child's small blood volume makes even small blood losses significant.

       3) Shock in the multi-injured child is most often due to intra-abdominal bleeding. It is frequently underestimated and difficult to diagnose early. The child's pulse and blood pressure can remain normal for some time owing to his great sympathetic reaction causing vasoconstriction; then

there is a sudden, rapid, and drastic fall in blood pressure. Pallor and restlessness are significant early clues. The child will have lost considerable blood before shock is obvious.

4) Infants and young children are very susceptible to "cold stress" (heat loss) because of a large surface area relative to size. When resuscitative measures take priority, the child is often left uncovered in a cold environment for extended periods of time. Rapid infusions of cold blood can produce significant hypothermia as well.

h. Brain

1) A child's head is more often injured than an adult's.[12] A head injury makes the evaluation of any multi-injured patient difficult, but neurological testing and assessment in a young child is particularly difficult.

2) Many children with just a mild head injury are prone to a focal, lateralized, or generalized convulsion within the first 24 hours. This may be transient or it may present a long-term management problem.

3) Bloody discharge from the nose and/or ears following a significant head injury is common in children. One has to consider the possibility of a cerebrospinal fluid leak.

i. Bowel

1) The abdomen is the most common area for blood loss; a common injury is a ruptured spleen injured by the overlying ribs.

2) Gastric and intestinal dilation are very common in injured children. Excessive gastric dilation can severely compromise the already small lung volumes.

3) Gastrointestinal bleeding often occurs in the child with severe head injury, owing to vagal stimulation or therapy with steroids or aspirin.

j. Bladder

1) The bladder can easily distend beyond the protection of the bony pelvis and rupture when there is abdominal trauma.

2) The kidneys are not well shielded by the rib cage, and the peritoneum covering the kidneys is thin and easily torn. However, the renal arteries and veins are not easily torn because of vessel elasticity and the small weight of the kidney.

k. Bone

1) There is more rapid healing of fractures than in the adult because of a stronger and more active periosteum.

2) The bony pelvis is less rigid than in the adult; it doesn't fracture as easily but provides less protection for the viscera.

Signs and Symptoms	Possible Diagnoses	Medical/Nursing Actions
1. Breathing		
a. Slack jaw, displaced tongue. Secretions, blood, vomitus in airway. Dyspnea, tachypnea, stridor, wheezing, grunting, indrawing, air hunger. Retractions, tracheal tug. Color pale, gray, cyanosed. Restlessness, confusion, decreased response, apnea. Decreased air entry, decreased PO_2, increased PCO_2.	a. Airway obstruction.	a. Position head to side, lift jaw, extend neck (Use caution when possible cervical injuries). Suction, insertion of oral airway. Provide O_2 by face mask (start with 100%). Vital sign monitoring. Nasogastric tube to alleviate gastric distention. Repeated blood gas analysis. Intubation, artificial ventilation. Bronchoscopy and tracheostomy may later be necessary.
b. Chest pain, decreased air entry on affected side. Collapse of lung, tracheal deviation, mediastinal shift, subcutaneous emphysema as shown on X-ray. Herniation of abdominal contents up into chest as shown on X-ray (interferes with breathing).	b. Pneumothorax. Hemothorax. Ruptured diaphragm (mortality rate high).	b. O_2 therapy, chest X-ray to confirm diagnosis. Chest tube insertion with closed drainage system and suction. Observe degree of air leak. Measure and replace blood losses. Intubation and artificial ventilation. Thoracotomy if a major bronchial or vascular tear or a ruptured diaphragm.
c. External bruising and abrasions. Subcutaneous emphysema. Limited inspiration and difficulty in coughing due to pain.	c. Fractured ribs.	c. Analgesics for pain (avoid respiratory and neurologic depression). Intercostal nerve block.

d. Flail chest.
    Several ribs fractured.
    Fractured ribs separated from sternum.
    Fractured sternum.
    Paradoxical chest movements.

    d. Intubation and artificial ventilation.

e. Lung contusion.
    Atelectasis, pneumonia.
    Dyspnea, decreased PO_2, increased PCO_2.
    X-ray shows "clouding" of lung areas.

    e. Humidified O_2 and inhalations.
        Suctioning, chest physiotherapy (with caution if ribs, sternum are fractured).
        Broad spectrum antibiotics.

f. Pulmonary edema.
    Excessive, frothy, blood-tinged secretions.

    f. Ventilation with high pressures, high volumes, FIO_2, and PEEP.
        Sit upright with support if condition allows.
        Fluid control, diuretics.

2. Blood
    a. Obvious bleeding.
        Hypovolemic shock due to external or internal bleeding.
        Pallor, cyanosis, cold and clammy skin.
        Decreased BP, decreased CVP, increased heart rate; weak; thready pulse.
        Increased respirations, may be irregular.
        Oliguria, vasoconstriction, acidosis.
        Thirst if awake, confusion, disorientation.

        a. Pressure to obvious bleeding sites.
            Give 100% O_2 initially, may have to ventilate.
            Vital sign monitoring; use a Doppler to pick up a thready pulse and weak BP.
            Establish an IV line, preferably a central venous line for rapid fluid administration and pressure monitoring.
            Rapidly infuse (may have to pump) crystalloid, colloid solutions and then blood when available.

Signs and Symptoms	Possible Diagnoses	Medical/Nursing Actions
2. Blood (*Continued*)		Blood samples for cross and type and hemogram; coagulogram, electrolytes, BUN, and sugar later. Insert urinary catheter to monitor output and specific gravity and test for blood. Keep child warm, filter and warm blood transfusions, give sodium bicarbonate for acidosis, give calcium if large volumes of blood administered. Insertion of Swan Ganz catheter to measure pulmonary artery wedge pressures.
b. Signs of shock out of proportion to blood loss. Increased central venous pressure, decreased blood pressure, decreased heart sounds. Pulsus paradoxus (i.e., weaker on inspiration), neck vein distention. Abnormal cardiac shadow and widened mediastinum on X-ray. Absent femoral pulses. Decreased cardiac index (if cardiac output being measured).	b. Cardiac tamponade. Blood in pericardial sac causing decreased cardiac output. Aortic aneurysm or rupture.	b. Pericardiocentesis, perhaps thoracotomy. Replacement of blood losses. Arteriogram, surgical repair using cardio-pulmonary bypass. Insertion of a left atrial line at the time of thoracotomy to monitor left atrial pressures and assess cardiac output.

c. Bruises and abrasions on chest. Cardiac arrhythmias. Decreased cardiac output.	c. Cardiac contusion, penetration injury.	c. Electrocardiogram monitoring, cardiac catheterization. Thoracotomy for penetration injury. Drugs to treat cardiac arrhythmia and improve cardiac function.
d. Distended neck veins. Petechiae of head, neck, upper extremities. Conjunctival hemorrhages.	d. Traumatic asphyxia.	d. Cardiopulmonary and neurologic support.
e. "Milky" fluid from chest drain.	e. Chylothorax.	e. Chest tube with suction. Restrict protein in diet, replace drainage with plasma or albumin. Check serum proteins daily. Thoracotomy to repair if drainage persists.

3. Brain

a. Decreased level of consciousness, increased blood pressure, decreased heart rate and respiratory rate. Lateralizing signs: Dilated pupil. Progressive paralysis of contralateral limbs. Facial "droop."	a. Extradural hematoma (usually a rapid deterioration) or Subdural hematoma (may be a slower change).	a. Repeated neurologic assessment (do not give sedation; avoid restraining child if possible). Computed tomography, (CT scan), "burr holes," craniotomy. Subdural taps in the infant.

Signs and Symptoms	Possible Diagnoses	Medical/Nursing Actions
Brain *(Continued)*		
b. Generalized neurologic deterioration.	b. Cerebral edema.	b. Keep child well oxygenated, avoid hypoxemia. Attend to patient position to avoid airway obstruction; semiprone is best. Elevate head of bed. Suction to clear airway. Ensure good ventilation to control PCO_2. Hyperventilation to decrease PCO_2 may be used.
		Restrict fluid intake, maintain electrolyte balance. Give steroids; Mannitol may be necessary but repeated use can cause "rebound" edema. Temperature control, hypothermia to decrease cerebral O_2 requirements. Surgical decompression of skull.
c. Pathologic posturing (decortication, decerebration).	c. Brainstem injury.	c. General supportive measures. Diuretics, hypothermia may help. Drugs to prevent shivering and assist with cooling. May be necessary to heavily sedate or paralyze to control ventilation and temperature.

d. Spinal cord injury.

Discomfort, tenderness, pain in the spinal column (can be missed in the unconscious patient). Neurologic deficit below the injured area:
Decreased sensation, movement.
Impaired breathing, coughing.
Bladder distention.
Decreased bowel tone.

Careful positioning and moving of the child: turn as a unit, apply traction to head and feet and use several people when lifting child.
Spinal x-rays, myelogram.
Cervical collar, sand bags, halter traction, skull tongs and traction, Stryker frame, CircOlectric bed.
Laminectomy and cervical fusion.
Attention to respiratory status and bladder function.

e. Compound skull fracture(s).
Linear.
Basal.

Scalp laceration (may cause significant blood loss).
Foreign body penetration.
"Raccoon eyes," scleral hemorrhages.
Drainage from nose or ears.

Pressure dressing, protection from further injury.
Replacement of blood loss, monitoring of hemoglobin.
Surgical debridement, antibiotics, tetanus immunization.
Monitor closely for increased cerebral edema.

f. Cerebrospinal fluid fistula.
Rhinorrhea.
Otorrhea.

Bloody or "watery" looking nasal or aural discharge.

Observation of discharge to determine if it is cerebrospinal fluid.
No suctioning through the nose and no cleaning of the ear, to avoid introduction of bacteria.
Antibiotics, surgical repair later if leak doesn't heal over spontaneously.

g. Scalp hematoma.

Bruising, swelling of scalp.

Observe for increase in size.
Monitor hemoglobin.
May need blood if anemic.

Signs and Symptoms	Possible Diagnoses	Medical/Nursing Actions
3. Brain *(Continued)*		
h. Seizures.	h. Meningitis. Post-traumatic epilepsy.	h. Documentation of seizure activity. Protection of the patient; anticonvulsant therapy (do not force objects into child's mouth during a seizure). Antibiotic therapy.
i. Oliguria, increased specific gravity of urine. Overhydration, decreased serum Na, decreased serum osmolality.	i. Inappropriate antidiuretic hormone (ADH).	i. Restrict fluid intake. Urinary catheter, careful recording of intake and output, testing of specific gravity of urine. Frequent testing of blood and urine electrolytes.
j. Polyuria, polydipsia. Decreased specific gravity of urine, dehydration.	j. Diabetes insipidus.	j. Replacement of fluid and electrolyte losses. Use of pitressin to decrease diuresis.
4. Bowel		
a. Signs of hypovolemia or shock. Restlessness, decreased hemoglobin. Distended, tense, tender abdomen. Decreased bowel sounds. Blood as shown by rectal exam.	a. Hemorrhage into abdomen: Spleen (most common). Liver (high morbidity and mortality). Retroperitoneal (i.e., kidney).	a. Check abdomen frequently for distention and rigidity (best done by the same person). Abdominal girth measurement every hour. Vital sign monitoring, serial hemograms. Abdominal x-rays, ultra sounds, scans, computed tomography, angiography Nasogastric tube drainage and/or suction, IV therapy, blood loss replacement. Abdominal paracentesis, laparotomy. Hold sedation to avoid masking symptoms.

b.	Gastrointestinal perforations leading to peritonitis.	b. Care as for hemorrhage, with antibiotic therapy and monitoring of white blood cell count. Resection and anastomosis, sometimes an ileostomy.
	Shock, free intra-abdominal air on X-ray film. Fever, leukocytosis.	
c.	Injury to pancreas, duodenum.	c. Serum amylase studies. Total parenteral nutrition. Surgical repair.
	Increased serum amylase. Air or "double bubble" appearance on X-ray film.	
d.	Trauma to gastrointestinal tract, bowel. Stress ulcer due to effects of trauma (particularly with head injury) or to steroid or aspirin therapy.	d. Transfusions to replace blood losses and maintain normal hemoglobin level. Iced saline gastric irrigations. Give antacids and cimetidine. Discontinue steroid and aspirin therapy. Surgical repair.
	Gastrointestinal bleeding: Hematemesis, blood in gastric drainage. Melena stools or frank blood. Decreased hemoglobin.	

5. Bladder

a.	Kidney contusion.	a. Urinary catheter, monitoring of output, testing urine for blood. Pyelogram, cystogram, urethrogram after resuscitation and treatment for shock.
	Bruises, abrasions on trunk. Abdominal and flank pain. Lower abdominal distention, difficulty voiding. Hematuria.	
b.	Pelvic decompression: Kidney rupture. Tear of renal artery or vein. Ruptured urethra, bladder.	b. Treatment of shock; blood transfusions and antibiotics. Laparotomy, removal of torn kidney, surgical repair of surrounding areas.
	Palpable mass. Signs of shock. Urgency but inability to void. Blood at the meatus.	

Signs and Symptoms	Possible Diagnoses	Medical/Nursing Actions
5. Bladder *(Continued)* Peritonitis.	Escape of blood into peritoneal cavity, leading to shock, peritonitis.	
6. Bone a. Bruising, tenderness, localized pain, swelling. Deformity of the limb(s). Muscle spasms, crepitations. Impaired motion, inability to use part.	a. Fractured femur: usually the shaft, occasionally the neck. Can bleed into surrounding thigh tissues.	a. Careful positioning of the limb, initial splinting. Use of the Thomas splint with skin traction or skeletal traction. Frequent assessment of sensation, movement and circulation of the limb(s). Attention to skin care and pressure areas, exercising of the ankle and foot. Hip spica after suitable alignment. Internal fixation usually necessary for fractures of the femur neck.
	b. Open fractures.	b. Tetanus immunization and antibiotics. Debridement and reduction.
	c. Fractured pelvis.	c. Bed rest, careful positioning and turning. Observation for signs of organ, nerve, and vascular injuries.
	d. Fractured clavicle.	d. Careful positioning, figure-of-eight bandage to support area. Analgesics if allowed. Avoid area during chest percussion.

7. Special complications

a. "Shock" lung.

Tachypnea, grunting respirations, flaring of nares.
Wet, wheezy breath sounds.
Copious secretions, fever.
Decreased PO_2, increased PCO_2, increased cyanosis despite treatment.
Increased opacity of lungs shown by x-ray.

a. Serial chest x-rays and blood gas studies.
Fluid restriction, steroids, and diuretics.
Volume cycled respirator using high FIO_2, pressures, volumes, and PEEP.
Vigorous chest physiotherapy and antibiotics.
Decrease O_2 needs by controlling fever, pain, and activity.
Nurse in upright position if condition allows.
Filter and warm all blood transfusions.
Good supportive therapy.

b. Fat emboli.
Most likely with fractures of the long bones (e.g., femur).

Increased respiratory distress, cyanosis.
Tachycardia, decreased blood pressure, increased fever.
"Snow storm" appearance of chest x-ray film.
Multiple petechiae, mainly of the conjunctiva, upper chest, and axilla.
Decreased hemoglobin and platelets, increased serum fatty acids.
Fat globules in urine and sputum.

b. Keep fractured femur in good alignment (no pillows behind knees) and avoid movement of fracture sites.
Vigorous respiratory care: frequent change of chest position, breathing and coughing exercises, suctioning, test airway secretions for fat globules.
Intubation and artificial ventilation.
Use of anticoagulants, steroids, Dextran solution.
Test urine for fat globules.
Good supportive therapy.

c. Renal failure.
Acute tubular necrosis (ATN) secondary to hypotension.

Oliguria or anuria.
Blood: increased potassium, blood urea nitrogen, and serum creatinine, metabolic acidosis.

c. Early treatment of shock.
Monitor fluid intake and urine output carefully.
Frequent urine and blood chemistry.

Signs and Symptoms	Possible Diagnoses	Medical/Nursing Actions
7. Special complications (Continued) c. Oliguria or anuria. (Continued) Urine: fixed specific gravity, increased osmolality, creatinine, and urea, decreased sodium. Fluid retention resulting in body edema, particularly of eyes, hands, and feet; weight gain. Cardiac arrhythmias because of increased potassium.	c. Renal failure (Continued)	Careful regulation of fluid and electrolyte balance, diuretics. Restrict fluid intake, weigh child daily, amino acid intake. Electrocardiogram monitoring, particularly for effects of increased potassium. Insulin along with IV dextrose and Kayexalate enemas to decrease potassium. Calcium to assist in preventing cardiac arrhythmias due to increased potassium. IVP, renal scan to assess kidney function. Peritoneal dialysis or hemodialysis.
d. High prolonged fever. Peripheral vasoconstriction, acrocyanosis. Decreased central venous pressure, blood pressure, and cardiac output. Acidosis, increased urea and potassium. Decreased platelets, increased prothrombin time and partial thromboplastin time (disseminated intravascular coagulation). Oliguria (prerenal failure).	d. Sepsis: often gram-negative.	d. Establish satisfactory circulation first. Fluid replacement: plasma, Dextran, fresh frozen plasma for clotting factors, platelets. Close monitoring of cardiovascular status, respiratory support. Sodium bicarbonate for acidosis, Kayexalate to decrease potassium. Lumbar puncture; blood, airway, urine, and wound site cultures. High doses of antibiotics to which organisms are sensitive. Steroids may be of help.

e. Malnutrition.

   e. Severe weight loss.
Inability to tolerate feedings, diarrhea.
Skin breakdown, susceptibility to infections.
Poor healing of wounds.

   e. Daily weight, careful recording of food intake, particularly caloric content.
Frequent, small amounts of high calorie, high protein, and low fat feedings by nasogastric tube.
Medication to control diarrhea.
Control of activity, fever, and hypoxia which increase metabolic processes and calorie consumption.
Total parenteral nutrition, using aseptic technique.

f. Irreversible coma.

   f. Neurological status is neither improving nor getting worse.
Decorticate or decerebrate posturing continues.
No lateralizing signs.
May or may not require ventilatory support.

   f. General supportive care aimed toward preventing infection (particularly pneumonia and urinary tract infection), skin breakdown, and severe weight loss.
Try to "wean" patient from respirator.
May need long-term tracheostomy tube to keep chest clear.
Establish a bladder and bowel routine.
Parents will need much support and assistance.
Long-term placement and care may be a problem.

Signs and Symptoms

7. Special complications (*Continued*)

g. Excessive fear, inability to sleep. Depression, passivity, complete withdrawal. Unreasonable guilt, anger, hostility, uncontrollable behavior. Fear of punishment, bizarre fantasies.

Possible Diagnoses

g. Psychological, emotional disorder. May involve parents as well. Contributing factors: Suddenness of illness. Multiplicity of injuries. Multiservice treatment program with many people examining the child. Prolonged sleep deprivation, sensory overload, and immobilization. Frequent exposure, lack of privacy. Fear of mutilation and permanent disability.

Medical/Nursing Actions

g. Assign a primary nurse who can establish a rapport with the child and his family. Try to arrange for the parents to communicate with just one doctor. Attempt to control noise and the number of people handling the child. Reasonable rather than excessive use of restraints. Cover the child as much as possible and provide some degree of privacy despite complex care. Encourage parents and child to express their fears and frustrations. Allow liberal visiting whenever possible; include other members of the child's family. Make use of other support service such as the clergy, psychiatrists, play therapists.

BIBLIOGRAPHY

1. Bolanowski, P.J.: The chest. Emerg. Med., *8*(2):74, 1976.
2. Carey, L.C.: And then worry about shock lung. Emerg. Med., *8*(2):97, 1976.
3. Cook, W.A.: Shock lung: etiology, prevention and treatment. Heart Lung, *3*:933, 1974.
4. Craver, W.L.: Blunt chest trauma. Am. Oper. Room Nurs., *16*:54, 1972.
5. Cullen, P., et al.: Ventilation for flail chest: controlled mechanical vs intermittent mandatory. R.N., *39*(5) ICU/CCU:1, 1976.
6. del Bueno, D.J.: Recognizing fat embolism in patients with multiple injuries. R.N., *36*(1):48, 1973.
7. Del Guerico, L.: Hemorrhage shock. Emerg. Med., *8*(2):42, 1976.
8. Downes, J.J., and Raphaely, R.C.: Pediatric intensive care. Anesthesiology, *43*:238, 1975.
9. Durkin, D.M.: Pulmonary fat embolism a complication of fracture. Heart Lung, *5*:477, 1976.
10. Groff, D.B.: The injured child. Emerg. Med., *8*(2):58, 1976.
11. Grosfeld, J.L. (ed.): Symposium on childhood trauma. Pediatr. Clin. North Am., *22*:267, 1975.
12. Haller, J.A.: Pediatric trauma treated in a unique unit: Johns Hopkins. Amer. Oper. Room Nurs., *19*:1273, 1974.
13. Jones, R.S., and Owen-Thomas, J.B.: Care of the Critically-Ill Child. London, Edward Arnold, 1971.
14. Keen, G.: Closed chest injuries. Parts I and II. Nurs. Mirror, *134*(24):14, 25, 1972.
15. Larkin, J., and Moylan, J.: Priorities in management of trauma victims. Crit. Care Med., *3*:192, 1975.
16. Love, J.W.: Chest injuries. Emerg. Med., *8*(4):156, 1976.
17. Moncreif, J.A.: Sepsis. Emerg. Med., *8*(2):104, 1976.
18. Mueller, C.B.: Renal failure. Emerg. Med., *8*:(2):102, 1976.
19. Pagliero, K.M.: Chest injuries.–I. Immediate consideration. Nurs. Times, *71*:252, 1975.
20. Seehode, J.J.: The kidneys. Emerg. Med., *8*(2):91, 1976.
21. Shaftan, G.: Bone and muscle. Emerg. Med., *8*(2):82, 1976.
22. Simpson, J.S.: Trauma: the leading childhood killer in Canada and elsewhere. Clin. Pediatr., *15*:313, 1976.
23. Smith, C.A.: The Critically Ill Child: Diagnosis and Management, 2nd ed. Philadelphia, W. B. Saunders, 1977.
24. Stein, A.M., et al.: Multiple fractures: how to prevent pulmonary complications. Nursing 74, *4*(11):26, 1974.
25. Strichen, F.M.: The abdomen. Emerg. Med., *8*(2):79, 1976.
26. Surgical Staff, Hospital for Sick Children: Care for the Injured Child. Baltimore, Williams and Wilkins Co., 1975.
27. Wagner, M.M.: Assessment of patients with multiple injuries. Amer. J. Nurs. *72*:1822, 1972.
28. Wagner, M.M. (ed.): Symposium on emergency nursing. Nurs. Clin. North Am., *8*:377, 1973.
29. Webb, K.J.: Early assessment of orthopedic injuries. Amer. J. Nurs., *74*:1048, 1974.
30. Wilson, R.F., and Sibbald, W.J.: Acute respiratory failure. Crit. Care Med., *4*:79, 1976.
31. Worth, M.H.: Abdominal trauma. Emerg. Med., *8*(4):160, 1976.
32. Young lungs and injured. Emerg. Med., *5*(1):95, 1973.

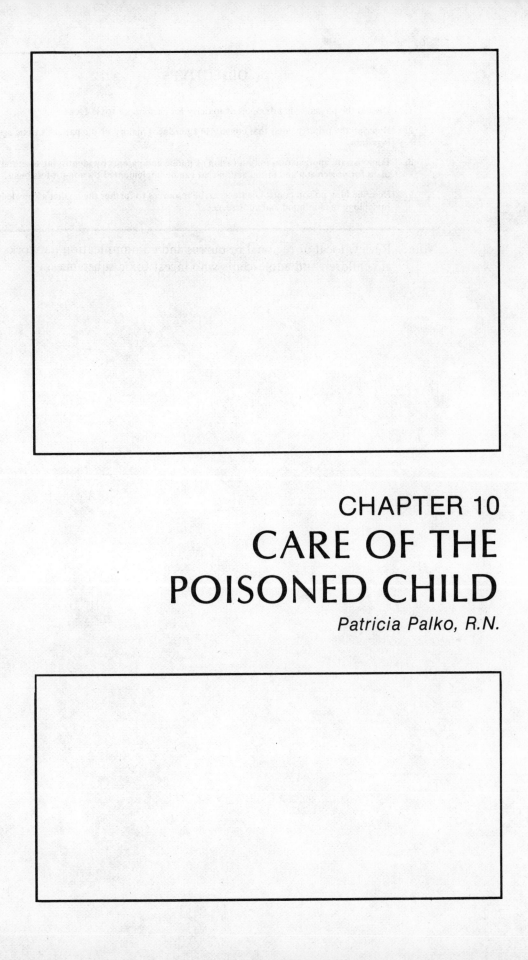

CHAPTER 10
CARE OF THE POISONED CHILD
Patricia Palko, R.N.

OBJECTIVES

1. Discuss the physiologic principles of toxicity for each major toxic agent.

2. Describe the priority areas that constitute a pertinent history of the patient's toxic agent ingestion.

3. Demonstrate appreciation for education of public and parents by identifying essential plans for prevention and initial action that can be implemented by non-professionals.

4. Describe how poison control centers can be resources to further the learner's knowledge of toxicology in childhood and adolescence.

Note: Review local or regional resources and communication networks that aid children and adolescents who ingest toxic substances.

INTRODUCTION

Prevention: the most effective treatment of poisonings

1. Manufacturer's role:
   a. Child-proof containers, safety caps.
   b. Number of tablets in bottle limited to 36.
   c. Increased use of warning on labels.
   d. Clear information as to package content.
   e. Recommended treatment for accidental ingestion or overdose included on container labels.
   f. Identification of drugs by imprints from manufacturers and coding of tablets.
2. Poison control centers:
   a. More than 600 throughout United States.
   b. Function as vital resource centers to disperse information to physicians and public:
      1) Signs and symptoms of poisoning.
      2) Methods of treatment.
      3) Complications.
   c. Sources of information utilized by centers:
      1) National Clearinghouse for Poison Control Centers: has on file approximately 20,000 reference cards, which are continually updated and sent to poison control centers.
      2) Gleason, Goslin, and Hodges: Clinical Toxicology of Commercial Products — 25,000 trade name products.
      3) Toxifile—a microfile system like the card system.
      4) Posindex—a microfiche system with ingredient lists and toxicologic data on more than 150,000 items.
   d. Introduction of Mr. Yuk:
      1) A nationally promoted, green, circular sticker with a frowning face.
      2) Attached to household items to discourage youngsters from ingesting toxic substances.
   e. National Poison Prevention Week:
      1) A March promotional effort to teach prevention of poisoning, distribute Mr. Yuk stickers, and distribute syrup of ipecac samples with instructions in how to implement emergency treatment in case certain substances are ingested.
3. Public and parent education.
   a. Pharmacist's role:
      1) Distribute literature.
      2) Remind parents to keep medication out of children's reach.
      3) Be available as a speaker to community groups.
   b. Nurse's role:
      1) Be available to schools and preschools to establish preventive programs.
      2) Be aware of toxicology; function as a resource counselor to the family and physician.

3) Support legislation for requiring safe packaging.
4) Refer families to social services in the event of high-risk or repeated ingestions.
5) Teach parents and patients about their medications, effects, and the side effects.

  c. Parents' role:
1) Store toxic household items away from curious children who crawl and climb.
2) Have ipecac available in home.
3) Keep medicines out of reach or locked up.

General Information about Poisoning

1. Liquids are more easily taken in quantity than powders or solids.
2. A "bad taste" does not affect the amount ingested.
3. Dirty or contaminated particles do not deter ingestion.
4. Colorful, attractively packaged medications seen to be taken and used by parents are enticing to the young child. However, any medication or drug used even occasionally in front of the child is potentially a source of poisoning.
5. Dispensing or packaging techniques make a difference; e.g., less perfume from a spray bottle will be ingested than antacid from a wide-mouth bottle.
6. Most poisonings occur in children under the age of 5 years; this does not include drug abuse.
7. Children with known allergies may be more susceptible to poisonings of all varieties, particularly inhalation and absorption.

INITIAL HISTORY

A calm and confident approach to the parent will assist in obtaining necessary information.

1. If initial contact is by phone, obtain patient's or informant's phone number immediately in case you are disconnected.
2. Ask for a patient profile: age, sex, weight.
3. Establish time of ingestion and what was ingested:
    a. Correct spelling.
    b. Whether substance is in original container.
    c. How much was ingested.
    d. Whether any was spilled.
    e. How full the container was before ingestion.
    f. Whether the child has received anything since ingestion.
4. Establish presence of any symptoms:
    a. Airway obstruction or change in respirations.
    b. Vomiting.
    c. Cramping.
    d. Sleepiness.

e. Irritation around or in mouth.
f. Skin color change.
g. Focal or systemic seizures.

SUBSTANCES MOST COMMONLY INGESTED _____

Salicylates (Including aspirin and oil of wintergreen)
1. Incidence.
    a. Accidental ingestion in the toddler group has decreased owing
        to:
        1) Limitation of the number of baby aspirins to 36 tablets per
            bottle.
        2) Use of other antipyretics (Tylenol, Datril).
        3) Public awareness of danger and realization of the fact that a
            safety cap does not guarantee a poison-proof container.
    b. Therapeutic ingestion is 50% of the toxic ingestion.
        Uninformed, alarmed parents may begin feeding frequent
        doses of aspirin to the already febrile child.
    c. Infants are more susceptible than older children.
    d. Fever, for which aspirin is most frequently given, tends to
        aggravate the effects of the drug.
2. Physiological effect.
    a. Aspirin causes a metabolic confusion in carbohydrate
        metabolism.
    b. Fat becomes mobilized and is converted to ketone bodies.
        Increase of ketones causes acidosis. resulting in Kussmaul
        respirations. Salicylates decrease the level of prothrombin by
        interrupting the utilization of vitamin K in the liver.
3. Identification of component.
    a. Tablet coding.
    b. Container.
    c. Tablet description.
    d. Rubbing compound ingredients.
4. Presenting symptoms.
    a. Hyperventilation; rapid and *deep* breathing is the first and most
        dependable sign of aspirin poisoning.
    b. Vomiting (may be the "coffee ground" type), dehydration.
    c. Fever, sweating.
    d. Acute abdominal pain.
    e. Dizziness and tinnitus.
    f. Convulsions.
5. Principles of treatment.
    a. Induce emesis with syrup of ipecac for immediate emptying of
        stomach. May follow with gastric lavage, using magnesium
        oxide as a neutralizing agent.
    b. Give activated charcoal.

    c. Utilize intravenous therapy to:
      1) Maintain adequate hydration.
      2) Correct acid-base imbalance.
    d. Laboratory tests.
      1) Blood salicylate level.
      2) Toxicology screen of urine.

6. Common complications.
    a. Tetany, convulsions.
    b. Hemorrhage into various tissues and organs (commonly gingival bleeding), gastritis.
    c. Renal failure due to less effective physiologic mechanisms for excreting salicylates in children.
    d. Respiratory alkalosis, then later metabolic acidosis.
    e. Skin rash.
    f. Hypoprothrombinemia.

7. Nursing management.
    a. Establishment and maintenance of patent airway.
    b. Careful intake and output measurement.
    c. Guaiac test of all emesis and stools.
    d. Oral care; especially if there is vomiting, bloody drainage from buccal trauma during seizures, or inflamed irritation.
    e. Vitamin K therapy.
    f. Dialysis.

Iron

1. Incidence.
    a. An estimated 2000 cases of iron poisoning per year occur in the United States.
    b. Lethal dose: 40 mg/kg.

2. Physiologic effect.
    a. Gastrointestinal: The initial lesion, which is formed either in the stomach or in the intestinal tract, is a necrotizing hemorrhagic reaction.
    b. Cardiovascular: Iron in the serum in amounts that exceed the normal binding capacity of serum protein causes a toxic effect of syncope and tachycardia. Edema and swelling occur in the heart owing to excessive deposit of iron.
    c. Neurologic: Areas of hemorrhage occur owing to the necrotizing effect, producing a lesion that causes the central nervous system symptoms.

3. Identification of components.
    a. Tablets are small and easily ingested; the lack of enteric coating makes the resemblance to candy an outstanding factor in attracting the child.
    b. Iron can be identified by container, breakdown of tablet, and medication history obtained from parents.
    c. Problem of quantity exists.
    d. Radiographic studies can be performed after initial treatment to assess opaque tablets.

4. Presenting symptoms.
   a. Abdominal cramping within 30 to 40 minutes of ingestion.
   b. Emesis: brownish in color, with a few obvious tablets.
   c. Diarrhea: dark green.
   d. Profound shock.
5. Principles of treatment.
   a. The stomach should be emptied by lavage tube (preferably not by emetics such as ipecac).
   b. Lavage with phosphate salts or sodium bicarbonate to cause the contents of the gastrointestinal tract to be more alkaline, thus preventing absorption of the ferrous sulfate.
   c. Maintain adequate intravenous administration of isotonic saline.
   d. Laboratory tests:
      1) Iron-binding capacity.
      2) Total iron level.
      3) Electrolytes.
      4) Blood glucose.
      5) Fischer test: indicates presence of unbound serum iron.
   e. Desferoxamine (Desferal) administration:
      1) Indications:
         a) Prophylactically, to reduce iron absorption after overingestion.
         b) Hypotension or preliminary symptoms of shock.
         c) Positive Fischer test.
      2) Action:
         a) Desferoxamine blocks absorption of iron, binds it, and excretes it. Normal dosage *if patient not in shock:*
            (1) Intramuscular: 90 mg/kg every 8 hours; may follow with up to 1 g every 8 hours.
            (2) Intravenous: in cardiovascular collapse use the IV route and administer medication very slowly. The rate should not exceed **15 mg/kg/hr** and may need to be given in a much less concentrated solution.
   f. Patient should be hospitalized for at least 24 hours; recovery should be cautiously observed, because some victims appear to improve rapidly during the 12 to 24 hours after ingestion and then suddenly collapse.
6. Common complications.
   a. Immediate:
      1) Convulsions.
      2) Circulatory collapse.
      3) Shock due to iron toxicity or too rapid IV infusion of Desferal.
      4) Coma.

b. Long-term:
1) One to two months after ingestion, scarring of sites in gastrointestinal tract occur. Pyloric or duodenal obstruction often requires surgical intervention.

7. Nursing Management.
   a. Establish and maintain patent airway.
   b. Protect patient from further injuries during convulsions.
   c. Monitor isotonic IV fluids during pending circulatory shock.
   d. Monitor all vital signs q 15 minutes until patient is stable.

Hydrocarbons

1. Incidence:
   a. Account for approximately 10% of all poisonings in preschool children.
   b. One of the most common liquids in the child's environment in the form of kerosene, charcoal lighter fluid, mineral seal oil, turpentine, and gasoline.
   c. Southern states have a greater prevalence of kerosene ingestion because it is utilized there for cooking.
   d. Northern states have a greater prevalence of furniture polish ingestion.

2. Physiologic effect.
   a. Pulmonary system: Direct inhalation of fumes during ingestion and during regurgitation and sucking in of actual liquid stomach contents predisposes to lung congestion, pneumonia (predominately aspiration type), and eventually respiratory distress syndrome.
   b. Central nervous system: Depression of consciousness followed by various levels of coma depending on amounts of material ingested and time lapse since ingestion.
   c. Cardiovascular system: Shunting of circulating volume into capillary beds, stagnation of extracellular fluid shifts causing a decrease of cardiac output and profound vasogenic/ hematogenic shock.

3. Identification of component.
   a. Difficult task; liquids are often removed from their original containers.
   b. Area where child was playing, odor on clothes or hands, complaints of irritation of mouth or burning sensation in stomach.
   c. Vomitus will have the characteristic odor of gasoline or kerosene.

4. Presenting symptoms.
   a. Pulmonary:
1) Cough and choking.
2) Rales.
3) Cyanosis.
4) Breath-holding; may appear to be strangling.
5) Pulmonary edema.

      b. Central nervous system:
         1) Irritability.
         2) Convulsions.
         3) Lethargy to total depression.
      c. Cardiac system:
         1) Cardiac arrhythmias with change in ST segment and T wave depression.

5. Principles of treatment.
    a. Whether to use ipecac-induced treatment or cautious lavage depends on the risk of aspiration. Most authorities advise against inducing vomiting unless the ingested amount of hydrocarbon distillate is very large.
    b. If there is a risk of aspiration owing to deteriorating neurologic signs, age, or ingestion of a large quantity, a cautious lavage can be performed.
    c. Oxygen therapy if patient is cyanotic or dyspneic.
    d. Antibiotic therapy if patient is febrile or has an infectious condition.
    e. Steroids initiated as supportive treatment for 48 to 72 hours (may establish lung capillary membrane integrity and reduce risk of respiratory distress syndrome).

6. Complications.
    a. Aspiration pneumonia.
    b. Pulmonary edema.
    c. Death if toxic course is not altered.
    d. Inadequate or inappropriate restoration of circulating volume.

Heavy Metals: (lead, mercury, arsenic, thallium, cadmium, gold, copper)

1. Occurrence.
    a. Lead: most commonly ingested heavy metal; rate may be as high as one child dying every 36 hours from lead poisoning.
    b. Average age: 12 to 36 months.
    c. May be associated with bizarre, compulsive eating habits (pica).

2. Physiological effect.
    a. Central nervous system: possibility of encephalopathy causes the most clinical concern. Children who survive lead poisoning often have residual damage consisting of mental retardation, visual impairment, cerebral palsy, convulsive disorders, and learning disabilities.
    b. Renal system: toxic effects on the nephron create a change in ultrafiltrate reabsorption and ultimately insufficient urine production.
    c. Soft tissues and bone: alterations of blood-forming sections of long bones.

3. Identification of component.
    a. Lead.
       1) Lead-glazed ceramic pieces.
       2) Chips of paint and putty from older homes and furniture.

       b. Mercury.
          1) Contaminated fish.
       c. Arsenic, cyanide, strychnine.
          1) Rodent poisons.
          2) Ant and roach preparations.

4. Presenting symptoms.
   a. Irritability.
   b. Vomiting.
   c. Anorexia and constipation.
   d. Iron-deficiency anemia (almost always present).
   e. Lethargy.
   f. Ataxia.
   g. Seizures, and opisthotonos posturing.
   h. Facial muscle spasm accompanied by excruciating pain (risus sardonicus).
   i. Pyrexia.
   j. May have intermittent laryngotracheal spasms with commensurate vital sign changes—tachycardia, apnea.
   k. Hemorrhage.
   l. Garlic-like breath odor (smell in exhaled vapor like vomitus or feces)

5. Treatment.
   a. Establish and maintain patent airway and ventilations.
   b. Maintain adequate hydration.
   c. Establish urine flow.
   d. Begin chelation therapy:
      1) Functions to absorb and hold the respective metal within the extracellular space.
      2) BAL and Ca Na EDTA are the two drug treatments of choice and are given IM over a period of 2 to 3 days.
      3) Monitor calcium, electrolytes, urine output.
   e. Give iron supplement to replace excessive iron lost.
   f. Control seizure activity.
      1) Valium, Dilantin, or anesthesia if required.
      2) Mannitol to lower intracranial pressure.
      3) Hypothermia to decrease metabolic activity.
   g. Eliminate primary source of lead.
      1) Control or change environment.
      2) Parent and patient education.
   h. Tests to show lead in quantities that exceed normal levels:
      1) 24-hour urine specimen.
      2) Complete blood count and differential.
      3) X-ray film to show lead in the gastrointestinal tract.

6. Nursing interventions.
   a. Reduce environmental stimuli to decrease seizure risk.

b. Careful intake and output measurements; appropriate bedside urine tests—specific gravity, hematologic assessment, bilirubin level, ketone level.

Other Types of Poisoning

1. Contact nearest poison control center for information on specific toxic agents.
2. Antidotes.
   a. Syrup of ipecac.
      1) An emetic drug available over the counter.
      2) Amount of drug is 30 ml; instructions on dosage for age of child are on bottle.
      3) At the direction of physician or poison control center, ipecac is given and followed by two to three 8-ounce glasses or bottles of clear fluid; juices are second choice.
         a) Do not use carbonated beverages.
         b) Bouncing, rocking, moving will augment emesis.
      4) Time and amount given should be recorded by parent.
      5) Approximately 20 minutes later, emesis should occur.
      6) Dose can be repeated once.
         a) Inability to vomit will necessitate lavage, as ipecac has cardiogenic toxic effects if retained.
      7) Patient should remain on side or sitting to prevent aspiration.
      8) Caution: evaluate adequate return of liquid through emesis so as to prevent ipecac toxicity.
   b. Activated charcoal.
      1) Inhibits the gastrointestinal absorption of potential poisons if given within 30 minutes of ingestion.
      2) Activated charcoal is usually mixed with water in a 5:1 ratio and given to the patient to drink.
      3) No contraindications to repeated doses.
      4) Should be stored in black bottles.
   c. Gastric lavage.
      1) Lavage is utilized in the event of:
         a) Deteriorating level of consciousness.
         b) Hydrocarbon ingestion, to prevent aspiration (this treatment is controversial).
         c) Hyperactivity.
         d) Lack of response to emetic therapy.
         e) Ingestion of corrosive agents.
      2) Technique of lavage:
         a) Head and neck should be lowered.
         b) Stomach tube should be passed through nose to avoid excessive gagging and choking.
         c) Stomach contents should be removed prior to lavage, as most lavage fluids do not mix with the hydrocarbons.

BIBLIOGRAPHY

1. Children's Orthopedic Hospital and Medical Center, Seattle, Wash.: Poison Control Center Protocol and Procedure Manual and Files, 1979.
2. Coleman, A., and Alpert, J. (eds.): Poisoning in children. Pediatr. Clin. North Am., *17*:471, 1970.
3. Fischer, D., et al.: Acute iron poisoning in children. J.A.M.A., *218*:1179, 1971.
4. Pascoe, G.: Quick Reference to Pediatric Emergencies. Philadelphia, J.B. Lippincott Co., 1973.
5. Reimold, W., et al.: Salicylate poisoning. Am. J. Dis. Child., *125*:668, 1973.
6. Shirkey, H.: Pediatric Therapy. St. Louis, C. V. Mosby Co., 1975.
7. Smith, C.: The Critically Ill Child: Diagnosis and Management, 2nd ed. Philadelphia, W. B. Saunders Co., 1977.

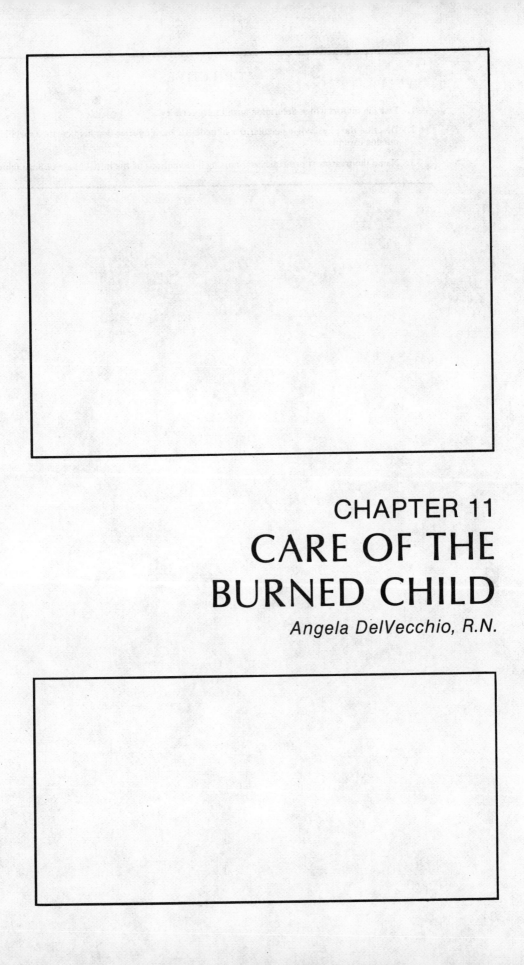

CHAPTER 11
CARE OF THE BURNED CHILD

Angela DelVecchio, R.N.

OBJECTIVES

1. List the factors which determine burn injury severity.

2. Describe the physiologic peculiarities of pediatric burn injuries that help create a specific nursing care plan.

3. Name the treatment principles and nursing interventions of the initial phase of burn injury.

INTRODUCTION

DEFINITION OF BURN INJURY

Burn injury refers to tissue destruction that results from exposure to thermal (flame and hot liquid), chemical, electrical, and radiation energy.

GENERAL CONSIDERATIONS

Pediatric burn care combines the specialties of pediatrics and intensive burn care in an attempt to successfully treat the burned child. Because a major burn injury affects all major systems of the body, a multidisciplinary "burn team" approach to care is essential. Members of the burn team include the medical staff (pediatricians, surgeons, anesthesiologists, psychiatrists), nursing staff, physical and occupational therapy staff, dietary staff, recreational therapists, laboratory technicians, and housekeeping staff. The nurse who is in constant contact with the child coordinates the care and services delivered by each discipline.

The aim of pediatric burn care is the permanent closure of the burn wound in as short a time as possible, since the longer the burn wound is open, the greater are the chances of complications. In so doing, the burn team endeavors to attain as normal a functional and cosmetic result as possible, because the physical and psychologic effects of a severe burn injury last a lifetime.

The severity of burn injury depends upon a number of factors:

1. The percentage of body surface area burn.
2. The depth of burn.
3. Age of the child.
4. The child's past medical history.
5. The area of the body burned.
6. The presence of concomitant injuries (inhalation injury, fractures, trauma.)

The classification of burn severity developed by the American Burn Association reflects these factors.[2]

MAJOR BURN INJURY

Second degree burns of greater than 20% body surface area (BSA) in children (25% in adults); all third degree burns of 10% BSA or greater; all burns involving the hands, face, ears, eyes, feet, perineum; all inhalation injuries, electrical burns, and complicated burn injuries involving fractures or other major trauma; and all poor-risk patients.

MODERATE UNCOMPLICATED BURN INJURY

Second degree burns of 10 to 20% in children (15 to 25% in adults), with less than 10% third degree burns which do not involve eyes, ears, face, hands, feet, and perineum. Excludes electrical injuries, complicated injuries such as fractures, inhalation injuries, and all poor-risk patients.

MINOR BURN INJURY

Second degree burns of less than 10% BSA in children (15% in adults) with less than 2% third degree burns, not involving eyes, ears, face, hands, feet, and perineum. Excludes electrical injuries, complicated injuries, inhalation injuries, and all poor-risk patients.

PSYCHOLOGIC CONSIDERATIONS

Psychologic support is just as vital to a child's overall well-being and survival as the physiologic support demanded by the burn injury. The isolation, pain, grief, and in some cases, guilt and rejection that the child experiences during his hospitalization must be recognized and dealt with by the burn team and by the child's family and friends.

The needs, fears, likes, and dislikes of the child who suffers a severe burn injury must be recognized. Once the burn team, particularly the nurse, can look beyond the severely burned body and recognize that the mind and spirit of a child are still present, the child can then more openly express his fears and needs. Time should be set aside every day when the child is free from medical and nursing treatments to permit visitation with family and friends. Play therapy, in whatever form allowed by the child's physical condition, should be a part of every day. The creation of a relaxed, cheerful, psychologically stimulating environment is very important for the physical and emotional well being of the child.

After wound healing is achieved and the child is discharged from the hospital, continued psychologic support is vitally needed. The child leaves the protected environment of the burn unit, where he has been accepted and supported, to reenter a society where those who look "different" are often not easily accepted. The child's family, friends, and schoolmates are key people in providing the support and acceptance vitally needed by a child who has to deal with an altered body image and in some cases with functional losses.

In the months after wound closure has been achieved, the development of contractures and hypertrophic scarring, which is especially common in children, may necessitate subsequent hospitalizations over a period of years for reconstructive surgery. The purpose of this surgery is to provide functional or cosmetic improvement. Discomfort, pain, and memories of the original incident are heightened with each return to the hospital. The recent practice of primary excision and immediate grafting of deep dermal and full thickness burn injuries greatly reduces scar formation and thus the need for reconstructive surgery.

INCIDENCE, ETIOLOGY, AND PRECIPITATING FACTORS _____

1. The National Safety Council reports burn injuries as the third leading cause of accidental death in childhood. Children less than three years old are at greatest risk.
2. Burn accident patterns in children are related to developmental stage in the same way that burn injury hazards are specific to age.

MOST COMMON AGENTS OF BURN INJURY ACCORDING TO DEVELOPMENTAL STAGE[14]

Infants and Children Less Than One Year of Age

Scald burns from tap water and bath water that is too hot for the child's delicate skin. Contact burn injuries from the child's touching hot stoves, radiators, and hot floor furnace grates while crawling.

Toddlers

Toddlers are particularly prone to burn injuries resulting from their curiosity and exploration of their environment. Scald burns occur when the child pulls down electrical cords of hot liquid-containing appliances, overturning pots and cups containing hot liquids onto themselves, and turning on hot water faucets. The young toddler tends to put everything he finds into his mouth. Chemical burns result from the ingestion of lye and drain openers. Electrical injuries of the corner of the mouth result from the child's chewing or sucking on electrical cords.

Preschool Children

The preschool child is physically more coordinated and active. The child attempts to be more self-reliant. Flame burns may occur when the child climbs and reaches for something near the stove, which in turn ignites the clothing, particularly the frilly gowns worn by girls. Other flame injuries are caused by playing with matches and by open outdoor fires of burning leaves and trash.

School-age Children

Peer involvement and acceptance, and the need for self achievement, are important with the schoolage child. Flame burns from stove accidents and playing with candles that drip hot wax onto flesh or ignite clothing are frequent events among girls of this age. Young boys sustain injuries from a variety of other causes, including playing with gasoline, burning leaves, and exploding firecrackers. Boys and girls may try to imitate adults in some work situations for which they do not have the skills and in so doing accidentally sustain burn injuries. The most common categories for this group include homemaking chores and agricultural and shop duties.

Adolescents

Boys tend to be injured more often than girls in this age group. Accidents result from risk-taking behavior or work-related injuries. Firecrackers, chemistry lab experiments, and fast-order cookery are common causes. Flash flame burns of face, hands, and chest are seen with explosive ignition of outdoor fires where gasoline, kerosene, or some other highly inflammable starter fluid is used.

Most accidental burn injuries may be prevented through closer supervision of the young child and burn prevention education of children of all ages. Children should be taught to drop to the ground and roll to smother the fire if their clothing ignites, as the extent and degree of the injury may be minimized in this way. Quick removal of clothing soaked by scalding water also decreases the severity of tissue injury.

PHYSIOLOGIC ASPECTS OF PEDIATRIC BURNS

Integumentary System
1. The dermis of an infant and child is thinner than that of an adult, so children are more prone to full-thickness injury.[1]
2. Children are prone to the formation of hypertrophic scarring and contracture that may require skin releases to allow complete mobility and normal structural growth.

Pulmonary System
1. The diameter of a child's airway is normally narrower than that of an adult and is more easily occluded by secretions and edema.
2. Infants are nosebreathers and are unable to breathe through their mouths.
3. If intubation is necessary, intubate by oral or nasal routes. A tracheostomy should be avoided if at all possible in a burned patient.[9]
    a. In burned or edematous tissue, the trachea is difficult to define clearly, and a tracheostomy may be easily malpositioned.

b. Tracheostomy performed through infected burn tissue causes pneumonia, as the burn exudate enters the tracheostomy site.

4. Full thickness circumferential trunk injuries restrict thoracic excursion, and escharotomies may be needed to relieve the pressure on the chest wall and allow normal lung expansion.

Cardiovascular System

1. Myocardial function is good but peripheral compensation is poor in the infant. Therefore, vasoconstriction to raise the effective circulating volume and vasodilation to release body heat do not occur quickly.
2. The percentage of water composition to body weight in the infant and child is greater than in the adult, so there is a greater danger of fluid overload and deficit.
3. Children have a relatively larger body surface area per kg of body weight than adults and thus a greater potential for evaporative water loss.[15] The average evaporative fluid loss is greater than 4000 ml per square meter of burn for a child as compared to 2500 ml per square meter of burn in an adult.[18]

Renal System

1. Because infants have immature renal function and decreased ability to concentrate urine, they excrete hypotonic urine, which may contribute to hypovolemia and electrolyte imbalance.
2. Severe burn injury produces hypovolemia and decreased cardiac output, which if severe and prolonged may cause renal failure.
3. In monitoring the child's response to fluid therapy, urine output is one of the easiest parameters to monitor but can be misleading owing to:
    a. Depression of the glomerular filtration rate, a common occurrence in burned patients.
    b. Osmotic diuresis, which may be present if dextrose is given in intravenous fluids if the child has hyperglycemia due to stress or if mannitol has been given.
    c. The oliguric or diuretic phase of renal failure.

Metabolism

1. The metabolic rate of a child is approximately two times that of an adult.[5]
2. Burn injury, with the loss of fluids, electrolytes, protein, and energy through the open wounds causes a hypermetabolic state. The exact cause of this phenomenon is unknown.
3. The insensible water loss of the infant occurs relatively faster than that of an adult, owing to:
    a. The infant's higher metabolic rate.
    b. The hypotonic urine excreted by the infant kidney.
    c. The relatively greater surface area of the child.[15]
4. Children lose proportionately larger amounts of sodium, chloride, and nitrogen than adults.
5. Infection causes an increased loss of electrolytes from the wound surface.

Gastrointestinal System

1. The infant has a weak gastroesophageal sphincter and can easily regurgitate gastric contents, increasing the risk of aspiration.
2. The functioning of the gastrointestinal tract is one of the major factors in the survival of the severely burned child. The nutritional state of the child becomes the principal determinant in healing.
3. The nutritional needs of the burned child are great, but the child may have an intolerance for the high osmolarity feedings frequently used in burn therapy. Advancement to high protein diets may be slow owing to poor assimilation.

Musculosketal System

1. A position of comfort most often desired by the burned patient is likely to be one that leads to flexion contractures.
2. Immobilization of body parts during grafting or critical periods leads to pressure areas, decubiti, and muscle atrophy.

Neurologic System

1. Possible causes of cerebral symptoms are hypoxia with anoxic cerebral injury, septic foci in the brain, or fluid and electrolyte abnormalities. Hypovolemia with cerebral ischemia, hyponatremia, and hypoproteinemia may cause additional neurologic deficits in the patient with burns.

CLINICAL PRESENTATION

General Signs and Symptoms

1. Compromised ventilation if thermal burns with inhalation of carbon products have occurred or if circumferential full thickness burns are present.
2. Hypoxia, hypoxemia.
3. Voice changes—"crowing" noises—when glottic swelling is present.
4. Denuding of skin, loss of protective covering.
5. Labile body temperature.
6. Varying burn wound appearances according to burn depth:
    a. Dry, elastic red tissue with first degree burns.
    b. Moist, blistered with color varying from mottled white to red with second degree burns.
    c. Dry, inelastic, leathery tissue with color varying from white to dark brown with third degree, full thickness burns.
7. Massive swelling.
8. Massive fluid shifts and losses.
9. Tachycardia and normal or elevated systemic blood pressure initially. Lowered systemic blood pressure with ensuing shock.

Laboratory findings

1. Normal arterial blood gases or changes with lowered Pao_2, elevated $Paco_2$.
2. Hemoglobinuria (frequently accompanies extensive inhalation injury and resulting pulmonary involvement).

3. Oliguria, occasionally anuria.
4. Myoglobinuria (common with extensive electrical burns and deep full thickness burns with muscle involvement).
5. Hyperkalemia.
6. Hypoproteinemia.
7. Elevated hematocrit.
8. Leukocytosis with "left shift."

THERAPEUTIC MANAGEMENT

Generally, the clinical management of pediatric patients with burns is very similar to that of adults with burns except for the physiological peculiarities of children that were noted earlier. It is imperative to obtain a thorough history of events related to the patient's burns. In areas where prehospital emergency intensive care is utilized, the paramedic or nurse can provide a good description of where the patient was found and the specific aspects of burn components. If the patient is admitted to the emergency department by nonmedical personnel, direct and very specific questions must be asked of all associated persons in order to determine the approaches for immediate and long-term care.

Objectives of Therapy
1. Establish and maintain adequate airway and ventilation.
2. Oxygenate to level of preinjury state.
3. Avoid complications, especially infection and further organ dysfunctions.
4. Maintain full and active mobility.
5. Attain permanent wound closure as quickly as possible.
6. Help patient to establish effective coping mechanisms and good mental health.

Initial Phase (first 24 to 72 hours)

Assess Adequacy of Ventilation, Establish and Maintain Patent Airway
1. Suspect impending respiratory problems in the following patients:
   a. Burned in an enclosed space.
   b. Burns involving the "respiratory areas" of the head, face, and neck.
   c. Altered mental status or unconsciousness.
2. Initial pulmonary evaluation should include checking for:
   a. Presence of singed nasal hair.
   b. Erythema of the palate.
   c. Soot in the mouth, larynx, or sputum.
   d. Nasal flaring.
   e. Respiratory crowing or stridor.
   f. Chest retractions.

  g. Anxiety, agitation, combativeness, which are often the first signs of respiratory insufficiency and should be considered such until proven otherwise.

  h. Change in character of the child's voice.

3. As fluid resuscitation is given, watch for the development of massive neck edema and airway obstruction. This can occur quickly and dramatically in children. Prophylactic intubation should be considered before complete obstruction occurs and makes intubation traumatic and very difficult.

4. Obtain baseline arterial blood gases and chest x-ray. Do not expect to necessarily see abnormalities immediately on admission. Do not rule out pulmonary injury on the basis of admission results. It may take hours to days for the clinical manifestations of inhalation injury to occur.

5. Administer humidified oxygen and elevate the head of the bed to reduce the degree of edema formation.

6. Continue to monitor the respiratory status at least hourly; intervene appropriately.

Assess Cardiovascular Status; Prevent and Treat Burn Shock

1. Establish large bore IV line and immediately begin infusing fluid (lactated Ringer's, normal saline).

2. Obtain patient's preburn weight (Needed in estimating the fluid requirements, medication dosages, and body surface area).

3. Insert Foley catheter. Measure and record urine output every hour. Monitor specific gravity of urine and check for heme and myoglobin.

4. Estimate the per cent and depth of burn on burn diagram (see Fig. 11–1). The immediate definitive determination of depth is not essential and may not be immediately apparent, but the correct estimation of extent is important in estimating fluid requirements for the first 24 hours.

5. Calculate the estimated fluid requirement and *adjust to patient response*. Various burn formulas are available, all of which are intended to avert hypovolemic shock. Some contain just crystalloids, others a combination of colloid and crystalloid.

6. Monitor vital parameters every hour. (Apical pulse, blood pressure, urine output, central venous and pulmonary capillary wedge pressures)

7. Laboratory studies at admission should include sodium, potassium, hematocrit, osmolality, total protein, blood urea nitrogen, creatinine, glucose, and bleeding time.

Decompress the Gastrointestinal Tract

1. Insert a Levin tube and connect to suction for the first 24 to 48 hours or until bowel sounds are present.

2. Avoid oral feedings, as paralytic ileus is common in the postburn period from a combination of factors: decreased splanchnic blood-flow, fluid and electrolye imbalance, and metabolic derangements.

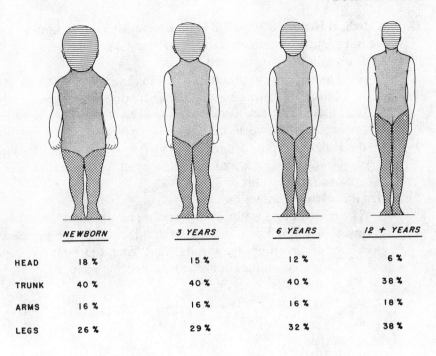

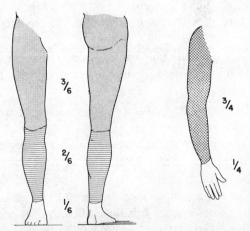

Figure 11-1. The percentage figures in the chart refer to front and back. For example, if an individual suffered a burn of the whole anterior chest, this would comprise 10 per cent of his body surface. (From Talbot, N., Richie, R., and Crawford, J.: Metabolic Homeostasis. Cambridge, Harvard University Press, 1959. After Lund, C., and Browder, N.: The estimation of areas of burns. Surg. Gynecol. Obstet., 79:352, 1944. Reprinted by permission.)

3. Burn patients are prone to the development of stress ulcers with the prolonged stress of the burn injury. Anatacids should be administered to alkalinize gastric contents.

Perform a Physical Examination

1. The burn patient is a trauma victim and should be treated as such.
2. Identify and treat any additional physical trauma.

Obtain Medical History of the Child and History of Present Injury
1. Burn injury exacerbates any preexisting illnesses.
2. Burn injury history should include:
   a. Time of injury: needed for estimating fluid replacement rate.
   b. Causative agent: may influence treatment regimen.
   c. Where the injury occurred: to evaluate whether the child is likely to have an inhalation injury.
   d. How the injury occurred: to help evaluate further trauma.
   e. Child's conception of what happened: to evaluate the child's neurologic status.

Minimize Burn Wound Infection
1. The burn wound is initially avascular and prone to bacterial invasion. Minimize transmission of infection by the use of cap, mask, and gown by the hospital staff when the wound is exposed.
2. The potential sources of autocontamination include:
   a. Hair follicles.
   b. Sweat glands.
   c. Respiratory flora.
   d. Gastrointestinal tract flora.
   e. Urinary tract flora.
3. Wash the child's entire body with sterile saline and pHisoDerm, starting with the burn wound. Shave hair in and around the burn wound.
4. Shampoo the hair and examine the scalp for burn or trauma.
5. Debride loose, nonvitalized skin, as bacteria can get under the loose skin.
6. Do not disturb intact blisters. They provide a good biologic dressing.
7. Administer tetanus toxoid as a precaution against the development of tetanus. Necrotic burn tissue is a perfect medium for anaerobic bacterial growth.
8. Dress the wound with the prescribed antimicrobial agent and wrap with loose gauze bandage, allowing for edema formation.

Evaluate Blood Circulation to Involved Extremities
1. Vascular occlusion from edema beneath an inelastic burn eschar in full thickness circumferential burns of the extremities can compromise blood flow to its distal part. If this goes untreated it can cause pressure necrosis.
2. Check capillary filling by exerting digital pressure on the nail beds of the involved extremities and evaluating capillary filling time. Also observe color, warmth, and motion, and evaluate sensation. Check for the presence and strength of distal pulses.
3. Elevate involved extremities to minimize edema formation.
4. If capillary perfusion is poor, the doctor may perform an escharotomy. An incision is made through the full thickness burn eschar to immediately relieve the pressure.

Minimize Contractures and Joint Deformities
1. Splint all involved joints as soon as the splints are available. Remove splints periodically to allow active motion.

2. Wrap fingers separately to allow for movement.

Provide Emotional Support and Comfort

1. Explain procedures to the child and his family; answer questions as honestly as possible.
2. Medicate the child for pain with IV analgesia as ordered for the first 24 to 48 hours, since the uptake of IM medication is uncertain and uncontrollable during this time. Medicate only after establishing adequate blood pressure and circulatory volume and after evaluating respiratory function.
3. Keep the child comfortably warm because evaporative cooling may be great.

Recovery Phase (ongoing burn care until complete wound closure is achieved)

Provide Needed Nutritional Support

1. Utilize the gastrointestinal and, if necessary, parenteral routes.
2. It is essential that the child be in positive nitrogen balance to heal the burn wounds.

Treat the Burn Wound

1. There are different methods of achieving wound closure; they all are basically attempts to:
    a. Prevent the conversion of a partial thickness burn to a full thickness injury.
    b. Remove exudate and devitalized tissue.
    c. Protect the wound from mechanical trauma and infection.
    d. Promote spontaneous epithelialization in areas of partial thickness injury.
2. In full thickness or deep dermal injury the aim of wound care is to:
    a. Remove necrotic tissue and cover the wound with autograft as soon as possible.
    b. Protect the wound from mechanical trauma and infection until such time as the wound can be covered with autograft.
    c. Prepare the granulation bed for the acceptance of autograft.

Minimize the Development of Joint Contractures

Prevent and Observe for Complications

1. Nearly every major organ system can be affected by the stresses of thermal injury.
2. Patients must be reevaluated at least daily, sometimes hourly, to recognize and intervene in impending organ failure or malfunction.

Provide Psychological Support to the Child and his Family

Reconstructive Phase (after full wound closure)

Correct Cosmetic and Functional Deformities

Help with Long-term Psychologic Adjustments

BIBLIOGRAPHY

1. Abramson, D.: The care and treatment of severely burned children. Surg. Gynecol. Obstet. *122*: 855, 1966.
2. American Burn Association. Specific Optimal Criteria for Hospital Resources For Care of Patients with Burn Injury. April, 1976.
3. Antoon, A., et al.: Burn encephalopathy in children. Pediatrics, *50*:609, 1972.
4. Bernstein, N.: Emotional Care of the Facially Burned and Disfigured. Boston, Little, Brown & Co., 1976.
5. Blake, F., et al.: Nursing Care of Children. Philadelphia, J.B. Lippincott Co., 1970.
6. Burke, J., et al.: Patterns of high tension electrical injury in children and adolescents and their management. Am. J. Surg., *133*:492, 1977.
7. Burke, J., et al.: Primary excision and prompt grafting as routine therapy for the treatment of thermal burns in children. Surg. Clin. North Am., *56*:477, 1976.
8. Burke, J., and Quinby, W., Jr.: Treatment of burns. *In* Cave, E., et al. (eds): Trauma Management. Chicago, Year Book Medical Publishers, 1974.
9. Eckhauser, F., et al.: Tracheostomy complicating massive burn injury: a plea for conservatism. Am. J. Surg., 127:418, 1974.
10. Feller, I., and Archambeault, C.: Nursing the Burned Patient. Ann Arbor. Institute for Burn Medicine, 1974.
11. Herrin, J., and Crawford, J.: The seriously burned child. *In* Smith, C. (ed.): The Critically Ill Child, 2nd ed. Philadelphia, W. B. Saunders Co., 1977.
12. Jacoby, F.: Nursing Care of the Patient with Burns, 2nd ed. Saint Louis, C. V. Mosby Co., 1976.
13. Kunsman, J.: Nursing care after primary excision. R.N., *37*:25, 1974.
14. McLaughlin, E., and Healer, C.: Patterns of burn accidents. Emergency Product News, June 1977. pp. 28–33.
15. Pickrell, K., and Mladick, R.: A brief guide to fluid therapy for infants and children on a plastic surgical service. Plast. Reconstr. Surg. 49:404, 1972.
16. O'Neill, J.: Continuing care of the acutely burned child. R.N., *37*:93, 1974.
17. Sheehy, E.: Primary excision: innovation in pediatric burn care. R.N., *37*:22, 1974.
18. Wilson, R.: Anesthesia and the burned child. Int. Anesthesiol. Clin., *13*:203, 1975.

CHAPTER 12
CARE OF THE ABUSED AND NEGLECTED CHILD (BATTERED CHILD SYNDROME)

Donalda Parkes, R.N., B.Sc.N. and
Carmelle Sylvestre-Simon, R.N., B.Sc.N.

OBJECTIVES

1. List five types of child abuse and neglect.

2. Understand the child abuse formula by all of the following sub-objectives:

   a. List five characteristics of the high-risk parent.

   b. List five characteristics identifying the "at-risk" child.

   c. Note five possible "triggering" factors that lead to child abuse or neglect.

3. Develop a list of five agencies that could become involved in a case of child abuse.

4. Describe ten clinical findings suggestive of a case of child abuse.

5. Compare the objectives of and the difficulties in the treatment program of an abused child.

6. State the nursing actions appropriate to each response to question 5.

INTRODUCTION

The use of physical force in the disciplining of children has long been sanctioned in our society. This force can reach the level of physical abuse, which is an extreme form of a child-rearing style quite prevalent in our culture.[13] It is a widespread, complex, multidimensional social and psychological problem, not easily resolved, and it presents a great challenge to health care workers in the areas of prevention and therapy.

DEFINITION OF CHILD ABUSE AND NEGLECT

"Child abuse and neglect means the physical or mental injury, sexual abuse, negligent treatment, or maltreatment of a child under the age of eighteen by a person who is responsible for the child's welfare under circumstances which indicate that the child's health or welfare is harmed or threatened thereby."[18]

CLASSIFICATION

Acts of Commission and Acts of Omission
1. Physical: "the battered child."
   a. Bruises, hematomas, fractures, dislocations, and burns.
   b. Head trauma: especially common in the younger child.
   c. Bizarre types of injuries may occur.
2. Nutritional.
   a. Failure to thrive, extreme dehydration, malnutrition, and cachexia.
   b. Infected sores and bites.
3. Emotional.
   a. Lack of mothering, complete rejection.
   b. Hostility, constant belittling or overprotection.
4. Sexual.
   a. Poorly reported because of its nature; it is usually "hushed up."
   b. Most incidents involve people known to the child and occur in or near the child's or the offender's home.
   c. Usually involves girls about 11 1/2 years of age who have also undergone other forms of abuse.[8]
5. Drug.
   a. Impact in recent years of the drug culture and illicit drug traffic.
   b. Infants born of addicted mothers suffer serious withdrawal and possibly permanent effects.
   c. May be victims of habitual addiction or of sustained doses of depressant drugs to keep the child quiet and easy to manage.
   d. Child is neglected because addicted parents are unable to cope and provide care.
   e. Must be considered in the child with repeated "accidental" poisonings.

INCIDENCE

1. Impossible to be accurate, owing to incomplete reporting; many cases go undetected.
2. Occurs in every geographic area and on all socioeconomic levels.[9]
3. More likely to be reported in low income and minority groups; occurs in the public domain, schools, and other child care settings.[11]
4. Majority of cases involve children under 3 years; these are considered most at risk and in danger of death.[9,11]
5. Children of both sexes are equally abused, although sexual abuse usually involves girls.
6. Statistics vary from center to center, study to study, and author to author; those given here provide a general view of the incidence of child abuse.
7. In United States.
   a. Estimated incidence is 380 per million urban population yearly.[4]
   b. 325,000 cases of child abuse and neglect reported in 1975.[16]
   c. 10% of all injuries in children under 5 years are presumed not to be accidents.[4]
8. Morbidity.
   a. 30 to 50% of abused children who are not reported will be severely abused again.[4]
   b. 15 to 20% are rebattered even when there is close supervision.[3]
   c. 15% are left with some type of permanent neurologic damage.[28]
   d. 10 to 15% of children who fail to thrive have been nutritionally deprived, and there is a high incidence of nutritional neglect along with physical abuse.[4] In one large pediatric center, 50 to 60% of children who failed to thrive have been found to be nutritionally neglected.
   e. 100,000 children yearly are subjected to sexual abuse, 27% by someone in their own household and 11% by someone closely related.[8]
9. Mortality
   a. May range from 2 to 11% (as high as 55% in some studies).[26]

ETIOLOGY AND PRECIPITATING FACTORS

1. Race, color, creed, sex, income, education, social strata do not determine child abuse.
2. However, there is a prevalence of reported battering in families of low socioeconomic status.[3]
   a. Lower class: tends more to physical abuse.
   b. Upper class: tends more to emotional neglect and abuse.

3. The female parent was said to be the most frequent abuser,[13] but the current ratio of male to female abusers is generally equal.
4. Alcohol and drug addiction are not major factors.[3]
5. Majority of abusers are not psychotic nor criminals.[13]
6. Significant factor is that the basic pattern of child rearing is poor.[13]

CHILD ABUSE FORMULA

HIGH-RISK PARENT + AT-RISK CHILD + TRIGGERING FACTORS = CHILD ABUSE

1. High-risk parent: although a specific abusive personality does not exist, some characteristics are:
   a. Lack of mothering and subjection to abuse as a child, leading to an inability to mother and poor child-rearing practices as an adult.
   b. Low self-esteem, emotional immaturity, dependency; looks to child as a source of love, comfort, and reassurance; "role reversal" occurs whereby the child exists to satisfy parental needs and little thought is given to the child's needs.
   c. Youth, loneliness, isolation, lack of spousal support and family cohesiveness; does not trust people, expects to be disappointed, is reluctant to get help from others, has few friends or outside interests.
   d. Sets extremely high standards for the child at an inappropriately early age; has unrealistic expectations of a child's ability to understand, respond, and perform (e.g., insists on toilet training at 6 months, thinks baby should eat without "messing" clothes).
2. At-risk child: usually one child in the family is singled out, although more than one may be abused. Some characteristics are:
   a. Unplanned, unwanted, or illegitimate child.
   b. Difficult pregnancy and/or delivery.
   c. Prematurity, failure of the "bonding" process: a close mother-child relationship fails to develop owing to separation during the early postnatal period.
   d. The "difficult" child: colicky, irritable, hyperkinetic, retarded.
   e. The "different" child: a "look-alike" reminder of an abusive parent, congenital abnormalities, unpleasant personality traits.
   f. The adolescent who is asserting independence and entering into heterosexual relationships.
3. Triggering factors: a crisis, major or minor, can "set things off," some crises would seem trivial and would be managed well by the stable, well-adjusted individual.
   a. Child vomits, "messes his pants," "acts up," won't eat, cries a lot.

  b. Social, economic problems: breakdown of a partner relation-
      ship, illness, loss of employment.
  c. Environmental stress: crowded living conditions, lack of
      privacy, noise, poverty, crime.

LEGAL CONSIDERATIONS

The first priority is to protect the child and to serve his or her best
interests. Every state and Canadian province has statutory laws concerning
child abuse, primarily to compel reporting and provide protection.[5]

  1. Reporting of child abuse cases.
      a. Mandatory reporting in effect in each state since 1961.[26]
      b. Primary responsibility lies with the physician, but others,
          particularly nurses, have a moral, professional, and now in many
          states a legal obligation to report.
      c. Suspicion of abuse is grounds enough to report, and the
          informant is protected from civil and criminal liability pro-
          vided he or she acts in good faith.
      d. If a child's life is at risk owing to parental religious beliefs and
          practices, a report must be made and protection provided.
      e. Reluctance to report must be tempered by a concern for the
          child's welfare.
      f. To whom the report is made varies from state to state; it may
          be a law enforcement or social welfare agency, a juvenile court,
          a local prosecutor, a child abuse team, or a hospital
          administrator.
      g. It is not up to the informant to determine guilt or determine
          who inflicted abuse.
      h. Many states now have penal sanctions for failure to report.
      i. Despite reporting laws there is gross underreporting owing to
          ignorance and misunderstanding of laws, an unwillingness to
          recognize and face the problem, and fear of getting involved.
  2. Central registries.
      a. Community or state-wide central registries for child abuse
          reports now exist in many states.
      b. Provide stastical data for research, maintain information con-
          cerning prior reports that may help those dealing with suspected
          cases and aid in recognizing and keeping track of abusive
          parents who "hospital shop."
      c. Access to their files, confidentiality, and privacy are issues.
      d. Important to remove disproved cases from the files to avoid
          stigmatizing families or prejudicing decisions.
  3. Child protection services.
      a. Aim is to investigate complaints and referrals and to evaluate
          and improve the child's environment.

    b. Can offer services, but if refused are obligated to bring a situation to the attention of a law enforcement agency, an appropriate court, or another community agency.[13]

    c. An experienced social worker may be the best person to determine whether court action or social services will be most effective.[13]

4. Law enforcement agencies.

    a. Police are available 24 hours a day and can provide immediate custody of suspected abusers, although admission of the child to the hospital for protection is thought to be better.

    b. Skilled in investigative work and court case presentations, have elaborate and sophisticated photography and laboratory services.

    c. Involving the police is controversial; many feel the orientation to the criminal and punitive aspects of child abuse is not therapeutic.

5. Other support services.

    a. Community Health Nurses: can investigate home situations, help in followup care.

    b. Parents Anonymous: a self-help group for potentially or already abusive parents.[21]

    c. Family resource centers, parent aid groups: multiservice neighborhood centers that help break down the wall of isolation with families.

    d. Crisis nurseries: provide temporary care for young children.

    e. Therapeutic day care centers: help parents learn nurturing skills.

    f. Lay therapists: provide support to parents.

    g. Pediatric Bill of Rights: not a law, but subscribed to by many hospitals and agencies.[19]

    h. Child advocacy programs: have begun in some hospitals and agencies; someone is appointed to "represent the child."

6. Juvenile courts.

    a. Laws exist to provide child protection through the juvenile courts.

    b. These courts have power over abused and neglected children, and make dispositional decisions.

    c. The judge has wide powers and may act quickly in an emergency; he or she may warn or counsel parents, order medical and psychiatric treatment for the child and parents, place the child under supervision in the home, temporarily remove the child, or rule a permanent change of custody.[13]

    d. The attempt to balance the parent's rights to their child against the child's right to live makes court decisions difficult.[13]

    e. Parents often view court action as coercion and respond poorly.

7. Criminal courts.

    a. Laws exist that forbid cruelty to children, establish child abuse as a criminal offense, and punish the offender(s).

b. Proceedings take a long time, guilt is hard to prove.
c. Acquittal may encourage offenders to think behavior is acceptable.
d. Legal action is a poor means of preventing abuse or rehabilitating offenders, does little to help the child.

CLINICAL PRESENTATION AND ASSESSMENT

A common problem is that the child is often too young or fearful to speak for himself. The nurse must rely on objective evidence. All injuries to young babies are highly significant and should be investigated. Nursing personnel need to be aware of many clues and suggestive signs in order to assist in the recognition and diagnosis of child abuse.

1. History.
   a. Parents vague, evasive, defensive, hostile.
   b. Contradictory, inappropriate, confusing statements, with a story unrelated to actual injuries or age of the child.
   c. Delay in seeking medical attention, neglect of health care (e.g., immunization not done).
   d. Child's behavior is reported to be unusual.
   e. Repeated incidents and visits, "hospital shopping."
   f. Statements revealing home and family problems.
2. Physical examination.
   a. Multiplicity of injuries in various stages of healing.
   b. Bruises, lacerations, burns, scars, unusual skin markings (some take the shape of a weapon, e.g., cigarette tip, electrical cord, hand print).
   c. Unexplained soft tissue swelling, fractures of the ribs, arms, or legs.
   d. Head trauma, particularly in the infant; retinal and galeal hemorrhages (can be caused by severe shaking).
   e. "Failure to thrive," malnutrition, dehydration, cachexia.
   f. Inappropriate clothing, dirty unkempt appearance, infected skin lesions, bites.
   g. Signs of emotional deprivation: "blank" look, under- or hyper-reactivity, great fearfulness, language retardation.
   h. Signs of drug intoxication: erratic or inappropriate behavior, excessive drowsiness, coma.
   i. Injuries to genitourinary structures (venereal disease in the young child must arouse suspicion).

3. Diagnostic procedures.
   a. Total body x-ray films (skeletal survey).
      1) Radiologic signs are specific in the battered child syndrome and are the physician's most important diagnostic tool; x-rays should be repeated in two or three weeks to note type of healing.
      2) Multiple fractures at different stages of healing and repair, trauma to soft tissues and viscera can be seen.
      3) Unusual locations and types of fractures are significant; fractures primarily involve the metaphyses and epiphyses of the long bones with subperiosteal new bone formation.
      4) Separation of cranial bones and widened sutures suggest possible subdural hematoma.
      5) Subdural hematoma and long bone fractures are a frequent combination, owing to twisting and yanking of the infant.
      6) Skull fractures are often irregular, multiple, and comminuted.
      7) Pre-existing bone disease must be ruled out.
   b. Hematological study.
      1) Hemogram and coagulogram to rule out bleeding disorders that may account for bruising.
      2) Test for anemia caused by internal bleeding and malnutrition.
   c. Toxicologic examinations.
      1) Look for exogenous poisons or overdoses of therapeutic drugs such as aspirin, cough medicine, barbiturates.
   d. Developmental assessment.
      1) Pediatric consultation and charting of growth and development (height and weight records are very important).
      2) Psychologic and intelligence testing (age is a factor here).
   e. Photographs.
      1) Photos help to document findings to law enforcement agencies and courts, are valuable in teaching programs.
      2) Colored photos are best but not admissible in some courts; black and white are also needed.
      3) Child's general appearance, specific skin markings, limb deformities, and injuries.

PATIENT CARE MANAGEMENT

Objectives of Therapy.
1. Protect the child and possibly the siblings from further abuse or neglect.

2. Treat the child's injuries or health needs.
   a. Save the child's life.
   b. Prevent neurologic damage and permanent physical and emotional disability.
3. Support, rehabilitate, and educate the parents to enable an early return of their child to a safe, healthy environment.
   a. Examine the total pattern of parent/child/family interaction.
   b. Help alleviate the stresses in the family unit.
   c. Improve the basic pattern of child rearing.

General Considerations

1. The physician determines the severity of injuries and, if nonaccidental, prescribes treatment, reports to authorities, ensures immediate protection, collects data for a disposition conference, informs and counsels the parents, consults and coordinates support services, and arranges for medical and social followup.[13]
2. The approach must be an interdisciplinary one. Ideally a child abuse team made up of experts in dealing with this problem should be involved.
3. The critical care nurse plays a major role as liaison between child and parents and the rest of the health care team.
4. The long-term program depends on community facilities and how long it will be before the home is safe. A dependency petition and foster placement may be needed.

Medical/Nursing Actions

1. Attend to the child's immediate injuries and health needs.
   a. The "battered," severely malnourished, or dehydrated child is the most likely one to need admission to a critical care unit.
   b. Assess and treat emergency physical needs involving airway, ventilation, bleeding, and level of consciousness.
   c. Ensure appropriate hydration and nutrition.
2. Observe closely and document objectively the child's and parents' behavior and their interactions.
   a. Information is important to the physician, the agencies, and the courts making decisions for the child.
   b. Use a standardized report and observation form to simplify documentation. Keep all records confidential.
3. Provide emotional support for the child.
   a. Consider culture, age, level of response, and extent of injuries.
   b. Assign a primary nurse with total patient care responsibilities and promote continuity of care between personnel on all tours of duty.
   c. Encourage the child to verbalize and act out fears and fantasies.
   d. Recognize that unusual fears and withdrawn or unmanageable behavior may be a result of abuse and neglect. The critical care environment can exacerbate problem behavior and make support difficult.

e. Do not discuss the parents in front of the child; remain with the child during their visits.

4. Provide emotional support for the parents.

    a. Use experienced medical and nursing staff, limiting the numbers who will be communicating with the parents.

    b. Converse with the parents, using a nonjudgmental approach, and focus on them and their concerns rather than on the child.

    c. Listen attentively and gather information to help identify the parents' needs and assess the home situation.

    d. Keep parents well informed even if they are resentful of what is being done. They need to know any legal implications and their rights; they may need to obtain legal counsel.

    e. Recognize that some parents will be submissive and cooperative, doing what they think is wanted, while others are belligerent, uncooperative, and resistant.[13] Subconsciously, most of them want help.

    f. Encourage parents' participation in their child's care, suggest appropriate modifications in child/parent interactions. Begin teaching appropriate child-rearing skills within the limitations of a critical care environment.

5. Utilize and communicate effectively with other disciplines and community agencies.

    a. This must begin in the critical care unit with members of the child abuse team and representatives of law enforcement and protective agencies.

    b. Participate in disposition conferences.

6. Provide support for critical care staff members working with abused children and their parents.

    a. Recognize the unique emotional impact of the problem.

    b. Encourage discussion and resolution of feelings about child abuse.

    c. Seek professional counseling and encourage the use of outside resources and the literature.

7. Communicate information to other caregivers when the child is transferred from the critical care unit.

    a. Provide complete documentation of all information gathered as well as that given to parents, details of present care, plans for followup care, those disciplines already involved, and the behavior of the child and parents.

SPECIAL NURSING SKILLS REQUIRED

1. Thorough knowledge of normal growth and development, as presented in this text.

2. Understanding of the child abuse syndrome and one's own feelings toward it.
3. Skill in caring for the child with multiple trauma, severe malnutrition, or dehydration.
4. Communication skills using a nonjudgmental approach, particularly in working with abusive parents.

COMPLICATIONS OF CHILD ABUSE _____

1. Death, particularly in the infant age group, from head injury.
2. Repeated injuries, neglect.
3. Morbidity: permanent neurological damage, long-term disability, retardation.
4. Emotional, psychologic, and learning disorders.
5. Failure of parent rehabilitation.
6. Emotional effects on staff who work with these children and their parents.
7. Financial expense to society and waste of potential human resources.

BIBLIOGRAPHY

1. Akbarnia, B., et al.: Manifestations of the battered-child syndrome. J. Bone Joint Surg., 56A:1159, 1974.
2. Avery, J.C.: The battered baby. Nursing Mirror, 134 (June 9):32, 1972.
3. Bates, R.P.: Child abuse. In Surgical Staff, Hospital for Sick Children: Care for the Injured Child. Baltimore, Williams & Wilkins Co., 1975.
4. Bates, R.P.: Child abuse and neglect: the pediatrician's role. CPS News Bulletin Supplement, 7:1, 1976.
5. Ebeling, N.B., and Hill, D.A.: (eds.): Child Abuse: Intervention and Treatment. Littleton, Mass. Publishing Sciences Group, 1975.
6. Fontana, V.J.: The maltreated child: the maltreatment syndrome in children, 2nd ed. Springfield, Ill., Charles C Thomas, 1974.
7. Fontana, V.J.: The diagnosis of the maltreatment syndrome in children. Pediatrics, 51:780, 1973.
8. Fontana, V.J.: Somewhere a Child is Crying: The Battered Child. New York, Macmillan, 1973.
9. Friedman, A.L., et al.: Nursing responsibility in child abuse. Nurs. Forum, 15:95, 1976.
10. Gelles, R.J.: Child abuse as psychopathology: a sociological critique and reformulation. Am. J. Orthopsychiatry, 43:611, 1973.
11. Gil, D.F.: Violence Against Children: Physical Child Abuse in the United States. Cambridge: Harvard University Press, 1970.
12. Green, F.C.: Child abuse and neglect: a priority for the private physician. Pediatr. Clin. North Am., 22:329, 1975.
13. Helfer, R.E., and Kempe, C.H. (eds.): The Battered Child, 2nd ed. Chicago, University of Chicago Press, 1974.
14. Hopkins, J.: The nurse and the abused child. Nurs. Clin. North Am., 5:589, 1970.

15. Kempe, C.H., and Helfer, R.E., (eds.): Helping the Battered Child and His Family. Philadelphia, J.B. Lippincott Co., 1972.

16. Kevles, B.: In her own words: Judge Lisa Richette says victims of child abuse should not be throwaway children. People Weekly, 6(21):87, 1976.

17. Learoyd, S.: Nursing care in the battered child syndrome. Nurs. Mirror, 140 (June 12):54, 1975.

18. Mindlin, R.L.: Child abuse and neglect: the role of the pediatrician and the academy. Pediatrics, 54:393, 1974.

19. National Association of Children's Hospitals and Related Institutions Inc.: The pediatric bill of rights. In: J. Assoc. Care Child. Hosp., 3(2):21, 1974.

20. O'Neill, J.A., et al.: Patterns of injury in the battered child syndrome. J. Trauma, 13:332, 1973.

21. Parents' Anonymous: Parents' Anonymous: daily goals and guidelines. J. Clin. Child Psychol., 2(3):41, 1973.

22. Pemberton, D.A., and Benady, D.R.: Consciously rejected children. Br. J. Psychiatry., 123:575, 1973.

23. Sanders, R.W.: Resistance to dealing with parents of battered children. Pediatrics, 50:853, 1972.

24. Shore, M.F.: Child advocacy. Address to the American Association for the Care of Children in Hospitals, Montreal, May 1972.

25. Shydro, J.: Child abuse. Nursing 72, 2(12):37, 1972.

26. Smith, S.M.: The battered child syndrome: some research findings. Nurs. Mirror, 140 (June 12):48, 1975.

27. Van Stolk, M.: The Battered Child in Canada. Toronto, McClelland & Stewart, 1972.

28. Wolman, I.J. (ed.): The Possibly Abused Child (The Battered Child Syndrome). Clinical Pediatrics Handbook II. Clin. Pediatr. 15:589, pp. 217-220, July, 1976.

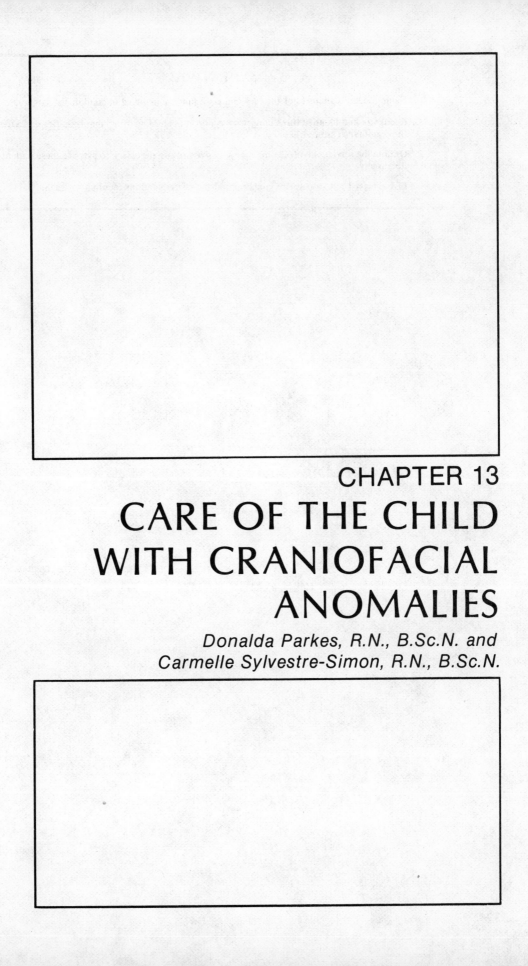

CHAPTER 13
CARE OF THE CHILD WITH CRANIOFACIAL ANOMALIES

Donalda Parkes, R.N., B.Sc.N. and Carmelle Sylvestre-Simon, R.N., B.Sc.N.

OBJECTIVES

1. Name the key structures of the face and skull that are involved in craniofacial surgery.

2. Recognize and identify three congenital syndromes and five other abnormalities that affect the craniofacial structures.

3. Outline the services involved and the extensive workup necessary to prepare these patients for surgery.

4. List at least 10 postoperative concerns and the nursing actions required for each.

INTRODUCTION

DEFINITION OF CRANIOFACIAL ANOMALIES

1. Malformations of the cranial and maxillofacial areas.

GENERAL CONSIDERATIONS

1. Craniofacial reconstruction is one of the newest and most constantly expanding specialties in plastic surgery.
2. Reconstruction of severe malformations was thought to be surgically and biologically impossible up until this past decade.[21]
3. Almost all skull and facial bones can now be repositioned and reconstructed to provide correction of complex and grotesque craniofacial anomalies. This will allow more radical treatment of head and neck tumors and of severe post-traumatic and even more complex congenital deformities in the future.
4. Correction of complex anomalies has considerable risk and demands both medical and nursing expertise.

ANATOMY

For detailed anatomy and physiology of the cranial, orbital, maxillary, mandibular, and eye structures, consult the references.[1,19]

Key Structures

1. Bones: frontal, ethmoid, sphenoid, zygoma, maxilla (these make up the orbit margins), cribriform plate, nasal, mandible.
2. Cranial nerves: olfactory (I), optic (II), oculomotor (III), trochlear (IV), trigeminal (V), abducens (VI), facial (VII).
3. Arteries: superficial temporal, supraorbital, branch of ophthalmic, internal maxillary, external maxillary, inferior alveolar.
4. Veins: superior sagittal sinus, diploic, superior ophthalmic, cavernous sinus, angular, maxillary, anterior facial.
5. Muscles: frontalis, corrugator supercilii, orbicularis oculi, orbicularis oris, platysma, buccinator, masseter, temporalis.
6. Paranasal sinuses: frontal, sphenoidal, ethmoidal, maxillary.

TYPES OF ANOMALIES

1. There are specific well-recognized syndromes, which vary in their severity.
2. A combination of the well-defined syndromes and other anomalies often occurs.

Mandibulofacial Dysostosis: Treacher-Collins Syndrome: (autosomal dominant):

1. Arises from the gill cleft phase of embryologic development, giving the child a fishlike facial appearance characterized by:
   a. A downward and outward slant of the eyes.
   b. Notching of the lateral aspects of the lower eyelids (coloboma).
   c. Absence of eyelashes on the medial two thirds of lower eyelids.
   d. Underdevelopment or absence of cheek bones.
   e. Small or deformed ears.
   f. Tonguelike hair projections in front of ears.
   g. Occasionally, ear anomalies, a small lower jaw, and a cleft palate.

Craniofacial Dysostosis: Crouzon's Syndrome (autosomal dominant)

1. The child's face has a froglike appearance characterized by:
   a. A wide skull due to early fusion of cranial sutures.
   b. A shortened forehead.
   c. Eye orbits wide apart and too shallow.
   d. Protruding eye balls (exophthalmos), causing limited visual field.
   e. An arched nose, giving a "parrot beak" appearance.
   f. An underdeveloped receding upper jaw, causing dental malocclusion.
   g. V pattern of strabismus.

Craniofacial Dysostosis with Syndactyly: Apert's Syndrome (autosomal dominant)

1. Syndactyly, a skin (occasionally bony) fusion of the fingers and toes, differentiates this syndrome from Crouzon's.
2. Characterized by the craniofacial deformities of Crouzon's, syndactylism, and some or all of the following:
   a. An anterior open bite and bow-shaped upper lip.
   b. A cleft palate.
   c. V pattern of strabismus.

Orbital Hypertelorism

1. Congenital or traumatic, occurring alone or with other anomalies.
2. Premature fusion of the cranial and facial sutures characterized by:
   a. An abnormally wide distance of varying degrees between the eye orbits.
   b. A broad, flat nasal bridge, making the nose look small.
   c. Eyesight not affected except for strabismus.

Retrognathism and Prognathism

1. Congenital or traumatic, occurring alone or with other craniofacial anomalies.
   a. Retrognathism: a mandibular deformity characterized by a receding lower jaw and protruding upper teeth.
   b. Prognathism: a mandibular deformity characterized by a protruding lower jaw and receding upper teeth.
2. These cause severe dental malocclusion with subsequent dental, nutritional, and psychosocial problems.

Cleft Lip and Cleft Palate

1. Congenital anomalies occurring alone or with other anomalies.
   a. Cleft lip: a unilateral or bilateral fissure of the upper lip extending to the nostril.
   b. Cleft palate: a longitudinal fissure involving the hard and soft palate.

INCIDENCE

1. Except for cleft lip and cleft palate, these anomalies occur rather infrequently but in all racial groups.
2. No higher incidence in males or females.
3. Not all cases are suitable for surgery.
4. Estimated number of candidates suitable for surgery in the United States is 1200 per year.[7]
5. There is a significant risk of morbidity and mortality with surgery.

ORBITOCRANIOFACIAL CASES IN UNITED STATES[7]

Types	Incidence (in live births)	New cases per year
Treacher-Collins syndrome	1: 10,000*	325
Crouzon's syndrome	1: 10,000*	325
Apert's syndrome	1:160,000	20

*rough estimate

ETIOLOGY AND PRECIPITATING FACTORS

1. Strong hereditary factor in many of the anomalies.
2. Altered embryology in early stages of fetal development.
3. Trauma may also cause significant deformities.

CLINICAL ASSESSMENT

1. A multidisciplinary team is necessary for extensive and precise data collection, diagnosis, operative design, and preoperative preparation. Team members may include:

   a. Pediatrician
   b. Plastic surgeon
   c. Neuro-ophthalmologist
   d. Neuroradiologist
   e. Dentist
   f. Orthodontist
   g. Speech pathologist
   h. Geneticist
   i. Anthropologist
   j. Medical illustrator
   k. Psychologist
   l. Psychiatrist
   m. Social worker
   n. Neurosurgeon
   o. Anesthetist
   p. Ward nurse
   q. Operating room nurse
   r. Critical care nurse

2. Physical examination is performed with particular attention to eye position and muscle movements, visual acuity, fields, and fundi. Potential intubation and upper airway problems are determined.
3. Skull and face x-ray films, cerebral arteriograms, pneumoencephalograms, brain scan, CT scan, radioisotope studies of cranial sutures.
4. Dental, orthodontal, and speech assessments.
5. Measurements of skull and face, stereophotographs, and design drawing.
6. Chromosome studies, identification of a syndrome and genetic counseling.
7. Intelligence testing to determine mental retardation (children with gross facial deformities are frequently misunderstood to be mentally retarded).
8. Assessment of the deformity's effect on the child's psychosocial development.
    a. Help is given the child and parents to adjust to the realities of surgery and to the possibility that it may not produce a normal appearance or may be so drastic that the child will be unrecognizable.
9. Laboratory tests: cross and type, hemoglobin, hematocrit, coagulogram, electrolytes, blood sugar, and blood urea nitrogen.
10. Preoperative teaching by ward, operating room, and critical care nurses, with special attention to airway management, mouth care, feeding, swelling and pain to be expected, and changes in body image.
    a. Preoperative visit to critical care unit by parents; include the child if he or she is of an appropriate age.

PATIENT CARE MANAGEMENT

Objectives of Surgical, Medical, and Nursing Therapy
1. To achieve functional and aesthetic improvement of the deformed craniofacial structures.
2. To lessen the psychosocial maladjustments the child may have.
3. To provide the emotional support so greatly needed by the child and family preoperatively and postoperatively.
4. To prevent, recognize, and treat complications of the surgery.

Preoperative Preparation
1. This must include both the child and his parents. Since most of this surgery is still performed on the adolescent, independence, self image, and peer relationships are important.
    a. Observe the child's relationships with his or her parents and with others on the ward. Note the degree of independence of the teenager.

    b. Encourage the child to express feelings about his or her appearance and expectations of the surgery.
        1) These patients are often shy and withdrawn, or defensive and attention-seeking.
    c. Give a thorough explanation, appropriate to age, of the surgery and the postoperative care involved.
        1) This is particularly important, because there is considerable fear and anxiety following surgery.
    d. The child should practice:
        1) Deep breathing and coughing exercises.
        2) Cleansing the mouth with a Water Pik.
        3) Using the mouth suction equipment.
        4) Drinking fluids using a syringe with catheter tip and a straw, all with teeth held closed if surgery will involve the jaw.
    e. The child should talk with others who have had similar surgery and see what it is like to have teeth wired together for some weeks.
    f. Parents and the adolescent patient should visit the critical care unit and see what the facilities and postoperative care will be like. The young child may not benefit from such a visit.

Surgical Therapy
    1. Factors affecting time of surgery:
      a. Age of the child
        1) Recent trend is to operate on younger and younger children in order to prevent serious functional disability secondary to the deformity, to relieve parents of some of the stress in raising them, and to prevent lasting psychosocial problems.
      b. Bone growth
        1) Although regeneration of the young child's skull is remarkable, the effect of extensive surgery on young growing bones remains a concern and an unresolved issue.[8]
      c. Increased intracranial pressure
        1) A significant rise in pressure necessitates early surgery to protect the growing brain from this pressure.
      d. Extreme exophthalmos
        1) There is a possibility that the eyes may prolapse from their orbits if the deformity is not corrected soon enough.
    2. Surgical procedures:
      a. Attempt is made to correct as much of the deformity as possible at one time.
      b. Detachment of the entire facial skeleton from the cranium is now possible, and most of the cranial and facial bones can be repositioned in any direction.
      c. Extracranial and/or intracranial approaches are used, which involve a combination of any of the following procedures:
        1) Craniotomy and cranioplasty.
        2) Multiple osteotomies.

        3) Frontal, orbital, and maxillary augmentation bone grafts using iliac and rib bones.

        4) Tracheostomy.

  3. Factors contributing to the complexity of surgery:

    a. The length of surgery, 2 to 10 hours, demands anesthetic expertise.

    b. A combination of complex deformities increases the risk of morbidity.

    c. Stripping bones of their blood vessels can cause significant blood loss but is controlled by hypotensive techniques.

    d. An intracranial approach involves dura and brain repositioning, which requires brain decompression using hyperventilation, Mannitol, and steroids.

  4. Characteristics of the infant and young child:

    a. Small airway structures require skillful, experienced intubation and airway management.

    b. Small anatomical structures of skull and face make surgical manipulation difficult.

    c. Temperature regulation, fluid control, and blood loss estimation and replacement need to be extremely precise.

Special Nursing Skills Required

1. An awareness and appreciation of the dangers and complications of craniofacial surgery.

2. An ability to take an active part in the preoperative preparation of the child and his parents.

3. Airway management.

4. Recognition of the signs of increased intracranial pressure.

5. An ability to communicate effectively with the intubated or tracheotomized child or one that has limited to total visual impairment.

6. An ability to assess and alleviate the child's fear, pain, and depression and parental anxiety that are so characteristic of craniofacial surgery.

Postoperative Medical and Nursing Therapy

1. When surgery has been done on their maxilla and/or mandible these children are nasally intubated and have their teeth wired together.
2. If the nasal bones are extensively involved, a tracheostomy rather than an endotracheal tube will be inserted. Oral intubation is not suitable.
3. If only the eye orbits and cranial bones are involved, intubation is usually unnecessary and concern for the eyes and brain is primary. The following outline is given with the intubated child in mind; not all statements will apply to each child having had craniofacial surgery.

Concerns	Medical Actions	Nursing Actions
1. Airway		
a. Obstruction Blockage of endotracheal (ET) or tracheostomy (trach) tube because of copious, thick sanguineous secretions from nasal and oral pharynx.	a. Warmed humidification of all inspired gases to loosen secretions.	a. Make certain that humidifier is warm and misting effectively. Deep breathing and coughing exercises (DB/C) q1–2h despite pain from the rib graft donor sites. Frequent but careful suctioning of nasal and oropharynx (N/OP) and trachea. Will need small catheter for the N/OP because of swelling. (Nasal suctioning is contraindicated if nasal bones have been repaired.) Take care not to dislodge dental wires; guide catheter around back of teeth. Use long curved catheters to ensure deep tracheal suction; child is afraid to cough so stimulate this reflex often.
b. Hypoxia May be due to airway obstruction or hypoventilation from pain and sedation. Anemia will contribute.	b. O_2 administration. Serial blood gas monitoring. Hematology studies.	b. Test FIO_2 of inspired gases q2–4h. Accurate blood gas sampling, interpretation of results. Report low hemoglobin, hematocrit. Encourage DB/C, change of position. Sedate prn.

Concerns	Medical Actions	Nursing Actions
1. Airway (Continued)		
c. Dislodging of ET or trach tube. Difficulty in keeping the tapes dry with the oozing of blood and mucus. Child may cough excessively, is often restless. Oxygenation equipment may drag on tube.	c. Secure taping of ET or trach tube, with daily retaping if necessary (best done by experienced medical staff).	c. Keep tapes as dry as possible, report when loosened. Suction frequently, sedate adequately. Position oxygenation equipment carefully to allow freedom of movement.
d. Aspiration High risk of aspiration when teeth are wired and there is a constant drooling of mucus, blood, saliva. Inability to swallow for first 48 to 72 hours owing to pharyngeal swelling. A tendency to nausea and vomiting due to blood collected in the stomach.	d. Use of a cuffed ET or trach tube (if no leak around tube because of postoperative swelling, cuff can be left deflated). Nasogastric (N/G) or orogastric (O/G) tube with low suction initially, then to straight drainage. Antiemetic prn.	d. Follow cuff deflation routine, being careful to suction airway thoroughly before and during deflation. Elevate head and shoulders 45°. Instruct older child in use of mouth suction equipment, leave it with him or her to use prn, helps child feel more secure. Maintain patency of N/G tube with saline irrigations, be sure that suction is working. Remove N/G tube when child able to swallow and peristalsis is satisfactory. Make certain dental wire cutters are always at the bedside to use should significant vomiting occur.

e. **Extubation**
ET intubation is usually for 48 to 72 hours (trach tube often in place longer).
If bilateral mandibular osteotomies, the considerable edema and hematomas cause serious laryngeal obstruction (may then have ET tube 4 to 7 days).

Extubations can be difficult and may require immediate reintubation.

e. Plan for and carry out extubation when:
There is an adequate air leak around the ET or trach tube, indicating minimal pharyngeal swelling.
Child is able to swallow his saliva and secretions.
Chest x-ray film is clear and blood gases are normal.

Blood gases, chest X-ray film after extubation.

e. Withhold sedation at least 2 hours and stop feeding at least 1 hr prior to extubation.
Prepare for and assist with extubation.
Explain procedure and reassure the frightened child.
Aspirate and remove N/G tube if still in place. Be sure stomach is empty.
Suction N/OP and trachea thoroughly.
Have oxygenation and reintubation equipment ready.

Observe child and monitor vital signs closely for several hours after extubation.
Report significant dyspnea, changes in color and vital signs.

2. **Fluid Balance**

a. **Hypovolemia**
Excessive bleeding may occur from N/OP in first 24 hours.

a. Insertion of arterial (art) and central venous pressure (CVP) lines.
Frequent hematology studies.
Blood transfusions as needed.

a. Maintain patency of lines, monitor and interpret vital signs, particularly pressures.
Estimate losses from N/OP and through suctioning.
Interpret lab results.
If hemorrhage, put child in shock position, increase blood or fluid IV rate, monitor pressures, suction to keep airway clear, call MD stat.

b. **Dehydration**
Excessive loss of body fluid through blood, mucus, saliva, and N/G tube drainage.

b. IV therapy.
Replacement of fluid losses.
Electrolyte studies.

b. Maintain patency of IV line, carefully regulate maintenance and replacement fluids.
Record intake and output (can only estimate N/OP losses).
Interpret lab results.

Concerns	Medical Actions	Nursing Actions
3. Neurologic Status		
a. Cerebral edema if the brain has been involved in the repair. Level of consciousness will be difficult to assess when eyes are swollen and teeth are wired, making communication difficult.	a. Avoidance of fluid overload. Steroids. Regular monitoring and control of PCO_2 to reduce intracranial pressure. Hyperventilation with a respirator may be necessary to decrease PCO_2. External cerebrospinal fluid drainage is occasionally used.	a. Diligent fluid regulation (CVP monitoring a great help). Elevate head of bed 30 to 45°. Frequent neurological assessment. Encourage change of position and activity, DB/C and suctioning to maintain normal PCO_2. Respirator care. Aseptic handling of CSF drainage system. Record CSF losses.
4. Pain		
a. Facial and neck swelling worsens over first 2 to 3 days.	a. Sedation by IV or IM route.	a. Administer sedation frequently but avoid respiratory and neurologic depression. Elevate head of bed, and turn child side to side frequently to decrease edema. ET or trach tube tapes should be adjusted as swelling increases. Ice packs may help.
b. Bone graft donor site If the iliac area was used, turning, sitting, and standing are very uncomfortable. If the rib area, DB/C is very painful.	b. Pressure dressings to donor sites. A chest drain to an underwater seal and suction is used if the pleura has been opened during removal of the ribs for bone grafting.	b. Examine dressings frequently and reinforce prn. Position child as comfortably as possible. Sedate prior to DB/C routine. Support rib graft donor site during DB/C. Chest drain care; ensure safety and measure losses.

5. Emotional and Psychological
    Needs
    a. Anxiety about breathing
        and frequent suctioning
        deprive the child of
        sleep.

    a. Child should have his own nurse, particularly his
        first postoperative night.
        Organize care as much as possible.
        Constant reassurance is needed.
        Remind child that a nurse is close by, leave a bell at his or
        her side.

    b. Child usually experiences
        considerable fear, frustra-
        tion, and even depression
        (can't see because of
        swollen or sutured eyes,
        can't talk because of
        wired teeth and being
        "tubed," worries about
        appearance).

    b. Provide a means of communication.
        Pencil and clipboard for writing (try to avoid IV in his or
        her writing hand).
        Word or picture board for young child if able to see.
        Ask mainly "yes or no" types of questions; explain
        everything you do.

    b. Inform child and parents of daily progress
        and plan of care.
        Reassure them that time will help
        appearance.

    c. Parents may experience
        great anxiety, even guilt,
        over having the surgery
        done and possible rejec-
        tion of their child's post-
        operative appearance.

    c. Support and encourage parents to help with their child's
        care, particularly to sit with, distract, and amuse him or
        her; can help nurses a great deal in interpreting child's
        needs and wants.
        Remind them that the child's appearance will improve
        greatly as swelling decreases.

Concerns	Medical Actions	Nursing Actions
5. Emotional and Psychological Needs (*Continued*) d. Nursing staff often find these children repulsive looking, very trying, and demanding of their time, may consider them mentally retarded when not so.	d. Explain expected outcomes of surgery to nursing staff.	d. Encourage staff to be patient and empathetic with these children, to examine "before and after" pictures of other cases, and to visit children postoperatively on the ward to see improvements. Early ambulation, attention to personal hygiene and appearance improves everyone's morale. Older child might request a face mirror, can be of help when swelling has decreased. Have ward nurses visit child in critical care unit. Older postoperative patients may be a help visiting adolescent.
6. Infection a. High risk of infection in various sites: Chest. Eyes. Sinuses. Gums, buccal mucosa. Meninges (meningitis). Bones (osteomyelitis). Skin.	a. Daily chest x-ray film. High prophylactic doses of antibiotics started 24 hours preoperatively. Cultures of airway secretions and other sites as indicated.	a. Encourage DB/C, use aseptic suctioning technique, encourage early ambulation. Cleanse eyes q2h if swollen or sutured. Diligent mouth care q2–4h with one-half strength hydrogen peroxide and sterile water, using a Water Pik. Although child has practiced using a Water Pik preoperatively, initially he or she will be frightened and there is danger of aspiration of cleansing solution. Sit child up, have suction on hand, hold basin under chin, have him lean forward and manipulate the Water Pik himself. Keep eyes, nose, and lips moistened with petroleum jelly. Keep rest of face, neck, and bone donor sites as clean and dry as possible. Report prolonged fever or any discharge suggestive of infection.

7. Nutrition
   a. Inability to swallow due to pharyngeal and neck swelling.

   a. IV therapy progressing to diet as tolerated. N/G or O/G tube feedings if prolonged inability to swallow.

   a. When able to swallow, start with water in small amounts frequently. Reduce IV intake accordingly.

   b. Teeth may be wired for weeks

   b. Allow only water by mouth for 3 weeks to minimize bacterial growth in the mouth. Sit up for feedings, have suction on hand. Use a large syringe with catheter attached; guide it in around back of teeth, pushing fluid slowly while encouraging child to swallow. Have child use syringe himself as long as nurse is present. General feeding tube care, if tube required. Progress to pureed diet after 3 weeks.

The child may be transferred out of the critical care unit when:
1. Facial and neck swelling have decreased.
2. He or she can swallow saliva, secretions, and water easily.
3. There is no respiratory distress after 12 hours of extubation.

BIBLIOGRAPHY

1. American Association of Critical-Care Nurses: Core Curriculum for Critical-Care Nursing. Irvine, Calif, American Association of Critical Care Nurses, 1975.
2. Chalk, B.A.: Surgical correction of craniofacial anomalies. J. Neurosurg. Nurs., 7 (Dec):123, 1975.
3. Converse, J.M.: Surgical Treatment of Facial Injuries, 3rd ed., Vol. 2. Baltimore, Williams & Wilkins, 1974. pp. 1013–1201.
4. Converse, J.M., et al.: Craniofacial surgery, Clin. Plast. Surg., 1:499, 1974.
5. Converse, J.M.: Reconstructive Plastic Surgery: Principles and Procedures in Correction, Reconstruction and Transplantation, 2nd ed., Vol. 2. Philadelphia, W. B. Saunders Co., 1977.
6. Crooks, L.: Correcting mandibular prognathism. Am. Oper. Room Nurs. 17 (5):66, 1973.
7. Davies, D., and Munro, I.: The anesthetic management and intra-operative care of patients undergoing major facial osteotomies. Plast. Reconstr. Surg., 55:50, 1975.
8. Edgerton, M.T., et al.: Craniofacial osteotomies and reconstructions in infants and young children. Plast. Reconstr. Surg., 54:13, 1974.
9. Edgerton, M.T.: New hope for the child with major craniofacial deformity. Birth Defects Original Article Series. 11 (7):297, 1975.
10. Fleming, J.: Improvement of the face in Crouzon's disease by conservative operations. Plast. Reconstr. Surg., 47:560, 1971.
11. Munro, I.: Orbito-cranio-facial surgery: the team approach. Plast. Reconstr. Surg., 55:170, 1975.
12. Obong, M.C.: Apert's syndrome: nursing care study. Nurs. Times, 68:1582, 1972.
13. Salyer, K., et al.: Difficulties and problems to be solved in the approach to craniofacial malformations. Birth Defects Original Article Series, 11 (7):315, 1975.
14. Tempest, M.: Correcting facial deformity. Nurs. Times, 71:1163, 1975.
15. Tessier, P.: The definitive plastic surgical treatment of the severe facial deformities of craniofacial dysostosis. Plast. Reconstr. Surg., 48:419, 1971.
16. Tessier, P.: The scope and principles, dangers and limitations and the need for training in orbito-cranial surgery. Melbourne, Transactions of the Fifth International Congress of Plastic and Reconstructive Surgery, February 1971, pp. 903–921.
17. Tuck, F.: Mandibular osteotomy for malocclusion. Nurs. Mirror, 141 (Nov. 13):51, 1975.
18. Wall, M.: Maxillary and mandibular osteotomy. Nurs. Mirror, 135 (Sept. 22):29, 1972.
19. Warwick, R., and Williams, P. (eds): Gray's Anatomy, 35th ed. Philadelphia, W. B. Saunders Co., 1973.
20. Whitaker, L., and Randall, P.: The developing field of craniofacial surgery. Pediatrics, 54:571, 1974.
21. Wood-Smith, D., and Porowski, P.: Nursing Care of the Plastic Surgery Patient. St. Louis, C. V. Mosby Co., 1967, pp. 234–285.

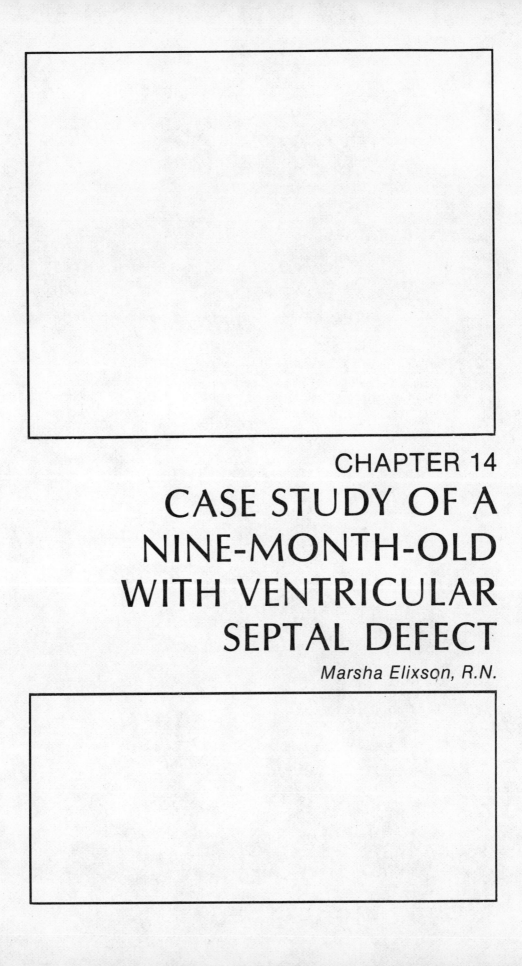

CHAPTER 14
CASE STUDY OF A NINE-MONTH-OLD WITH VENTRICULAR SEPTAL DEFECT

Marsha Elixson, R.N.

INTRODUCTION

Developmental disturbances occurring between days 20 and 50 of fetal life are responsible for congenital heart defects resulting in approximately 1% of all organic heart disease. Between the fourth and the eighth weeks of fetal life, as septal tissues develop, the heart partitions itself into four chambers. If the intraventricular foramen fails to fuse, a ventricular septal defect occurs.

Ventricular septal defects, the most common form of congenital malformation of the heart in children (about 30% of all lesions) is characterized by a ventricular septal communication that permits blood flow between the ventricles.[12]

The size of the septal defect ranges from single pinpoint defects through large multiple areas to absence of the entire septal wall. Many of the small septal defects close spontaneously in early childhood. Children with these defects usually are asymptomatic and do not require surgical intervention, owing to the relatively normal pulmonary blood flow and pulmonary artery pressure. Those children with moderate to large ventricular septal defects come to the hospital early in life for medical or surgical treatment or both, to relieve the congestive heart failure and increased pulmonary vascular congestion brought about by the left to right shunt.

Anatomical locations and types of septal lesions are:

1. Supracristal: smallest in size, rare, located under the crista supraventricularis.
2. Membranous: common, located in the membranous septum below the aortic valve, may extend posterior to the septal leaflet of the tricuspid valve.
3. Atrioventricular canal: endocardial cushion type of septal defect, located in membranous septum, anterior extends downward and forward across the septal wall of the left ventricular outflow tract; Posterior is located under the septal leaflet of the tricuspid valve.
4. Muscular: in muscular septum, tends to be of the multiple "Swiss cheese" type, all defects are difficult to find.[7]

PATIENT CASE STUDY

Nine-month-old Melissa, only child of a young, low-income, Italian couple, was noted to have a septal murmur at birth. Her progressive congestive heart failure was treated by digitalization while she was in the newborn nursery of the local hospital. Melissa's physical examination showed chronic congestive heart failure in a diaphoretic, thin, wasted, pale, irritable, orthopneic, tachypneic, frightened-looking baby. Her weight was 7.46 kg, approximately in the fifth percentile for her age. These findings, along with her failure of normal weight gain, concerned her local physician, who then consulted with the cardiology department of our center. It was decided to admit Melissa to the center for a complete diagnostic workup with the possibility of surgical correction.

Admission laboratory studies included a urinalysis, complete blood count, platelet count, electrolytes, blood urea nitrogen, total protein, calcium, and sugar; all data were within normal limits. A blood sample was sent to the blood bank for typing and crossmatching in preparation for cardiac catheterization and possible cardiac surgery.

Cardiac catheterization was done on the first day after admission, establishing that her diagnosis was a large ventricular septal defect. Pulmonary blood flow calculations showed a 4.3–1 left to right shunt.

Surgical repair of the ventricular septal defect, utilizing the deep hypothermia and circulatory arrest techniques, was performed on the following day. Recovery was fast. She remained in the cardiac intensive care unit for 2 days, then was transferred to the cardiovascular ward for 6 days prior to her discharge home. The total hospitalization time was 11 days.

The multidisciplinary team approach to care utilized staff members from the following groups: intensive care nursing staff, cardiac surgical and medical house staff, anesthesiology, radiology, respiratory therapy, operating room staff, cardiovascular ward staff, play therapy, social service, laboratory personnel, and chaplain. Total involvement of parents with child continued throughout her hospitalization.

Melissa's problem list included the following:
1. Congestive heart failure.
2. Parent reaction.
3. Cardiac catheterization.
4. Hypovolemia with resulting hypotension.
5. Right upper lobe atelectasis.

Her progess is outlined on the following pages.

Subjective/Objective Data

Day 1 — Admission Day, 4/20

1. *Congestive heart failure:*
Thin, pale, wasted baby girl appears frightened, irritable, and labors for breath. Pulse: 140, regular. Blood pressure: 120/68. Electrocardiogram: sinus tachycardia with right ventricular hypertrophy. Respiratory rate: 40, tachypneic, mild inter-costal and sternal retractions, orthopnea present. Lung fields essentially clear with basilar rhonchi. Chest x-ray: cardiomegaly with prominent pulmonary vasculature. Afebrile. Weight: 7.46 kg. Hepatomegaly demonstrated by downward systolic pulsation, palpable 3 cm below the costal margin. A septal murmur has been present since birth. She was digitalized at birth in the nursery. Slow to gain weight — 5th percentile for age, and slow in developmental task gains. She has been immunized for childhood diseases. She is an only child of a low income Italian family, who live 200 miles away. Initial laboratory data is within normal limits. A sample has been sent to the blood bank.

Assessment

Nine-month-old baby girl in respiratory distress due to congestive heart failure intractable to medical management.
Referred for cardiac catheterization to confirm diagnosis of ventricular septal defect and plan for possible surgical intervention.
Sodium and fluid restricted to lessen fluid overload.
Respiratory distress potentiates dangers of aspiration. Higher caloric intake due to increased metabolic needs.

Medical/Nursing Plan

Baseline assessment of all vital signs. Monitor electrocardiogram, especially for arrhythmias, potassium and digitalis effect, conduction delays. Alterations in rate of rhythm should be watched for.
Auscultation of heart and lung sounds with vital signs.
Keep comfortable with head elevated to prevent abdominal organs from impinging on diaphragm.
Keep calm — increased respiratory distress when stressed.
Accurate intake and output, daily weights. Positive balance would require diuretic therapy.
Restricted sodium and fluid intake. Feed solids prior to fluids, slowly.
Rest prior to feeding — fatigues easily.
Close observation of electrolytes, arterial blood gases.
Positive inotropic agents continued.
Two person medication check to decrease chance of error.
Hold evening dose prior to cardiac catheterization to decrease chances of arrhythmias.
Check daily chest x-ray results.
Vigorous respiratory support, clapping and vibrating all lobes.
Plan rest periods throughout day.

Subjective/Objective Data	Assessment	Medical/Nursing Plan
2. *Parent reaction:* Melissa is crying, parents are anxious and apprehensive, and cling to her.	Away from family and friends, overwhelmed by hospitalization, parents need referral to support services for financial and religious aid. Parents hear and retain only information they wish to retain.	Establish a trusting relationship. Constant reinforcement and explanation. Support and teach parents. Allow to help in care for, comforting of, and calming of child. Referral to social service for financial and to chaplain for religious support. Orientation to hospital situation.
Day 2 – 4/21 1. *Congestive heart failure.* Respiratory rate: 32.	Slight respiratory distress evident.	Continue regimen.
2. *Parent reaction:* Pacing the floor, anxious, asking many questions: How long will tests take? When can I see Melissa? Will she hurt? Will they do surgery?	Parents starting to build a relationship with staff. Reach out for help.	Provide a quiet place for them to wait. Assess understanding (medical terminology may be a problem with parents). Introduce the nurse liaison; explain her role with parents. She will keep them informed of progress of surgery and provide a quiet waiting place, utilizing her strengths at this stressful period. Orientation of parents to ICU staff and primary nurse. Help allay fears.

3. *Cardiac catheterization:*
NPO after 2 A.M.
Premedicated and calm baby.
Good peripheral pulses.

Cardiac catheterization showed a large ventricular septal defect with 4.3–1 left to right shunting with associated pulmonary hypertension. Peripheral pulses full and equal with no hematoma or bleeding noted from catheterization site. Vital signs stable. Temperature (rectal): 99^6.

Decision made for surgical repair of the ventricular septal defect.

Baseline vital signs established; stable at present

Combined medical–surgical cardiac conference to discuss the child's anatomic defect, physical status, failure of medical therapy, and prevention of irreversible pulmonary changes.

All factors considered; decided to have surgical repair in the morning.

Urge fluids till 2 A.M.
Adequate premedication. (Infants under 1 year not sedated).
Peripheral pulses marked.
To catheterization lab at 7:30 A.M.
Returned to ward at 11:45 A.M.
Note any alterations in peripheral pulses.
Continue hemodynamic monitoring.
Continue regimen from Day 1.

Hold evening Digoxin — see Day 1.
Comfort and console baby — crying will increase catabolic needs.
NPO after 12 midnight for surgery in A.M.

Day 3 — 4/22

Returned to ICU at 12 noon from the operating room after undergoing a ventricular septal defect repair, with Dacron patch closure, utilizing a transatrial approach. Deep hypothermia with circulatory arrest employed.

1. *Congestive heart failure:*
Cool to touch. Temperature (rectal): 97 to 99^2. Able to move all extremities. Good peripheral pulses. Pulse: 144, sinus tachycardia without dysrhythmias. No murmurs heard. Arterial blood pressure: 100/62. Pacing wires intact.

Awakening from anesthesia.
Tolerated procedure well.
Hemodynamically stable while congestive heart failure remains a problem.
Good aeration.
Unable to express herself in usual manner, confused at inability to cry.

Continue regimen from Day 1.
Monitor arterial blood pressure, left atrial, right atrial and pulmonary artery pressures, as well as electrocardiogram and urine output.
Meticulous care of sites.
Note irregularities or changes.
Make sure alarms are on!

Subjective/Objective Data

1. *Congestive heart failure: (Continued)*

Right atrial pressure: 6–7 Torr
Left atrial pressure: 12 to 14 Torr, Pulmonary artery pressure mean: 18. Urinary output 10 to 28 cc/hour. Nasogastric tube to regulated wall suction, draining clear yellow fluid. IV fluids: dextrose 5% in water at 18 cc/hour.
Potassium: 4.3 mEq/L with occasional potassium supplement. Chest tube to 20 cm negative pressure, patent, draining small amounts bloody drainage. Colloid replacement cc/cc. Intubated on MA_1 respirator.
FIO_2 100% tidal volume 75 cc. Respiratory rate 24/min. Aterial blood gases: PO_2 324 Torr, PCO_2 32 Torr.
Respiratory rate 24/min (to check Alveolar-arterial gradient). Pulmonary artery pressure mean: 18 Torr. Decreased FIO_2 40% with arterial blood gases: PO_2 138 Torr, PCO_2 39 Torr, pH 7.44. Equal and coarse breath sounds. Endotracheal tube suctioned for thin, clear, white secretions. Chest x-ray: residual cardiomegaly with prominent pulmonary vasculature. Invasive monitoring lines in good position, confirmed by chest x-ray.

Assessment

Medical/Nursing Plan

Maintain normothermia with hyper/hypothermic aids. Myocardium stressed with temperature changes. Low temperature causes acidosis and decreased cardiac output.
Close observation of arterial blood gases, electrolytes, hematocrit.
Accurate intake and output; regulate IV fluids carefully. Measure and record urine output with specific gravity every 4 hours.
Strip chest tube as needed to assure patency. Nasogastric tube irrigated every 4 hours to keep draining.
Medicate as indicated to reduce pain and apprehension.
Restrain prn; Constant bedside nursing. Parenteral antibiotics routinely for 3 days. Provide favorite toy or blanket for security. Continue vigorous respiratory support: Gentle vibration and percussion after invasive monitoring lines removed. Instill, Ambu, suction every 1 hour. Change position, side to side, if able. Always oxygenate before and after suctioning to prevent arrhythmias.
Head elevated to reduce pressure on diaphragm and for better ventilation.

Problem	Assessment	Intervention
		Note changes in airway pressure, any restlessness, or changes in ventilatory settings. Check daily chest x-ray results; use Ambu for a good inspiratory film. Note: If unable to ventilate through the endotracheal tube remove it and ventilate with an Ambu and mask. Be alert to obstruction, especially in children with small endotracheal tubes.
2. Parent reaction: Anxious, apprehensive, afraid to visit ICU, crying when in to visit. "Does she hurt?" "Why can't she cry?" "Take care of her for me."	Difficult for parents to view their baby with all the invasive monitoring devices. Much support needs to be given. Concern with the inability to be major provider.	Continue regimen as outlined. Maintain active primary nurse involvement. Encourage support team: social service, chaplain. Stimulate communications between parents and baby. While parents visit, cover baby with baby blanket. Much support needed. Encourage expression. Invite parents to visit for short, frequent visits.
3. Cardiac catheterization.	Resolved.	Omit from plan.
4. Hypovolemia with resulting hypotension: Hematocrit: 30, blood pressure: 70/50 mm Hg pulse: 146/min. temperature (rectal): 102.4, Right atrial pressure: 7.8 Torr, left atrial pressure: 8 to 10 Torr, pulmonary artery pressure mean: 15 Torr, urine output 6–10 cc/hour.	Small circulating blood volume in children; may come out of surgery in a slight negative balance. Needs more blood. Dopamine has a positive inotropic effect on myocardium, increases cardiac output, has a good effect on renal blood flow, increasing urinary output.	Replace blood samples and chest tube drainage cc/cc with colloid to keep hematocrit at 40 to 45. Keep accurate account of amount of blood samples. Repeat hematocrit in 2 hours. Careful labeling and constant infusion of dopamine through a central line.

Subjective/Objective Data

Blood cultures, tracheal aspirant sent. Additional colloid replacement.

Dopamine (Intropin) 1 mg solution, 4 mcg/kg/hour, instituted for 16 hours.

Day 4 – 4/23 (Postoperative Day 1)

1. *Congestive heart failure:*

Breath sounds clearer, with good aeration.

Weaned from respirator, extubated, and placed in Oxyhood. Pulse: 128 regular, respiratory rate 30.

Right atrial, left atrial, pulmonary artery, arterial lines removed.

Foley discontinued.

Chest tube removed without incident.

Assessment

Possible dehydration and/or infection.

Lungs most probable source (anesthesia).

Unlikely: transfusion reaction (no hives or hematuria).

Good progress.

Hemodynamically stable.

Cough reflex good.

Active bowel sounds.

Removal of lines allows for uncompromised breathing.

Medical/Nursing Plan

Tepid sponging to reduce temperature; may need hypothermia blanket.

Watch for chest infiltrates.

Active respiratory support as above.

Continue regimen from Day 3.

Decrease frequency of vital signs to every 2 hours, alert to changes.

Maintain accurate intake and output.

Obtain daily weights.

Weigh diapers.

Observe for fluid overload.

Progressive diet starting 4 hours after extubation.

Arterial line removed – steady direct pressure for 10 minutes followed by a nonencircling pressure dressing. Check distal circulation.

After removal of left atrial, right atrial, and pulmonary artery lines, observe for bleeding from chest tubes. Have colloid available.

Chest tube removed while child takes a full inspiration. Vaseline gauze occlusive dressing covers the pursestring closure of sites.

Observe for abnormalities on chest x-ray.

2. *Parent reaction:* Less anxious when in to visit. "She looks better without all the tubes sticking into her."	Parents seem comfortable with holding Melissa. Able to cope with situation and verbalize feelings much better.	Encourage further parent participation. Continue support. Anticipate home care plans, continue with teaching.
4. *Hypovolemia with resulting hypotension:* Hematocrit: 44, blood pressure: 108/64 mm Hg. Dopamine (Intropin) discontinued.	Resolved. Easily weaned from dopamine.	Continue monitoring vital signs and hematocrit. Omit from plan.
5. *Right upper lobe atelectasis:* Diminished breath sounds to right upper lobe; respiratory rate: 36/min. Chest x-ray shows infiltrate in right upper lobe. FIO_2: 40%; in Oxyhood. PO_2: 128–82 Torr PCO_2: 40–47 Torr, pH: 7.44–7.41.	Respiratory status slightly deteriorated after extubation.	Increase vigorous respiratory support. Frequent vibration, percussion, and clapping. Nasopharyngeal suctioning to stimulate cough and remove secretions. Always oxygenate before and after suctioning. Check arterial blood gases in 2 hours. Repeat chest x-ray in 12 hours. Frequent position changes. Head elevated. Assisted ambulation.

Day 5 – 4/24 (Postoperative Day 2)

1. *Congestive heart failure:* Chest x-ray improved. House diet. Transfer to cardiovascular ward.	Stable on present regimen. Resolving tachypnea, orthopnea. Good progress.	Continue regimen from Day 4. Decrease frequency of vital signs to every 4 hours. Ambulate.

Subjective/Objective Data	Assessment	Medical/Nursing Plan
2. *Parent reaction:* Glad to see baby progress to ward. "She's really getting better fast."	Parents able to remain with baby, giving care.	Parental support with weaning from ICU. Continue to check on progress after transfer. Continue parent demonstration of care; best time to evaluate and teach.
5. *Right upper lobe Atelectasis:* Breath sounds improved. Chest x-ray demonstrates marked decrease in infiltrate. Arterial blood gases stable; PO_2: 128 Torr in room air. Respiratory rate: 28/min.	Right upper lobe atelectasis resolving with present regimen.	Decrease frequency of chest physiotherapy to 4 times daily. Stimulate to cough. Continue antibiotics. Humidified room air to loosen secretions. Sedate as needed to allow for vigorous respiratory care.
Days 6–11 — 4/25–4/30 1. *Congestive heart failure:* Vital signs stable. Tolerating house diet. Good intake and output.	Ongoing recovery process. Stable on present regimen.	Continue regimen outlined. No modifications needed.
2. *Parent reaction:* "She's doing fine."	Healthy learning experience.	Less support needed. Continue with teaching.
5. *R.U.L. Atelectasis:* Respiratory rate 24 min; chest x-ray clear	Resolved.	Omit from plan.

Subjective/Objective Data

Day 12 – 5/1   Discharge home

1. *Congestive heart failure:*
Vital signs normal. Temperature: 98^6, pulse: 120 min, respiratory rate: 24/min.
Stable weight gain.
Incisions healed. Sutures and pacer wires removed.
Discharge home with follow up care by local physician.

2. *Parent reaction:*
Happy and anxious to go home.

Assessment

Ready for discharge.

Ready to assume care of their healthy baby. Have handled situation well.

Medical/Nursing Plan

Local physician informed of progress during hospitalization.
Referral forms filled out in detail by Primary nurse.
Visiting nurse to assess home situation.
Social service to follow with periodic checkup

Parents urged to call local physician or community health nurse should they have any problems.
Well-baby care to be continued through local physician.

BIBLIOGRAPHY

Books

1. Abramson, H. (ed.): Resuscitation of the Newborn Infant. St. Louis, C. V. Mosby Co., 1966.
2. Andreoli, K., et al.: Comprehensive Cardiac Care, 3rd ed. St. Louis, C.V. Mosby Co., 1975.
3. Austin, W.G., and Behrendt, D.: Patient Care in Cardiac Surgery. Boston, Little, Brown & Co., 1972.
4. Avery, M.E., and Fletcher, B.D.: The Lung and Its Disorders in the Newborn Infant, 3rd ed. Philadelphia, W. B. Saunders Co., 1968.
5. Barnett, H.L., (ed.): Pediatrics, 15th ed. New York, Appleton-Century-Crofts, 1972.
6. Castaneda, Aldo, et al.: Care of the Infant and Child in Cardiac Surgery. Boston, Little, Brown & Co., 1977.
7. Friedberg, C.K.: Diseases of the Heart, 3rd ed. Philadelphia, W. B. Saunders Co., 1966.
8. Guyton, A.C.: Textbook of Medical Physiology, 5th ed. Philadelphia, W. B. Saunders Co., 1976.
9. Hardgrove, C.B., et al.: Parents and Children in the Hospital. Boston, Little, Brown & Co., 1972.
10. Hurst, J.W., and Logue, R.B.: The Heart, 3rd ed. New York, McGraw-Hill, 1973.
11. King, Ouida: Care of the Cardiac Surgical Patient. St. Louis, C. V. Mosby Co., 1975.
12. Klaus, M.H., and Fanaroff, A.A.: Care of the High-Risk Neonate, 2nd ed. Philadelphia, W. B. Saunders Co., 1979.
13. Korones, Sheldon: High-Risk Newborn Infants. St. Louis, C. V. Mosby Co., 1972.
14. Moss, A.J., et al.: Heart Disease in Infants, Children, and Adolescents, 2nd ed. Baltimore, Williams & Wilkins Co., 1978.
15. Nadas, A.S., and Fyler, D.C.: Pediatric Cardiology, 3rd ed. Philadelphia, W. B. Saunders Co., 1972.
16. Perloff, Joseph K.: The Clinical Recognition of Congenital Heart Disease, 2nd ed. Philadelphia, W. B. Saunders Co., 1978.
17. Snow, J.: "Pediatric cardiac disorders." In Armstrong, M., et al. (eds.): Handbook of Clinical Nursing. New York, McGraw-Hill Book Co., 1979.

Periodicals

1. Barnes, C.M.: Working with parents of children undergoing heart surgery. Nurs. Clin. North Am., 4:11, 1969.
2. Belling, D.T.: Complications after open heart surgery. Nurs. Clin. North Am., 4:123, 1969.
3. Benzing, G., et al.: Immediate postoperative care after cardiac surgery. In Kaplan, S. (ed.): Symposium: the infant and child with cardiovascular disease. Heart Lung, 3:415, 1974.
4. Frater, R.W.M.: Postoperative care in the pediatric patient. In Kaplan, S. (ed.): Symposium: the infant and child with cardiovascular disease. Heart Lung, 3:903, 1974.
5. Hoffman, J.I.: Ventricular septal defects: indications for therapy in infants. Pediatr. Clin. North Am., 18:1091, 1971.
6. Kaplan, S., (ed.): Symposium: the infant and child with cardiovascular disease. Heart Lung, 3:390, 1974.
7. Motter, J., et al.: Congestive heart failure in children. Hosp Med, 9:34, 1973.
8. Shor, V.Z.: Congenital cardiac defects: assessment and case findings, Am. J. Nurs., 78:256, 1978.

CHAPTER 15
CASE STUDY OF A CHILD WITH MULTIPLE TRAUMA

Donalda Parkes, R.N., B.Sc.N. and
Carmelle Sylvestre-Simon, R.N., B.Sc.N.

Nine-year-old David, youngest of three boys, with no previous illness or hospitalization, was struck by a car and thrown a considerable distance. He was taken to a local community hospital, where initial resuscitation was carried out. After resuscitation, David was noted to have respiratory distress, a fixed, dilated right pupil, gross hematuria, and anemia. The diagnosis of multiple trauma was made. He was immediately transferred by ambulance to a large pediatric center, accompanied by his parents.

After his arrival at the emergency department, the parents, who were Jehovah's Witnesses, refused blood administration. An emergency court session was held in the hospital, and David was made a ward of the court for a 30-day period in order to allow blood transfusions and appropriate treatment.

The following problems were identified during the time he was in the emergency department:

Problem list	*Confirmed by*
1. Aortic aneurysm.	Arch aortogram.
2. Left hemopneumothorax.	Chest x-ray.
3. Fractured left ribs 3–6.	Chest x-ray.
4. Left lung contusion	Chest x-ray, blood gases.
5. Lacerated left kidney with retroperitoneal hematoma.	Abdominal aortogram.
6. Splenic tear.	Liver-spleen scan.
7. Cerebral contusion.	Skull x-ray, CT scan

Emergency treatment consisted of (1) intubation and artificial ventilation; (2) insertion of a central venous catheter and radial arterial catheter; (3) blood samples sent for pH and blood gases, cross and type, hemogram, coagulogram, electrolytes, blood urea nitrogen, creatinine, osmolality, calcium, and sugar; (4) administration of Ringer's lactate and whole blood; (5) insertion of a left chest drain; (6) insertion of a urinary catheter; (7) urine sample sent for routine urinalysis, electrolytes, and osmolality; (8) insertion of a nasogastric tube; (9) radiologic examinations.

A multiservice team, including staff members from cardiovascular surgery, general surgery; urology, nephrology, neurosurgery, anesthesiology, radiology, and critical care physicians and nursing staff, was responsible for David's care.

Two hours after his arrival in the emergency department, David was brought to the critical care unit, where he stayed for 9 days. He was then transferred to a general surgical ward. After 25 days of hospitalization, he was returned to the custody of his parents and discharged to his home.

During his stay in the critical care unit, the following were added to his original problem list:

8. Parent reaction.
9. Acute tubular necrosis.
10. Paralytic ileus.
11. Right hemiparesis.
12. Left recurrent nerve palsy.

Documentation of David's progress in the critical care unit is on the following pages.

Subjective/Objective Data	Assessment	Medical/Nursing Plan
Day 1 – 12 hours after admission to ICU		
1. *Aortic aneurysm:*		
Blood pressure: 110/70 mm Hg to 115/75 mm Hg, central venous pressure: 8 to 10. Heart rate: 100 to 110 minute, no murmurs or arrhythmias.	Vital signs stabilizing.	Electrocardiogram monitoring with attention to any arrhythmias. Continue recording David's vital signs q½ to 1h. Check femoral pulses qh. Report hypotension, increased heart rate, increased restlessness, decreased urine output. Routine arterial line care; note circulation to left hand, provide continual flushing with heparinized solution.
David is still restless, occasionally thrashes about.	Restlessness may be due to cerebral injury, respiratory distress, internal bleeding, fear, and pain.	Sedation should be given with caution to avoid masking symptoms.
	Since danger of aortic hemorrhage remains, stress, anxiety, and activity must be minimized.	Do not change David's position suddenly. Keep him flat. Stay with him, use no restraints. Scheduled for thoracotomy and aneurysm repair. Prepare David physically and emotionally for surgery; reinforce doctor's explanation to the parents.

2. *Left hemopneumothorax:* Air entry decreased to left lung. 280 cc sanguineous chest drainage in 12 hours. Considerable air bubbling in drainage bottle.	David is having chest pain; sedation may be necessary. Hemopneumothorax still significant.	Try to place David in a comfortable position. Repeat chest x-ray in 2 hours. Replace chest drainage with whole blood. Increase suction to chest drain from 15 to 20 cm water pressure. Continue monitoring amount of air leak and amount and type of chest drainage, with particular attention to color, temperature, and rate of bleeding.
3. *Fractured left ribs:* Obvious bruises on left chest. Very upset when left chest touched. Expands right chest more than the left.	David has a flail chest, which is painful and alters his chest movement.	Bennett respirator (FIO_2 40 Torr, rate 24/min, volume 300 cc, pressure limit 35, positive end-expiratory pressure [PEEP] 5 mm Hg) to prevent paradoxical chest movements and pulmonary collapse. Avoid direct pressure on fractured rib area, support chest well when turning.
4. *Left lung contusion:* Decreased air entry to left lower lobe. pH: 7.25, PO_2: 70 Torr, FIO_2: 40 Torr, PCO_2: 55 Torr; base exess: -9, Blood-tinged secretions with endotracheal suctioning.	Needs correction of mixed acidosis and improvement of ventilation.	Adjustments to Bennett respirator: increase FIO_2 to 60 Torr, rate to 30/min, volume to 400 cc, pressure limit to 45 cm H_2O, PEEP to 6 mm Hg. Give sodium bicarbonate to correct metabolic acidosis.

Subjective/Objective Data

Assessment

Medical/Nursing Plan

4. *Left lung contusion: (Continued)*

Repeat blood gases in 30 minutes.
Suction endotracheal tube frequently but cautiously, as excessive coughing may rupture aorta.
May need instillation of saline into endotracheal tube with suctioning if secretions difficult to remove.
No chest physiotherapy at this time (fractured ribs and danger of hemorrhage).
Start IV antibiotics q6h after secretions from endotracheal tube sent for culture.

5. *Lacerated left kidney:*

David gets upset and is guarding when left flank examined.
Rigidity and some distension of his lower abdomen, hemoglobin 8.2 gm/dl.
Gross hematuria.

Has retroperitoneal bleeding, could go into shock from kidney hemorrhage.

Close attention to signs of shock, maintain adequate blood pressure with blood and fluids.
Laparotomy scheduled to be done along with thoracotomy.

Hematuria could block catheter.

Catheter irrigation unwise with kidney injury, report absence of urine stat.

Decreased urine output, specific gravity: 1.035.
Blood urea nitrogen: 24 mg/dl, creatinine 3.8 mg/dl.

Possible renal failure, may need diuretics.

Measure urine volume, check specific gravity, and test for blood qh.
Save hourly urine samples for comparison.
Lasix given IV; report urine output over next hour.

6. Splenic tear: Pale, hemoglobin 8.2 mg/dl. Upper abdomen tense and tender to touch, no bowel sounds.	Concern that David is bleeding into abdomen.	Vital sign monitoring. Measure David's abdominal girth qh (mark abdomen to have a consistent point of measurement). Nasogastric tube to suction, measure drainage, test for blood qh, irrigate q2h with 10 cc normal saline. Replace gastric drainage with IV normal saline with KCl added. Blood transfusion to increase hemoglobin. Splenectomy may be necessary.
7. Cerebral contusion: David is drowsy but rouses easily when spoken to, nods his head to questions, eyes look frightened. Pupils equal and reacting briskly now. No spontaneous movement of right arm, weak right hand grasp.	Neurological status stable, although difficult to be sure when David is sedated. May have spinal or peripheral nerve injury.	Thorough neurological assessment qh. Spinal x-rays to be done. Plan repeat arteriogram, CT scan to rule out subdural hematoma.
Temperature: 38° C rectally.	Fever may increase cerebral edema.	Tepid sponging and Tempra (or Tylenol) to decrease fever (no aspirin because of bleeding), may need hypothermia blanket if sponging not effective. Prevent shivering, administer Largactil prn. David really dislikes being uncovered, can have a thin sheet.

Subjective/Objective Data	Assessment	Medical/Nursing Plan
8. *Parent reaction:* Parents very anxious, expressing fears of impending surgery. Reluctant to touch or talk to David. Said they resented the court action, very unhappy about the blood David is receiving.	Need a great deal of support, frequent explanations. Intimidated by David's condition and treatment.	Explain each nursing and medical procedure as it occurs. Permit parents to sit at bedside, encourage them to talk to David and hold his hand. Allow parents to talk about their resentment.
Day 2 David has had a repair of his aortic aneurysm with cardiopulmonary bypass, a left nephrectomy, and suture repair of his spleen.		
1. *Aortic aneurysm:* Blood pressure: 115/85 to 120/90, central venous pressure: 8 to 12. Heart rate: 110 to 115, strong and regular. Femoral pulses equal and strong. Less restless.	Possibility of a hemorrhage from the site of the anastomosis. Anxiety and activity must still be controlled.	Continue electrocardiogram monitoring, check vital signs and femoral pulses qh. Keep David flat, turn carefully side to side qh, avoid strenuous coughing. Explain activities and reassure, give mild sedation IV prn to settle David if other systems stable.
2. *Left hemopneumothorax:* David has two chest drains in left chest following thoracotomy. Air entry slightly improved to left lung. Minimal chest drainage (60 cc in 12 hours). No air bubbling in drainage bottles now.	Left hemothorax resolving. Left pneumothorax resolved.	

1 hour ago David coughed vigorously when turned and 100 cc dark blood suddenly drained from chest tube #1. Chest x-ray: small amount of blood remains in left pleural space, but no pleural air or subcutaneous emphysema.	Collection of blood in pleural space disturbed by David's coughing.	Continue with Day 1 plan.
3. Fractured left ribs: David not objecting so much when left chest examined. Less inequality of chest movement when off respirator for suctioning.	David is having less pain. Flail chest has stabilized with respirator.	Protect fractured left ribs as on Day 1.
4. Left Lung contusion: Decreased air entry to left lower lobe. Chest x-ray shows left lower lobe atelectasis. pH: 7.32, PO_2: 67 Torr, (FIO_2: 60 Torr) pCO_2:54 Torr; Base excess: -6.	Respiratory status has deteriorated, likely due to atelectasis. Possible fat embolus.	Alter David's respirator again, increase FIO_2 to 70 Torr, rate to 34/min, volume to 450 cc, PEEP to 7 mm Hg. Fractured ribs still prevent David from having chest physiotherapy, but continue suctioning qh. Collect tracheal secretions for culture and examination for fat particles.
5. Lacerated left kidney: Removed at the time of laparotomy.	No longer a concern.	Omit 5 from problem list. See problem 9, acute tubular necrosis.
6. Splenic tear: David's color has improved, hemoglobin now 11.2 gm/dl. Abdomen still tense and tender. No increase in abdominal girth. Bile-colored nasogastric drainage.	No signs of further abdominal bleeding.	Continue measuring David's abdominal girth qh.

Subjective/Objective Data	Assessment	Medical/Nursing Plan
6. *Splenic tear:* (Continued)		His nasogastric tube is prone to blockage, be sure to irrigate it thoroughly. Continue replacement of nasogastric drainage.
7. *Cerebral contusion:* Since surgery David has been slower to rouse but will nod head to parents' questions. Few spontaneous movements but reacts to touch.	David is tired after surgery. Subdural hematoma still possible.	Even though difficult, continue neurologic assessment qh, may have to inflict pain to test.
Will not try to grasp with hands or move his legs. Right arm and leg are weaker. Pupils equal and reacting briskly.	Unwilling to cooperate with neurologic testing, so it is difficult to be sure of neurologic status.	Persist in having David try to move his arms and legs himself.
Temperature: 37°C.	Fever under control, hypothermia blanket not yet needed.	Repeat tepid sponging and Tempra if fever increases, and investigate for sepsis.
8. *Parent reaction:* Will not leave bedside. Look exhausted, constant questioning.	Still very fearful and lacking trust in hospital staff.	Persuade David's parents to leave for meals, rest, and sleep. Allow them to sit in room near ICU when visiting is not appropriate. Be patient, continue with repeated explanations and much reassurance.
9. *Acute tubular necrosis:* Decreased urine output, specific gravity 1.028 to 1.034. "Puffy" eyes, positive fluid balance. Weight gain of 1.6 kg in 48 hours.	Developing renal failure due to hypotension at time of accident and decreased renal flow while aorta clamped during aneurysm repair.	Monitor David's urine output closely. Lasix and Edecrin IV to increase urine output. Watch for further edema, begin daily weighing. Watch electrocardiogram for arrhythmias due to

Na: 142 mEq/l K: 5.5 mEq/l Cl: 110 mEq/l creatine 4.2 mg/dl, blood urea nitrogen 55 mg/dl.

increased K, discontinue KCl in all IV fluids. Repeat electrolytes, blood urea nitrogen, and creatine in 4 hours.

Day 3

1. *Aortic aneurysm:*
   No changes.

   David could still rupture his anastomosis.

   Continue with Day 2 plan.

2. *Left hemothorax:*
   No chest drainage today.
   Chest x-ray shows no fluid in left pleural space.

   Hemothorax resolved.

   Both chest drains removed.
   David very upset with procedure, needed extra sedation.
   Omit 2 from problem list.

3. *Fractured left ribs:*
   David complains of pain only when he is moved, not when area is touched.
   Chest movement remains unequal when off respirator.

   Flail chest improving.

   May turn David onto his left side.

4. *Left lung contusion:*
   Decreased air entry to right lung today.
   Minimal air entry to left lung.
   Chest x-ray shows more atelectasis, now involving right upper lobe.

   Secretions very thick and difficult to clear.

   David will need chest physiotherapy despite fractured ribs.
   May be fluid overload from acute tubular necrosis.

   Start chest physiotherapy q2h using percussor on right chest, gentle hand clapping on left chest; sedate prior to physiotherapy.

   Instill normal saline into endotracheal tube during suctioning to loosen secretions.

Subjective/Objective Data	Assessment	Medical/Nursing Plan
4. *Left lung contusion: (Continued)* No spontaneous efforts to breath except when off respirator for suctioning. PO_2: 94 Torr, (FiO_2: 70 Torr), PCO_2: 58 Torr.	Lack of respiratory effort likely due to fatigue. Not ready to try weaning from respirator.	
6. *Splenic tear:* Abdomen less tense, girth unchanged. Hemoglobin 11.4 gm/dl.	David's splenic tear no longer a concern.	Omit 6 from problem list. See problem 10, paralytic ileus.
7. *Cerebral contusion:* David is alert, oriented today. Trying to talk, wants endotracheal tube out. Pupils equal and reacting briskly. Right hemiparesis persists.	Neurologic status satisfactory except for pronounced right hemiparesis.	Discontinue neurologic assessment except for right limbs. Begin physiotherapy to weakened limbs. Omit 7 from list. See problem 11, right hemiparesis.
8. *Parent reaction:* Parents are more relaxed, visiting frequently but for shorter periods. Starting to help with David's care. Still questioning the "why" of many procedures.	Parents are adjusting to David's condition and complex treatment.	Involve parents more in David's care, e.g., turning, skin care, reading to him.

9. *Acute tubular necrosis:*
Increased urine output after diuretics.
Negative fluid balance.
Decreased facial edema, weight loss of 1.45 kg in 24 hours.
K decreased to 3.0 mEq/L, blood urea nitrogen decreased to 30 mg/dl, creatinine decreased to 3.1 mg/dl

David has responded well to diuretics and fluid restriction but is still in some degree of renal failure.

Continue diuretics prn if urine output is decreased.
Maintain restricted fluid intake.

Restart KCl in IV fluids because K now 3.0 mEq/L. Repeat electrolytes, blood urea nitrogen, and creatinine in 4 hours.

10. *Paralytic ileus:*
Excessive bile-colored nasogastric drainage.

No bowel sounds.

David now has a paralytic ileus.

Continue nasogastric suction and replace nasogastric losses with normal saline.
Add KCl to the normal saline once again.

11. *Right hemiparesis:*
Gross movement of right arm but no hand grasp.
Unable to lift right leg from bed but will move it with considerable persuasion.

Right hemiparesis has worsened.

To have an arteriogram.

Continue assessment of right limb movement.
Encourage David to use his right arm.

Day 4

1. *Aortic aneurysm.*

No longer a concern.

Omit 1 from problem list.

3. *Fractured left ribs:*
David complains of pain only during chest physiotherapy.
Left chest now moving just slightly less than right when off respirator.

Flail chest not distressing David.

Continue to give David sedation prior to chest physiotherapy.
Turn from side to side q2h, encourage more activity.

Subjective/Objective Data	Assessment	Medical/Nursing Plan
4. *Left lung contusion:* Increased air entry to right upper lobe after a night of chest physiotherapy. Decreased air entry to left lower lobe but improved from yesterday. Chest x-ray shows right upper lobe reexpanded, left lower lobe still congested.	Chest condition improved.	
At 1200 hours David is resisting the respirator, trying to breathe "on his own."	Ready to try weaning from respirator.	Hold sedation, add an intermittent mandatory ventilation (IMV) circuit to the respirator, decrease rate to 10/minute, decrease FIO_2 to 60 Torr and PEEP to 4 mm Hg.
PO_2: 110 Torr, (FIO_2: 70 Torr), PCO_2: 42 Torr.	Gas exchange adequate.	Stay with David, remind him to take deep breaths, check air entry, heart rate, and respiratory rate q½h × 2 hours. Repeat blood gases in 2 hours, chest x-ray in 4 hours.
At 1630 hours David is increasingly agitated, respiratory rate increased to 42/min, heart rate to 144/min.	Attempt to wean has failed owing to atelectasis.	Increase IMV rate to 20/min, PEEP to 6 mm Hg. Leave David on respirator overnight.
pH: 7.23, PO_2: 72 Torr, (FIO_2: 60 Torr), PCO_2: 54 Torr, Base excess: -6	Acidosis needs correction.	Sodium bicarbonate given for acidosis. Needs more vigorous chest physiotherapy and suctioning.
8. *Parent reaction:* No problems today. Helped with David's bath, turning him and rubbing his skin.	Parents feeling more comfortable with nursing staff.	
Have requested that David's 15-year-old brother visit.	Brother's visit might cheer David up.	Arrange for brother to visit.

9. *Acute tubular necrosis:*
David is beginning to look "puffy-eyed" again, but no weight gain as yet. Decreased urine output, required Lasix twice.
Responded quickly and appropriately to diuretic. K: 4.2 mEq/l, creatinine: 2.1 mg/dl, blood urea nitrogen: 28 mg/dl.

Renal failure still a concern.

Continue as previously planned.

10. *Paralytic ileus:*
Still excessive nasogastric drainage and no bowel sounds.
David frequently nauseated.

Paralytic ileus unchanged.

Give antiemetic IM q4h prn (David prefers injection into right leg).

11. *Right hemiparesis:*
Arteriogram negative.
No change in limb movement.

David's right hemiparesis is due to original left cerebral contusion.

Arrange for physiotherapist to set up exercise program.

Days 5 through 8
3. *Fractured left ribs:*

Day 8
Chest movement still unequal, but possibility of a paralyzed diaphragm ruled out by fluoroscopy.

Unequal chest movement due to David guarding his left chest. Flail chest no longer a concern.

Can be more vigorous with chest physiotherapy.

No restrictions in moving David.

Subjective/Objective Data	Assessment	Medical/Nursing Plan
4. *Left lung contusion:*		
Day 5		
Increased air entry to left lower lobe. Chest x-ray shows right lung clear, left lung still congested. PO_2: 90 Torr, (FIO_2: 50 Torr), PCO_2: 44 Torr.	Vigorous chest physiotherapy and suctioning is clearing David's left lung.	Will try to wean David from respirator to spontaneous PEEP circuit.
Tracheal secretion cultures negative.	Has no chest infection.	Continue to send daily tracheal secretions for culture.
Day 6		
Tolerated spontaneous PEEP circuit overnight. Increased air entry to left lower lobe. Chest x-ray shows lungs have improved, blood gases are satisfactory.	David is ready for extubation.	Explain procedure to David and his parents. Assist with extubation. Assess David's air entry, check respirations and heart rate q½h until stabilized after extubation. David is to wear a humidified O_2 mask with FIO_2 40 Torr. Repeat blood gases in 2 hours, chest x-ray in 4 hours.
Day 8		
Increased air entry to left lower lobe. Chest x-ray shows residual left lower lobe atelectasis. PO_2: 82 Torr, (FIO_2: 40 Torr), PCO_2: 42 Torr.	Has tolerated extubation well but still has some left lung congestion.	Chest physiotherapy must continue q2h during the day, q4h at night to allow for more sleep. Give sedation prior to physiotherapy. David must try to do his deep breathing and coughing exercises, needs much persuasion. Suction him if he won't cough. Insist that he wear his O_2 mask, but he settles better with an O_2 hood at night. Check Day 6 tracheal secretion culture report.

Some fever at night.
Has now been on IV antibiotics for 1 week.

Should continue receiving antibiotics.

Get reorder for antibiotics; see if David can tolerate them orally.
Start getting David up in a chair for 10 minutes morning, afternoon, evening; increase as tolerated.
To be seen by ENT service.

David has unusually excessive nasal and oral secretions (not chest) today and is drooling his saliva.
Having some difficulty swallowing and chokes occasionally.
Cough is very weak.
Speech is rather slurred.

May have some nerve impairment affecting pharyngeal function.

Elevate David's head and shoulders 45°.
Make sure he is sitting up when drinking.

See problem 12.

8. *Parent reaction:*
Day 8

Father back to work.
Mother and brother visit daily, are relaxed with David, like doing things for him.
Pleased with his progress but worried about his weak right arm and leg.
Continue to express resentment of court order.

Parents handling David well.
Improved relations with hospital staff.

Will need help with home care and rehabilitation.

Arrange a conference with ward nursing staff before David is transferred to ward to discuss his care and parent involvement.

9. *Acute tubular necrosis:*
Day 8

Urine output satisfactory with daily diuretic dose.
No edema, slight weight loss over 3 days.
Na: 130 mEq/l, K: 3.8 mEq/l, Cl: 94 mEq/l, creatinine: 1.1 mg/dl, blood urea nitrogen: 16 mg/dl.

David's kidney is functioning well.

Stop diuretics to see how urine output will be affected.
Check serum electrolytes twice daily.

Subjective/Objective Data	Assessment	Medical/Nursing Plan
10. Paralytic ileus: _Day 8_ Nasogastric tube removed Day 7. Tolerating clear fluids. Active bowel sounds but no bowel movement as yet. IV removed this A.M.	Ileus resolved.	Start full fluids today, if tolerated, increase diet tomorrow. No bowel movement by A.M., give a glycerin suppository.
11. Right hemiparesis: _Day 8_ Gross movement of right arm, but cannot grasp or lift an object or perform fine motor movements with right hand. David is frustrated and angry with his disability, "afraid it won't get better." Has a right-sided limp when walking from chair.	Leg is stronger but arm has not improved. Will need much support and encouragement in his rehabilitation program.	Continue with right limb exercise program. Physiotherapist to continue David's program on the ward. Avoid putting David in frustrating situations, e.g., place his belongings near his left arm so he can pick them up.
12. Left recurrent nerve palsy: _Day 8_ David has been examined by Dr. Jackson of ENT service. Had a choking spell while drinking apple juice, ate pudding with less difficulty.	David has a left recurrent nerve palsy caused by the trauma to his aortic arch that occurred with his chest injury.	Have David sit up while drinking or eating. Encourage him to take his fluids slowly; he can't manage a straw. Give David puddings, custards, ice cream, gelatin; he manages these better than fluids. Leave oral suction tip with David so he can clear his mouth when he wants to.

Will need vigorous chest physiotherapy and persistence in getting him to breathe deeply and cough.

David will likely need deep suctioning to stimulate his cough.

Be patient and take time to understand David's speech, encourage him to speak slowly and loudly.

After a conference with the ward staff and an opportunity for them to meet David and his family, David was transferred to the ward on Day 9 with the following unresolved problem list:

3. Fractured left ribs.
4. Left lung contusion.*
8. Parent reaction.*
9. Acute tubular necrosis.
10. Paralytic ileus.
11. Right hemiparesis.*
12. Left recurrent nerve palsy.*

---

*of primary concern.

INDEX